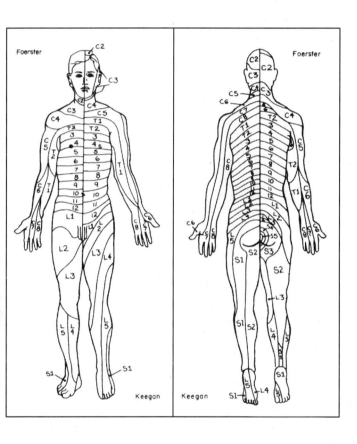

fourth
EDITION

THE LITTLE BLACK BOOK OF NEUROLOGY

Osama O. Zaidat, MD
Assistant Professor of Neurology
Case Western Reserve University School of Medicine
University Hospitals of Cleveland
Louis Stokes Cleveland VA Medical Center
Cleveland, Ohio

Alan J. Lerner, MD
Associate Professor of Neurology
Case Western Reserve University
School of Medicine
Cleveland, Ohio

Chief, Neurology Service
University Hospitals Health System
Heather Hill Hospital and Health Partnership
Chardon, Ohio

Illustrations by Sundee L. Morris, MD

 Mosby

An Imprint of Elsevier Science

St. Louis   London   Philadelphia   Sydney   Toronto

An Imprint of Elsevier Science

11830 Westline Drive
St. Louis, Missouri 63146

Third Edition 1995

Library of Congress Cataloging-in-Publication Data

The little black book of neurology.—4th ed. / Osama O. Zaidat, Alan J. Lerner.
    p.   cm
  Includes bibliographical references and index.
  ISBN 0–323–01415–1
  1. Nervous system—Diseases—Handbooks, manuals, etc. I. Zaidat, Osama O. II. Lerner, Alan J.
  [DNLM: 1. Nervous System Diseases—Handbooks. WL 39 L778 2002]
  RC355.L58 2002
  616.8—dc21   2002016682

Expo

Printed in the United States of America

Last digit is the print number: 9 8 7 6 5 4 3 2 1

CONTRIBUTORS

Ahmad Al-Khatib, MD

Ali Al-Mudallal, MD

Adeela Alizai, MD

Amer Al-Sheklee, MD

Marek Buzcek, MD

Kanokwan Boonyapasit, MD

Chere M. Chase, MD

Peter Cutri, DO

Joy Derwenskus, DO

Matthew Eccher, MD

Cony Esteban-Santillan, MD

Jose Fernandes-Filho, MD

Alexandros Georgiadis, MD

Sandra Kuniyoshi, MD

Shafqat Memon, MD

Zeyad Morcos, MD

Daniel Miller, MD

Svetlana Pundik, MD

Naiel Rahim, MD

Deborah Reed, MD

O. Adeltola Robert, MD

Gurwant Singh, MD

Anisa S.N. Ssengoba, BS

Eroboghene Ubogo, MD

Meg A. Varrees, MD

Neurology House Staff, Case Western Reserve University, University Hospitals of Cleveland, Cleveland VA Medical Center, Cleveland, Ohio

PREFACE

The Little Black Book of Neurology has become a dependable source of quickly retrievable, practical information for students, house staff and practicing neurologists. The first edition appeared in 1987, followed by revisions in 1991 and 1995.

The interval since the previous edition has seen many changes in both the publishing world and neurologic practice. Mosby-Year Book, Inc. has been incorporated into Elsevier Science and the Little Black Book continues under their aegis with the Mosby imprint. For the current edition I would like to specifically thank Delores Meloni at Elsevier and Berta Steiner for their patience and guidance. Neurology has changed from within and without—both by changes in access to care through managed care, and the emergence of technical gains and the first available treatments for a number of conditions. It is my sincere hope that despite all of these changes, the fundamental humanistic patient-centered approach to neurology prevails throughout this volume. We welcome comments and suggestions from our readers to help guide future improvements.

Alan J. Lerner, MD

With the turn of the new century, neurology evolves from a diagnostic field to a therapeutic field. With the effort of the founding neurologists behind them, the new generation of neurologists come with great energy to resolve old mysteries and discover new therapies. This makes it very hard to keep up with the pace of new knowledge. The fourth edition of the *Little Black Book of Neurology* is introduced to keep up with the ever-changing face of neurology. Many of the old chapters have been updated and some have been completely rewritten. New chapters have been introduced and the National Institutes of Health Stroke Scale has been added to the inside back cover of the book.

We hope that this book satisfies the needs of many physicians and those who work with patients with neurologic disease. Having used the Black Book myself as a medical student and a neurology resident, I am certain that it is of great help to medical students and residents in Neurology, Neurosurgery, Orthopedics, PMR, Internal Medicine, and Family Practice.

I would like to thank the neurology and neurosurgery residents at Case Western Reserve University/University Hospitals of Cleveland and Louis Stokes Cleveland VA Medical Center. I am very grateful to the faculty at the Department of Neurology, who provided their input and support, especially my co-editor Alan Lerner, Robert Ruff, Jose Suarez, Henry Kaminski, John Leigh, and Robert Daroff.

Preparation of this manuscript would not have been possible without the great effort of my editor Delores Meloni from Elsevier. Finally I would like to thank my family and my wife Sabreen Owais; without their help and support, this book would not have been produced.

Osama O. Zaidat, MD

CONTENTS

Abscess, Brain   1
Abscess, Epidural   3
Acalculia   3
Agnosia   4
Agraphia   4
AIDS   5
Alcohol   8
Alexia   10
Amaurosis Fugax   11
Aneurysms   12
Angiography   14
Angiomas   17
Antibody Testing in Neuromuscular Disease   18
Antidepressants   22
Aphasia   24
Apraxia   26
Asterixis   27
Ataxia   28
Athetosis   29
Attention Deficit-Hyperactivity Disorder (ADHD)   29
Autism   31
Autonomic Dysfunction   31
Benzodiazepines   34
Bladder   35
Brachial Plexus   38
Brain Death   39
Bulbar Palsy   40
Calcification, Cerebral   41
Calorics   42
Cardiopulmonary Arrest   43
Carpal Tunnel Syndrome   43
Cauda Equina and Conus Medullaris   44
Cerebellum   45
Cerebral Cortex   55
Cerebral Hemorrhage   56
Cerebral Palsy (CP)   58
Cerebrospinal Fluid   59
Chemotherapy, Neurologic Complications   64
Child Neurology   65

Chorea   71
Chromosomal Disorders   73
Coma   74
Complex Regional Pain Syndrome (Reflex Sympathetic Dystrophy)   80
Computed Tomography (CT)   81
Confusional State   83
Congenital Malformations of the Brain and Spine   83
Cramps   85
Cranial Nerves   87
Craniocervical Junction   88
Craniosynostosis   88
Degenerative Diseases of Childhood   89
Dementia   92
Demyelinating Disease   99
Dermatomes   101
Dialysis   103
Disseminated Intravascular Coagulation (DIC)   103
Dizziness   104
Dysarthria   105
Dyskinesia   105
Dysphagia   106
Dystonia   106
Electrocardiogram (ECG)   108
Electrocephalography   109
Electrolyte Disturbances   112
Electromyography and Nerve Conduction Studies (EMG/NCS)   117
Encephalitis   122
Encephalopathy   125
Encephalopathy, Perinatal, Hypoxic-Ischemic   126
Epilepsy   127
Evoked Potentials   144
Eye Muscles   148
Facial Nerve   150
Fontanel   153
Frontal Lobe   154
Gait Disorders   154
Gaze Palsy   155
Gerstmann's Syndrome   155
Glossopharyngeal Neuralgia   156
Glucose   156
Graves' Ophthalmopathy   158
Hallucinations   159
Headache   160
Hearing   165
Herniation   166
Hiccups (Singultus, Hiccoughs)   169

Horner's Syndrome   169
Huntington's Disease   171
Hydroicephalus   172
Hyperventiliation   173
Hypotonic Infant   174
Immunization   175
Impotence   177
Intracranial Pressue (ICP)   178
Ischemia   180
Lambert-Eaton Myasthenic Syndrome   200
Learning Disabilities   202
Limbic System   203
Lumbosacral Plexus   203
Lyme Disease   205
Macrocephaly   206
Magnetic Resonance Imaging (MRI)   207
Memory   212
Meningitis   213
Mental Status Testing   216
Metabolic Diseases of Childhood   218
Microcephaly   220
Motor Neuron Disease   221
Multiple Sclerosis   224
Muscle Diseases and Testing   226
Muscular Dystrophy (MD)   229
Myasthenia Gravis   235
Myelography   238
Myoclonus   239
Myoglobinuria   242
Myopathy   243
Myotomes   251
Mytonia   252
Neglect   254
Neurocutaneous Syndromes   255
Neuroleptics   258
Neuropathy   260
Nutritional Deficiency Syndromes   269
Nystagmus   270
Occipital Lobe   274
Ocular Oscillations   275
Olfaction   276
Opalski's Syndrome   277
Ophthalmoplegia   277
Optic Nerve   281
Optokinetic Nystagmus   283
Paget's Disease   284

Pain   284
Paraneoplastic Syndromes   288
Parietal Lobe   290
Parkinsonism   290
Parkinson's Disease   292
Periodic Paralysis   295
Peripheral Nerve   296
PET and SPECT   306
Pituitary   307
Porphyria   310
Pregnancy   313
Pseudobulbar Palsy   318
Pseudotumor Cerebri   319
Ptosis   320
Pupil   321
Radiation Injury   326
Radiculopathy   328
Reflex Sympathetic Dystrophy   330
Reflexes   330
Restless Leg Syndrome (Ekbom Syndrome)   332
Retinal and Uveal Tract   333
Rheumatoid Arthritis   335
Rigidity   337
Romberg Sign   337
Sarcoidosis   338
Sepsis   339
Shunts   339
Sickle Cell Disease   341
Sleep Disorders   343
Spasticity   345
Spinal Cord   346
Spinocerebellar Degeneration   351
Syncope   353
Syndrome of Inappropriate Antidiuretic Hormone (SIADH)   355
Syphilis   356
Taste   358
Temporal Lobe   359
Thyroid   359
Tourette's Syndrome: Gilles De La Tourette's Syndrome (GTS)   361
Transient Global Amnesia (TGA)   362
Transplantation—Neurologic Aspects   363
Tremors   365
Trigeminal Neuralgia (Tic Douloureux)   367
Trinucleotide Repeat Expansion   368
Tumors   369
Ulnar Nerve   373

Ultrasonography   374
Uremia   375
Vasculitis   376
Venous Thrombosis   379
Vertigo   380
Vestibulo-Ocular Reflex   383
Visual Fields   384
Wilson's Disease   386
Zoster   387

ABSCESS, BRAIN

Brain abscesses constitute less than 2% of intracranial masses and develop mainly in three clinical situations:

1. *Hematogenous* spread from distant sites of infection - common sources of metastatic brain abscesses are chronic infection of lungs and/or pleura (bronchiectasis, empyema, lung abscess), congenital heart malformations with right-to-left shunts (oral bacterial flora after dental procedures), or bacterial endocarditis (multiple small abscesses).
2. *Contiguous spread* via direct extension from local neighboring infection sites - nasal sinusitis (frontal lobe abscess), middle ear and/or mastoid cells infection (temporal lobe and cerebellar abscess), spread by local osteomyelitis or by septic thrombophlebitis of emissary vein.
3. *Penetrating head injury or neurosurgical procedures* - compound depressed skull fractures, basal skull fractures with cerebrospinal fluid (CSF) fistulae, and previous craniotomy can cause brain abscess formation, sometimes months/years after the acute event. Post-neurosurgical abscesses occur especially when surgery involves paranasal air sinuses.

Pathogens isolated from abscesses are related to the site of origin, as follows (organisms are listed in order of significance, many abscesses are polymicrobial):

1. Middle ear infection: Streptococci (aerobic and anaerobic), *Bacteroides fragilis*, and *Enterobacteriaceae (Proteus)* .
2. Sinusitis: as middle ear, plus *Staphylococcus* aureus, *Hemophilus* species, and mucormycosis (also seen with orbital cellulitis).
3. Penetrating head trauma: *S. aureus*, streptococci, *Enterobacteriaceae*, and *Clostridium* species.
4. AIDS is associated mainly with *Toxoplasma* species infection, although fungal abscesses may also occur.

Clinical features. Usually resemble other space-occupying lesions (focal signs, seizures in 50% of patients) with most symptoms related to increased intracranial pressure (ICP) (headache, nausea, vomiting, lethargy, and stupor). Fever occurs in only 50% of cases.

Histopathologic stages. (1) Days 1 to 3: Early cerebritis with a local inflammatory response around a necrotic center. (2) Days 4 to 9: Late cerebritis, which is characterized by increased necrosis and inflammation, with initial fibroblastic formation of the collagen capsule. (3) Days 10 to 13: Early encapsulation stage shows further development of the collagen capsule, which is typically thinner on the less vascular ventricular side. (4) Days 14 and later: Late capsular stage shows five distinct histologic layers – the necrotic center, inflammatory cells and fibroblasts, collagen capsule, neovascular layer, and surrounding reactive gliosis and edema.

Work up. Computed tomography (CT) scans correlate well with the histopathologic stages. In the cerebritis stage, CT without contrast shows the necrotic center as a hypodensity. Ring enhancement begins in the later stages of cerebritis. In the capsular stages the capsule becomes visible on CT without contrast as a faint ring of hyperdensity as compared to the hypodense necrotic core. Contrast produces a well-defined capsular ring, which is thinner on the ventricular side. Magnetic resonance imaging (MRI) appearance is bright on diffusion weighted images (DWI), T2 hyperintense ring of edema and hypointense capsule, enhances with gadolinium. MRI spectroscopy also reflects histologic changes and can add to differential between abscess, necrotizing tumor, or granuloma. Cerebral angiography demonstrates an avascular mass, "ring blush," or "luxury" collateral perfusion around an avascular mass and is especially helpful if mycotic aneurysms are suspected. Electroencephalography (EEG) abnormalities include focal slowing, seizure activity, and sometimes evidence of diffuse encephalopathy. If brain abscess is suspected, lumbar puncture (LP) should not be performed because organisms rarely grow from CSF and the risk of herniation seem greater with abscess than with other mass lesions.

Treatment. Combination of broad-spectrum antimicrobials, neurosurgical drainage or excision, and eradication of the primary infectious focus. If CT shows only cerebritis or abscess less than 2.5 cm and the patient is neurologically stable, antibiotics without surgery may suffice. Neurologic deterioration usually mandates surgery. Empiric antibiotics should be given based on the route of infection and adjusted based on the cultures. When the cause is unknown, the patient should receive a third-generation cephalosporin- e.g., ceftazidime 2 g IV q 8 hr (or penicillin (PCN) G 5 MU IV q 6 hr), and metronidazole 500 mg IV q 6 hr. For paranasal sinus sources administer PCN and metronidazole. In treatment of posttraumatic cases, nafcillin 2 g IV q 2 hr (or vancomycin 1g IV q 12 hr) and third-generation cephalosporin- e.g., ceftazidime 2 g IV q 8 hr. Treatment should be given for 6 to 8 weeks or until the resolution of neuroimaging findings. In patients who are positive for human immunodeficiency virus, coverage should be added for toxoplasmosis. Mucormycosis is treated with amphotericin B. Antiepileptic drugs may be given for up to 3 months. Routine corticosteroid administration is controversial.

Prognosis. Mortality rates range from 5% to 20%. Poor prognosis is associated with very young or old age, anaerobic pathogens, large abscess size, location in deep structures or cerebellum, acute clinical presentation with stupor/coma, metastatic abscess, rupture into ventricle or subarachnoid space, and concomitant pulmonary infection or sepsis.

REFERENCES

Greenberg MS: *Handbook of neurosurgery*, ed 5, Lakeland, FL, Greenberg Graphics, 2001.
Osenbach RK, Loftus CM: *Neurosurg Clin N Am* 3:403, 1992.

ABSCESS, EPIDURAL

Spinal epidural abscesses most commonly spread via a hematogenous route. Risk factors include intravenous drug abuse, diabetes, alcoholism, and chronic renal failure

Clinical features. Spinal and radicular pain that progresses to weakness over hours to days. Back pain, fever, spine tenderness, progressive myelopathy with bowel/bladder disturbance, and weakness progressing rapidly to para- and quadriplegia may occur.

Pathogens. Staphylococcus and gram-negative organisms.

Pathophysiology of spinal cord dysfunction. A combination of mechanical compression, vascular mechanisms leading to venous thrombosis, and infectious (myelitis) by direct extension. If diagnosis is suspected, *emergency imaging is indicated*.

Treatment. Adequate surgical drainage and broad-spectrum antibiotic coverage.

Prognosis. Poor, mortality can be as high as 25% of cases. Patients who are paralyzed before surgery rarely improve.

REFERENCE

Greenberg MS: *Handbook of neurosurgery*, ed 5, Lakeland, FL, Greenberg Graphics, 2001.

ACALCULIA

The acquired impairment of arithmetic skills typically occurs in three forms: (1) *number alexia*, an inability to read numbers; (2) *spatial acalculia*, a misalignment of numbers in appropriate columns that usually occurs with *right hemisphere* lesions; (3) *anarithmetria*, or loss of calculation skill, often associated with left parietal lesions.

Acalculia rarely occurs in isolation; it commonly accompanies aphasia and is a component of Gerstmann's syndrome.

REFERENCE

Mesulam MM: *Principles of behavioral and cognitive neurology*, New York, Oxford University Press, 2000.

AGNOSIA

Impaired recognition of sensory stimuli that cannot be attributed to sensory loss or language disturbance or global cognitive deficit.

I. *Visual agnosia* can be divided into the following:

A. The apperceptive type is a deficit of visual processing in which abnormal percepts are formed and may occur after *bilateral injury to the primary visual cortex*. Patients are unable to copy or match visually presented items.

B. The associative type is when the deficit lies after percept formation but before meaning has been associated. Patients are able to draw and describe the major meaning of stimuli with the exception of color. The majority of these patients have achromatopsia. Anomic aphasia should be excluded prior to diagnosing any visual agnosia. Object agnosia (inability to recognize objects), prosopagnosia (loss of recognition of specific members of a generic group; distinguishing and recognizing faces, cars, houses, etc.), and achromatopsia (inability to perceive color) are all visual agnosias occurring with *occipito-temporal lesions, usually bilateral*.

II. *Auditory agnosia* is an inability to recognize sounds that cannot be attributed to a hearing deficit. It may be restricted to non-speech sounds (selective auditory agnosia) or to speech sounds (pure word deafness) or involve both (generalized auditory agnosia).

III. *Tactile agnosia*, such as astereognosis (inability to recognize objects placed in the hand), is not well characterized in the absence of primary sensory loss and may not be a true agnosia. Less well understood problems are anosognosia (lack of awareness of a deficit), anosodiaphoria (failure of mood recognition), and simultanagnosia (inability to perceive more than one object at a time).

REFERENCE

Mesulam MM: *Principles of behavioral and cognitive neurology*, New York, Oxford University Press, 2000.

AGRAPHIA

The acquired inability to write, "aphasia of writing," occurs in five clinical forms:

1. *Pure agraphia* (no other language abnormality present) is seen with lesions of the *second frontal convolution* (Exner's area), *superior parietal lobule*, and the *posterior sylvian region*.

2. *Aphasic agraphia* is the writing disturbance of aphasics that usually resembles their spoken speech.

3. *Agraphia with alexia* is produced by a dominant angular gyrus lesion.

4. *Apractic agraphia*, in which production of letters and words is abnormal, usually occurs with a dominant superior parietal lobule lesion.

5. *Spatial agraphia* with abnormalities of spacing letters and maintaining a horizontal line is usually produced by nondominant parietal lesions.

Neuropsychologists have defined two systems of writing. The *phonological system* decodes speech sounds (phonemes) into letters. In phonological agraphia, produced by lesions of supramarginal gyrus or the insula medial to it, the patient is unable to spell non-sense words but is capable of spelling familiar words. The *lexical system* retrieves visual word images when spelling. Lexical agraphia is marked by errors in spelling irregular words, but these errors are phonologically correct (rough—ruf). Lexical agraphia occurs with lesions at the junction of the posterior angular gyrus and parieto-occipital lobule.

REFERENCES

Heilman KM, Valenstein E: *Clinical neuropsychology*, New York, Oxford University Press, 1993.
Mesulam MM: *Principles of behavioral and cognitive neurology*, New York, Oxford University Press, 2000.

AIDS

Acquired immunodeficiency syndrome (AIDS) is caused by the human immunodeficiency virus (HIV), a retrovirus. Neurologic manifestations can occur at any level of the neuraxis at any stage of infection and can be a result of direct HIV infection, HIV-induced immune dysregulation, or opportunistic infections. Specific syndromes tend to occur more frequently during particular phases of HIV infection, but can appear at almost any point during the course, and virtually all have been described as the initial presenting feature of HIV infection.

I. Early HIV infection

Initial HIV infection usually manifests as a nonspecific viral syndrome of fever, arthralgias, myalgias, and malaise lasting several days. Formed antibodies to HIV proteins take 6 months to appear. Prior to seroconversion, standard anti-HIV antibody assays are negative, and diagnosis can only be made by means of Western blot assay for viral antigen. Several syndromes can be associated with this early phase of infection, and their association with HIV may only be discerned if Western blot is obtained.

   A. HIV meningoencephalitis—a viral meningitis can accompany the syndrome of initial infection. In a few patients, this affects the brain parenchyma as well, resulting in a self-limited encephalopathy.
   B. Transverse myelitis rarely accompanies acute HIV infection.
   C. Acute inflammatory demyelinating polyneuropathy can occur upon or shortly after initial infection. It may be differentiated from Guillain-Barré syndrome (GBS) (also known as acute inflammatory demyelinating polyneuropathy [AIDP]) by the presence of cerebrospinal fluid (CSF) pleocytosis. Course and treatment are similar to those for idiopathic GBS.

    D. Sensory ganglioneuropathy.

    E. Brachial plexitis.

    F. Rhabdomyolysis can accompany initial infection. Steroids can be beneficial.

II. Midstage HIV infection (CD4 count 200 to 500/μl)

    A. HIV meningitis can recur at any point and may remain asymptomatic. The resulting elevated CSF protein and pleocytosis significantly complicates workup for other infections.

    B. CIDP is the chronic form of AIDP. Patients can benefit from intravenous immunoglobulin or plasmapheresis.

    C. Mononeuritis multiplex, when apparent in early or midstage HIV infection, is often self-limited.

    D. Nucleoside antiviral polyneuropathy—didanosine, zalcitabine, and stavudine can all cause a dysesthetic sensory neuropathy, especially at higher doses. Often of subacute onset over weeks, it gradually improves after change of offending agent; both features help to distinguish this from HIV-related distal sensory neuropathy (see below).

    E. Inflammatory myopathy—presents as proximal muscle weakness and sometimes myalgia. Biopsy shows inflammation. Steroids are beneficial, if immune status permits.

    F. Zidovudine (AZT) myopathy occurs because AZT is a mitochondrial toxin. Presentation is similar to inflammatory myopathy. Biopsy suggests mitochondrial dysfunction but may show inflammation as well. Clinical improvement after AZT withdrawal is the best means of diagnosis.

III. Late HIV infection (CD4 count <200/μl)

    A. Focal brain lesions

        1. Cerebral toxoplasmosis—caused by intracerebral reactivation of infection with the parasite *Toxoplasma gondii*, this syndrome is usually manifested in fever, headache, confusion, seizures, and focal neurologic signs, although any or all of these can be lacking. Neuroimaging typically reveals multiple ring-enhancing lesions. Antibiotics are usually quite effective.

        2. Primary CNS lymphoma (PCNSL) occurs in 2% of AIDS patients. PCNSL is the second most common etiology of ring-enhancing lesions on CT/MRI and is usually unifocal. It can be distinguished from *T. gondii* by single photon emission computed tomography (SPECT) or positron emission tomography (PET). Any patient with ring-enhancing lesions that are atypical for toxoplasmosis or do not respond to several weeks of anti-*Toxoplasma* therapy must undergo biopsy. Mean survival is 1 month from diagnosis without whole-brain radiotherapy and 4 to 6 months with it.

        3. Progressive multifocal leukoencephalopathy (PML) results from reactivation of JC virus, an infection generally of no consequence to the immunocompetent. Reactivation in oligodendroglia leads to

demyelinating white matter disease, focal neurologic deficits, and non–ring-enhancing white matter lesions on scan. Mean survival is 2 to 4 months. Ten percent of patients have enhancing lesions, which may be associated with increased survival. No specific therapy is known, although occasional patients have responded to treatment with cytarabine or cidofovir.

4. Stroke is not a complication of HIV per se, but 4% of AIDS patients have a symptomatic stroke during their life. Ischemic stroke may be caused by AIDS-related bacterial endocarditis, viral-associated vasculitis, or perivascular infection, or it may be a result of more traditional risk factors such as hypertension and hyperlipidemia; intracranial hemorrhage can complicate PCNSL, metastatic Kaposi's sarcoma, or (rarely) toxoplasmosis.

5. Focal brain lesions in AIDS patients can be due to any of the above, plus cysticercosis, fungal abscess (due to candida, aspergillus, mucormycosis, coccidiomycosis, etc.), bacterial abscess (mycobacteria, *T. pallidum*, *Nocardia*, *Listeria*, etc.), or other tumors (glioma, Kaposi's, other metastases). The usual approach in a patient with typical imaging findings such as a ring enhancing lesion and positive toxoplasma serology is to treat empirically for toxoplasmosis and proceed to biopsy if repeat scan shows no improvement. Those with negative serology or atypical scan should undergo biopsy immediately.

B. Cryptococcal meningitis develops in 10%. It often presents as a combination of cognitive impairment, personality change, lethargy, cranial neuropathies, and increased intracranial pressure, with or without typical signs and symptoms of meningismus. Fungal CSF culture is the gold standard, but results take weeks; CSF cryptococcal antigen is rapid and highly sensitive and specific. India ink smear is also rapid and increases sensitivity. Initial treatment should be amphotericin B with flucytosine. Unfortunately, response can be as low as 40%, and recurrence is common; however, in those surviving the initial infection, long-term suppression with daily fluconazole can be effective.

C. Syphilitic meningitis and meningovasculitis frequently complicate HIV infection, since *T. pallidum* shares some risk factors with HIV. Findings include meningismus, cranial neuropathies, and, with chronic infections, classic tertiary syphilis. Diagnosis depends on a combination of serology and clinical suspicion. Treatment is with penicillin.

D. Tuberculous meningitis is more common in AIDS patients than in the nonimmunosuppressed. Tuberculomas may also rarely occur. CSF polymerase chain reaction (PCR) can complement culture.

E. HIV encephalopathy (AIDS dementia complex, HIV-associated dementia) is a subcortical dementia of unclear pathogenesis characterized by cognitive slowing, emotional blunting, and motor impairment. Prevalence estimates vary widely (5 to 60%); in the pediatric population, the prevalence is much higher (90%). Workup consists of ruling out treatable infections (cryptococcus, syphilis, cytomegalovirus (CMV) encephalitis) and medical conditions (hypothyroidism, B_{12} deficiency). No specific treatment beyond antiviral therapy is known.

F. Vacuolar myelopathy is present in up to 55% on autopsy but symptomatic in far fewer. It is of uncertain pathogenesis and pathology shows vacuolization in the dorsal and lateral columns of the spinal cord. Symptoms, which develop late, include constipation, urinary disturbances, ataxia, and spastic paraparesis. There is no treatment. The process is painless and slowly progressive; pain or rapid progression should prompt evaluation for other causes, such as viral myelitis, metastatic cord compression, or epidural abscess. Other subacute myelopathies sometimes associated with AIDS include syphilis and B_{12} deficiency.

G. Mononeuritis multiplex in late HIV infection is often due to CMV and benefits from ganciclovir. CMV can also cause encephalitis, meningitis, retinitis, myelitis, or polyradiculitis. CSF PCR for central nervous system CMV infections has ~90% sensitivity.

H. Varicella zoster virus (VZV) can cause encephalitis, Ramsay-Hunt syndrome, myelitis, vasculitis, and segmental zoster rashes (shingles). Herpes simplex virus (HSV) can cause encephalitis or myelitis. Both HSV and VZV are treated with acyclovir.

I. Distal symmetrical polyneuropathy—axonal, predominantly sensory neuropathy with impairment of all sensory modalities, often with paresthesias, which can be painful. Tricyclic antidepressants and anticonvulsants can help dysesthetic symptoms, but some patients may require opiates. Capsaicin may also help.

REFERENCES

AAN Quality Standards Subcommittee: *Neurology*, 50:21–26, 1997.
Berger JR, Major EO: *Semin Neurol* 19:193–200,1999.

ALCOHOL

Neurologic effects of alcohol are due to a combination of its direct neuro-toxic effects or its metabolites, nutritional factors, and genetic predisposition. Complications include intoxication, withdrawal syndromes, Wernicke-Korsakoff's syndrome, nutritional deficiency states, and miscellaneous other conditions.

A. *Intoxication* with alcohol correlates roughly with blood concentrations. Cognitive dysfunction tends to occur early, while cerebellar, autonomic, and vestibular symptoms tend to occur at higher blood levels. Positional vertigo may result from alcohol diffusing into the cupula when the recumbent position is assumed. As the alcohol concentration rises to a certain level, the intoxication is greater than when it falls to the same level. Blackouts are periods of amnesia, usually during binge drinking, and occur in persons with and without alcohol dependence.

B. *Withdrawal* syndromes in individuals with alcohol dependency result from either decreased intake or cessation of drinking. The syndromes may be early or late. Most common are the early symptoms, which begin 12 to 24 hours after decreased intake. Tremulousness is common and may be accompanied by nausea, vomiting, insomnia, and *hallucinations (visual, tactile, or auditory)*. Treatment consists of benzodiazepines. Auditory hallucinations may persist, necessitating the use of neuroleptics. Withdrawal seizures are typically generalized tonic-clonic and begin within the first 24 hours but may occur after several days.

Focal seizures imply a structural lesion and should not be attributed to alcohol withdrawal. Treatment of withdrawal seizures is controversial since they are usually self-limited. Initial loading with phenytoin and slowly tapering off after several days is one approach. Thiamine is routinely given and hypomagnesemia, if present, is treated.

Late withdrawal symptoms, referred to as *delirium tremens*, are a serious complication and have a peak incidence 72 to 96 hours after decreased alcohol intake. Severe confusion, agitation, vivid hallucinations, tremors, and increased autonomic activity (tachycardia, fever, sweating, orthostatic hypotension) are characteristic. These symptoms can last 1 to 3 days and can be fatal (~10%). *Treatment* consists of sedation with benzodiazepines, hydration with IV fluids, and administration of thiamine, multivitamins, and magnesium (if indicated). Autonomic hyperactivity should be treated aggressively if present.

C. *Wernicke-Korsakoff's syndrome* is the most common deficiency syndrome due to chronic alcoholism. Wernicke's syndrome represents the acute phase and classically has the triad of *encephalopathy, ataxia, and ocular motor disturbance* (nystagmus, ophthalmoplegia, and gaze palsy). However, a complete triad of signs is often not present. Atrophy of the mammillary bodies is common. Korsakoff's syndrome is a more chronic condition and includes anterograde amnesia (the inability to incorporate ongoing experience into memory) leading to *confabulation*. Both syndromes are attributed to thiamine deficiency and can also be seen in nonalcoholic malnutrition states, although much less commonly. Treatment consists of thiamine, 100 mg per day for 3 days parenterally, followed by oral thiamine indefinitely. IV glucose should never be given without thiamine to a chronic alcoholic due to the risk of precipitating Wernicke's encephalopathy. As with most alcohol-related syndromes, supplemental vitamins and magnesium may be beneficial.

D. *Other alcohol-related syndromes* include cerebellar degeneration, peripheral neuropathy, optic neuropathy, and myopathy. Cerebellar degeneration invariably involves the *anterior vermis and paravermian regions* with resultant truncal and gait ataxia. A "dying back" sensori-motor neuropathy is usually heralded by complaints of numb, burning feet. Minor motor signs may evolve. *Nutritional amblyopia* (previously called tobacco-alcohol amblyopia) consists of gradual visual loss. It is due to poor nutrition and not a direct toxic effect of alcohol. In contrast, *alcoholic myopathy* is believed to be caused by the toxic effects of alcohol and improves with abstinence. It may occur as an acute necrotizing disorder with muscle pain and rhabdomyolysis, or as a more slowly progressive disease with proximal weakness. The combination of thiamine, multivitamins, and abstinence is the treatment of choice for these syndromes.

E. *Conditions of somewhat uncertain etiology occurring in chronic alcoholics* include central pontine myelinolysis, Marchiafava-Bignami syndrome, and cortical atrophy. *Central pontine myelinolysis* is a rare cerebral white matter disorder, associated with basis pontis lesions with resultant progressive quadriparesis, horizontal gaze palsy, and obtundation leading to coma. It occurs with excessively rapid correction of hyponatremia. *Marchiafava-Bignami syndrome* is a rare demyelinating disease of the corpus callosum and adjacent subcortical white matter, sometimes associated with excessive consumption of crude red wine. Patients can have cognitive impairment, spasticity, dysarthria, and impaired gait. *Cortical atrophy* causing dementia in chronic alcoholics, not explained by Korsakoff's syndrome, is not accepted by most authorities. The CT scan appearance of "atrophy" or "parenchymal volume loss" is probably related to fluid shifts in the brain and may reverse with abstinence.

Alcoholics have an increased incidence of stroke related to a variety of factors, including rebound thrombocytosis, altered cerebral blood flow, and hyperlipidemia.

REFERENCES

Adams RD, Victor M: *Principles of neurology*, New York, McGraw-Hill, 1997.
Victor M: *Can J Neurol Sci* 21:88–99, 1994.

ALEXIA

The loss of a previously acquired reading ability occurs in three forms: (1) *anterior alexia*, usually seen in association with Broca's aphasia, characterized by impaired comprehension of syntactic structure; (2) *central or aphasic alexia* (alexia with agraphia "acquired illiteracy"), usually seen in association with visual field deficit but may exist in isolation. It is seen with *angular gyrus lesions*; and (3) *posterior or pure alexia* (alexia without agraphia), seen with infarction of the *dominant occipital lobe and splenium of the corpus callosum*, which results in loss of visual input to the language areas. It is associated with right homonymous hemianopia.

REFERENCE

Mesulam MM: *Principles of behavioral and cognitive neurology*, New York, Oxford University Press, 2000.

AMAUROSIS FUGAX

Amaurosis fugax (AFx) or transient monocular blindness is a reversible loss of vision (partial or complete), classically from ischemia in the territory of central retinal or ophthalmic artery. Differential diagnosis includes "transient visual obscuration" resulting from increased intracranial pressure, arterial vasospasm, and ocular causes of transient visual loss. AFx has a short duration (seconds to minutes) and usually consists of negative symptoms (blackness or graying of the visual field) with an occasional positive phenomena (scintillating scotomas or points of light). Funduscopic examination may show the cholesterol emboli (*Hollenhorst*

TABLE 1
CAUSES OF TRANSIENT MONOCULAR BLINDNESS

I. Embolic.
    A. Carotid embolism.
    B. Cardiac and aortic embolism.
    C. Embolism related to intravenous drug abuse.
II. Hemodynamic.
    A. Hypoperfusion.
    B. Vasospasm.
    C. Inflammatory arteritides such as temporal arteritis, Takayasu's syndrome, and polyarteritis nodosa.
    D. Severe atherosclerotic occlusive disease of internal carotid or ophthalmic artery.
    E. Carotid dissection.
    F. Hypertensive crises.
III. Ocular.
    A. Anterior ischemic optic neuropathy.
    B. Central retinal vein occlusion.
    C. Intraocular causes such as hemorrhage, tumor, and glaucoma.
    D. Drusen.
IV. Neurologic disorders.
    A. Disease of the vestibular or oculomotor system.
    B. Optic neuritis (mainly demyelinating diseases).
    C. Optic nerve or optic chiasmal compression.
    D. Increased intracranial pressure.
    E. Migraine.
V. Psychogenic.
VI. Idiopathic.

Adapted from Amaurosis Fugax Study Group: *Stroke* 21:201–208, 1990.

plaques). Embolization from the internal carotid artery, aorta, or heart may be the cause (see Table 1).

Treatment of classical amaurosis fugax depends on the underlying etiology. Aspirin and warfarin may be indicated or endarterectomy in cases of hemodynamically significant carotid artery stenosis. AFx due to vasospasm (i.e., particularly in young adults), may respond to calcium channel blockers nifedipine or verapamil.

REFERENCES

Amaurosis Fugax Study Group: *Stroke* 21:201–208, 1990.
Winterkorn JM, Beckman RL: *J Neuroophthalmol* 15:209–211, 1995.

ANEURYSMS

Intracranial aneurysms are classified as saccular (berry), mycotic, arteriosclerotic, traumatic, dissecting, and neoplastic.

Clinical presentations include cranial nerve palsies (especially of nerve III, including the pupil, and nerves IV and VI), headache, mass lesion or "steal" phenomena effect (giant aneurysms), and thrombosis (athersclerotic aneurysms). Rupture with subarachnoid hemorrhage (SAH) is the primary manifestation. Ruptured saccular aneurysms account for 80% of nontraumatic SAH (most common after age 20); a severe headache of sudden onset is characteristic. The size and location of the bleed and the presence of intraparenchymal and ventricular extension (associated with a significantly higher mortality) affect the level of consciousness (lethargy to coma). Sudden loss of consciousness is the presenting feature in 20% of cases. Meningeal signs, papilledema, retinal hemorrhage, and seizures are common. Focal signs in the first 24 hours usually indicate parenchymal dissection, cerebral edema, or hypoperfusion distal to the ruptured aneurysm. After the first 48 to 72 hours focal signs may be due to vasospasm.

Diagnostic evaluation includes CT (results are negative in approximately 15% of cases) and LP if CT finding is negative. Angiography may locate and define the cause of SAH (aneurysm, AVM) and should be repeated in 5 to 15 days if results are initially negative. Magnetic resonance angiography is a promising alternative to conventional angiography.

The Hunt-Hess grading scale is commonly used for prognosis and timing of aneurysm surgery:

0: Unruptured aneurysm (symptomatic or incidental discovery).
I: Asymptomatic rupture or minimal headache and nuchal rigidity.
Ia: No acute meningeal or brain reaction, but fixed neurologic deficit.

II: Moderate to severe headache, nuchal rigidity, no neurologic deficit other than cranial nerve palsy.

III: Drowsiness, confusion, or mild focal neurologic deficit.

IV: Stupor, moderate to severe hemiparesis, possibly early decerebrate rigidity and vegetative disturbances.

V: Deep coma, decerebrate rigidity, moribund appearance.

Complications and sequelae of SAH result from systemic dysfunction (syndrome of inappropriate antidiuretic hormone [SIADH], cardiac arrhythmias, diabetes insipidus, pulmonary embolism, GI bleeding, respiratory depression, and cardiac arrest), vasospasm, rebleeding, seizures, herniation, and hydrocephalus. Cerebral ischemia or infarction is frequent in the first 4 to 14 days after the initial bleed because of arterial vasospasm. The amount of subarachnoid blood correlates positively with the rate of occurrence of vasospasm. The use of nimodipine (60 mg q 4 hr for 21 days) seems to reduce the occurrence of severe neurologic complications (death, coma, and permanent major motor deficits). The use of other agents such as aminophylline, dopamine, and isoproterenol remains controversial.

Lysis of the clot surrounding the aneurysm after the initial bleed results in rebleeding, which may become evident as development of new focal signs, or worsened clinical status. Slightly more than 20% of patients rebleed in the first 2 weeks; more than 30% rebleed in the first month. The mortality rate with rebleeding is over 40%, higher than with the initial bleeding. After the first 6 months the annual rebleeding rate is about 5%, with an annual mortality rate of 1% to 3%. Treating hypertension and maintaining the blood pressure in the normal range helps prevent rebleeding. In the acute phase, induced hypotension is associated with significant ischemic complications and should be avoided. The use of antifibrinolytic agents such as epsilon aminocaproic acid (Amicar), which are given by continuous IV infusion (at least 36 g per day) for up to 3 weeks and then tapered gradually, results in a decreased mortality rate for rebleeding. The decrease, however, is offset by an increased mortality rate for vasospasm. Side effects of epsilon aminocaproic acid include diarrhea, reversible myopathy, and thromboembolic disease.

Surgical clipping of the aneurysm, with intraoperatively induced hypotension and controlled ventilation, is the definitive therapy and should be performed as soon as possible, especially in stable patients (Hunt-Hess grades I to III), to avoid the risk of rebleeding. Late occurrence of hydrocephalus may require shunting.

The most common sites for aneurysms in adults are shown in Figure 1. A higher frequency of aneurysm has been reported in some familial cases and in patients with polycystic kidneys, coarctation of the aorta, and fibromuscular dysplasia.

A

ANEURYSMS

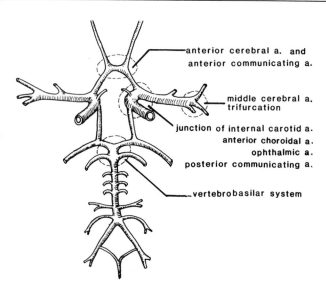

FIGURE 1

Most common sites of aneurysms.

REFERENCES

Schierenk WI: *N Engl J Med* 336(1):28–40, 1997.
van Gijn J, Rinkel GJ: *Brain* 124 (Pt 2): 249–278, 2001.
Wardlaw JM, White PM: *Brain* 123(Pt 2): 205–221, 2000.

ANGIOGRAPHY

Conventional cerebral angiography combines standard x-ray with injection of radio-opaque dyes directly into the arterial system of interest. This is done by threading a catheter (usually through the femoral artery in the groin) to the aortic arch or selectively to the carotid or vertebrobasilar systems. Computerized subtraction techniques improve the resolution of the image. Angiography also provides evaluation of the vessels in a given time frame ("ciné") following the distribution/dispersals of dye through arterial and venous phases.

It is indicated in the evaluation of suspected vascular malformations (aneurysms, angiomas), vasculopathies, and vasculitides, stenotic or ulcerative vascular lesions; and in delineating vascular anatomy and vascular supply to various tumors.

Local complications include puncture site hematomas, intimal tears, pseudoaneurysms, and AV fistulas. Systemic complications include

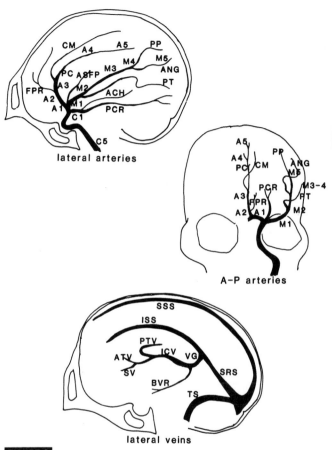

lateral arteries

A-P arteries

lateral veins

FIGURE 2

Internal carotid circulation.

A_1–A_5	Segments of anterior cerebral artery	ISS	Inferior sagittal sinus
ACH	Anterior choroidal artery	M_1–M_5	Segments of middle cerebral artery
ANG	Angular artery		
ASFP	Ascending frontoparietal artery	PC	Pericallosal artery
ATV	Anterior terminal vein	PCR	Posterior cerebral artery
BVR	Basal vein of Rosenthal	PP	Posterior parietal artery
CM	Callosomarginal artery	PTV	Posterior terminal vein
C_1–C_5	Segments of internal carotid artery	SRS	Straight sinus
		SSS	Superior sagittal sinus
FPR	Frontopolar artery	SV	Septal vein
ICV	Internal cerebral vein	TS	Transverse sinus
		VG	Great cerebral vein of Galen

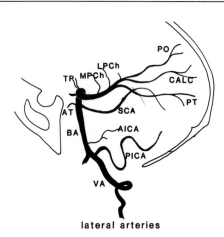

lateral arteries

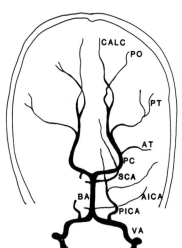

half-axial arteries

FIGURE 3

Vertebrobasilar circulation.

AICA	Anterior inferior cerebellar artery	PICA	Posterior inferior cerebellar artery
AT	Anterior temporal artery (branch of PC)	PO	Parieto-occipital artery (branch of PC)
BA	Basilar artery	PT	Posterior temporal artery (branch of PC)
CALC	Calcarine artery (branch of PC)		
LPCh	Lateral posterior choroidal artery	SCA	Superior cerebellar artery
MPCh	Medial posterior choroidal artery	TP	Thalamoperforate artery
PC	Posterior cerebral artery	VA	Vertebral artery

manifestations of anaphylaxis. Many forms of CNS (and ocular) dysfunction have been reported ranging from diffuse encephalopathy to focal ischemia. Most neurologic complications are transient. Complication rate is greater with increasing age and preexisting cerebrovascular disease. Permanent neurologic deficit occurs in approximately 0.5%.

Angiographic anatomy is depicted in Figures 2 and 3.

ANGIOMAS

Angiomas are congenital vascular lesions resulting from disordered embryogenesis. Histologic subtypes include the following (percentages refer to the frequency at autopsy): (1) *telangiectasias* (16%)—abnormal capillaries; (2) *venous angiomas* (59%)—anomalous veins; (3) *arteriovenous malformations* (AVMs) (14%)—clusters of abnormal vessels composed of arteries and veins without intervening capillaries; (4) *cavernous angiomas* (9%)—sinusoidal vessels without intervening neural tissue; and (5) *varices* (2%)—dilated veins. Angiomas are usually asymptomatic; symptoms usually are due to AVMs or cavernous angiomas. The most common intracranial locations are the cerebral hemispheres (75%) and basal ganglia (18%); posterior fossa angiomas are much less frequent (6%), occurring primarily in the pons; the spinal cord is a much rarer location (see Spinal Cord). Angiography detects most angiomas, with the notable exception of cavernous angiomas and telangiectasias. MRI is the preferred noninvasive neuroimaging modality.

AVMs are the most common symptomatic angioma. Eighty percent to 90% are supratentorial. Clinical manifestations include: hemorrhage (30% to 50%), seizures (approximately 30%), migraine-like headaches (20%), and gradually progressive focal neurologic deficits (10%). Hemorrhage occurs at a rate of 1% to 2% per year. Intraparenchymal hemorrhage occurs in two-thirds of cases, subarachnoid hemorrhage in one-third of cases. The short-term prognosis for patients with ruptured AVMs is better than that for patients with aneurysms, with lower rates of vasospasm (rare), mortality (10%), and rebleeding (6% in the first year, reverting to 1% to 2% subsequently). Recurrent hemorrhage is associated with higher rates of mortality and overall disability. The prognosis for patients with seizures alone is better than that after hemorrhage. Therapeutic modalities include surgical excision, embolization, and radiotherapy.

REFERENCES

Caplan LR: *Stroke: A clinical approach*, ed 2, Boston, Butterworth-Heinemann, 1993.
Mohr JP et al: In Barnett HJM et al, eds: *Stroke pathophysiology, diagnosis, and management*, ed 2, New York, Churchill Livingstone, 1992.

ANTIBODY TESTING IN NEUROMUSCULAR DISEASE

The presence of autoantibodies in certain neuromuscular diseases raises the possibility of immune-mediated pathophysiology and implies that immunosuppressive therapy might be effective. The antibodies may help in classifying the type of neuropathy in certain clinical syndromes and may predict the prognosis and response to treatment (see Table 2). The presence of the antibody does not define the clinical presentation and may be present in other clinical entities. In addition, the pathogenic role for the antibody is uncertain for many diseases.

ANTI-GANGLIOSIDE GM1 AND ASSOCIATED NEUROPATHIES

Autoantibodies directed against gangliosides are associated with multifocal motor neuropathy with conduction blocks, various lower motor neuron syndromes, and Guillain-Barré syndrome (GBS).

The anti-GM1 antibody is usually a low-affinity polyclonal IgM directed against the extracellular carbohydrate moiety of gangliosides. In 10% to 15% of patients, it is a monoclonal IgM, and rarely polyclonal IgG antibodies have been described. The clinical implications of these differences are unclear. Measurement of anti-GM1 antibodies in most laboratories involves ELISA methodology. Difference in techniques, methods of standardization between laboratories, and determination of "positive" titers makes it difficult to compare results.

Multifocal Motor Neuropathy (MMN)

MMN is rare and probably represents <1% of all patients presenting with a motor syndrome. Patients present with slow progressive asymmetrical

TABLE 2

NEUROPATHY SYNDROMES ASSOCIATED WITH AUTOANTIBODIES

Condition	Antigen	Antibody	% Positive
Ganglioside Antibodies			
Multifocal motor neuropathy	GM1	Poly IgM	60–80
Distal lower motor neuron syndromes	GM1	Poly IgM, IgG	50–60
Guillain-Barré syndrome	GM1, GD1a	Poly IgG, IgM	20–30
Miller-Fisher syndrome	GQ1b	Poly IgG	~95
Glycoprotein Antibodies			
Monoclonal IgM to MAG	MAG	Mono IgM	50
RNA-binding Protein Antibodies			
Paraneoplastic sensory neuronopathy	Hu	Poly IgG	> 95
Glycosphingolipid Antibodies			
Chronic sensory neuropathy	Sulfatide	Mono IgM	—
		Poly IgM, IgG	—

MAG = Myelin-associated glycoprotein.

weakness that follows peripheral nerve distribution with no sensory loss. The most distinctive and diagnostic feature of MMN are the electrodiagnostic findings, which demonstrate motor conduction blocks in multiple nerve distributions, allowing differentiation from other lower motor neuron disorders such as amyotrophic lateral sclerosis (ALS). High titers of IgM antibody to GM1 and other gangliosides are present in as many as 50% of patients with treatment-responsive MMN. There is no apparent difference between seronegative or seropositive MMN. The pathogenic role for GM1 antibodies in MMN is unclear.

GM1 antibody titers may be useful in patients with clinical features of MMN (slowly progressive course, asymmetric, distal > proximal weakness following nerve distribution) but who lack electrophysiologic evidence of conduction block. In a patient with the typical syndrome of MMN in the face of high GM1 antibodies, a trial of intravenous immunoglobulin (IVIg) is appropriate even if conduction block cannot be found.

Lower Motor Neuron Syndromes
The presence of anti-GM1 in lower motor neuron syndrome without conduction blocks implies that the disease process may be immune mediated. Seropositive patients have slow disease progression with potential response to immunosuppressive therapy when compared to ALS.

ALS
Although ~50% of patients with ALS will have detectable serum levels of anti-GM1, the titers are low compared to those with MMN. Immunosuppression in patients with the classic clinical and electrophysiologic picture of ALS is usually not effective, irrespective of GM1 antibody titers. At present, there is no clear role of testing for anti-GM1 in ALS.

Guillain-Barré Syndrome
A high proportion of GBS patients, particularly those with *Campylobacter jejuni* infection, have a high titer of IgM or IgG antibodies to GM1. The presence of anti-GM1b antibodies appears to be associated with rapid progression and severe course and predominantly distal weakness with slower recovery. However, the presence of anti-GM1 alone is not a significant prognostic factor in Guillain-Barré syndrome, but combination of *Campylobacter* and GM1 antibodies is more likely to predict axonal forms of GBS, e.g., acute motor axonal neuropathy (AMAN) and acute motor and sensory axonal neuropathy (AMSAN). The demyelinating form of GBS can also occur with *C. jejuni* infection and anti-GM1 antibodies.

Anti-Ganglioside GQ1B and Miller-Fisher Syndrome (MFS)
MFS accounts for less than 5% of patients with GBS. Clinically, it presents with a triad of ataxia, ophthalmoparesis, and areflexia. GQ1b is a minor ganglioside in both the peripheral and central nervous systems. The function of GQ1b is unknown. The antibody reactivity in MFS is

A

ANTIBODY TESTING IN NEUROMUSCULAR DISEASE

usually polyclonal IgG GQ1b. GQ1b epitopes can be found on some strains of *C. jejuni*, the antecedent infection in some cases of MFS.

IgG antibodies to GQ1b have been detected in >95% of MFS patients, including those with atypical variants and patients with GBS associated with ophthalmoplegia. Conversely, GBS patients without ophthalmoplegia are invariably IgG antibody negative, indicating a strong correlation between MFS and anti-GQ1b. The GQ1b is used to distinguish MFS from other diseases (such as brainstem encephalitis) that may present in a similar fashion. The assay may also be useful in patients who present with isolated "acute ophthalmoparesis," which may suggest a variant of GBS.

ANTI-MYELIN-ASSOCIATED GLYCOPROTEIN (MAG) AND ASSOCIATED NEUROPATHIES

MAG is a membrane glycoprotein that comprises <1% of peripheral nervous system proteins. It is found in periaxonal membranes. It may serve as a "membrane spacer" to prevent compaction of myelin and formation of major dense lines. Its functions in cell adhesion in Schwann cell/axon interactions during myelination.

Anti-MAG is typically associated with a slowly progressive, distal, symmetric, sensorimotor neuropathy. Sensory symptoms predominate early in the course. Paresthesia is present in ~75% of patients at presentation. Gait ataxia is common, and upper extremity tremor is prominent in 10% of patients. Motor involvement is eventually present in 65%. The cranial nerves are usually spared, and autonomic involvement is rare. In ~75% of cases, electrophysiologic studies show motor conduction velocities in the demyelinating range. Spinal fluid protein is frequently elevated, often >100 mg/dl. Many of these features are similar to those seen in the patients with neuropathies associated with IgG and IgA monoclonal gammopathy of unknown significance (MGUS), and with IgM-MGUS without reactivity to MAG. Seropositive patients tend to have a higher frequency and more severe sensory loss, more frequent ataxia and gait disturbance, and more severe nerve conduction abnormalities with distal accentuation of slowing in comparison to MAG-seronegative MGUS.

Anti-MAG reactivity is present in 50% to 65% of patients with an IgM monoclonal gammopathy and peripheral neuropathy. The anti-MAG IgM antibody is usually a MGUS; approximately 80% have kappa light chains. Rarely, patients with various hematologic malignancies, including lymphoma, chronic lymphatic leukemia, and Waldenström's macroglobulinemia will have MGUS with anti-MAG activity.

Although the presence of anti-MAG should be suggestive of immune-mediated pathogenesis, patients with neuropathy and anti-MAG tend to be more resistant to immune modulating treatments in comparison to patients with IgG or IgA MGUS. The main value of testing for anti-MAG is to help in better classification of clinical syndrome and prediction of response to treatment.

ANTI-HU AND PARANEOPLASTIC SENSORY NEURONOPATHY

Several conditions under a variety of names, including subacute sensory neuronopathy (SSN), paraneoplastic sensory neuronopathy, carcinomatous sensory neuropathy, and malignant inflammatory sensory polyganglionopathy are known to be associated with cancer (see Table 3).

Paraneoplastic sensory neuronopathy (PSN) is rare, affecting less than 1% of patients with small-cell lung carcinoma. The condition was also reported with prostate cancer, small-cell adrenal cancer, lung adenocarcinoma, neuroblastoma, and chondrosarcoma. In one series, 15% of the patients with anti-Hu antibody did not have cancer during the length of time of the study follow-up. Seventy-five percent of patients with anti-Hu have more widespread pathology that may include cerebellar degeneration and limbic or brainstem encephalitis (paraneoplastic encephalomyelitis/ sensory neuronopathy [PEM/SN]). Most patients with anti-Hu and PSN or PEM/SN are middle-aged or older, and 60% are women. In the majority, neurologic symptoms precede discovery of the tumor by months. In PSN, the typical onset of neurologic symptoms is subacute, usually over days to weeks. In some cases the onset is more abrupt. Numbness and parathesias are common presenting symptoms, usually accompanied by shooting pains and burning sensations. Gait ataxia, poor coordination, and loss of fine motor control follows. Autonomic neuropathy causing gastrointestinal dysmotility, intestinal pseudo-obstruction, postural hypotension, and neurogenic bladder. An associated limbic encephalitis may cause personality and mood changes, memory loss, confusion, hallucinations, and seizures.

Examination reveals a pan-modality sensory loss. Severely impaired proprioceptive sensation frequently results in severe gait ataxia and pseudo-athetosis. Pupils are irregular, with impaired reaction to light. Muscle strength is usually preserved or mildly decreased. Reflexes are usually absent.

The cerebrospinal fluid may have mild pleocytosis or elevated protein. EMG and nerve conduction studies show multifocal, decreased amplitude of sensory nerve action potentials with relatively normal motor conduction studies.

TABLE 3

AUTOANTIBODIES IN NEUROLOGIC PARANEOPLASTIC SYNDROMES

Syndrome	Cancer	Antibody	Antigen
Sensory neuronopathy, encephalomyelitis	Small-cell lung	Anti-Hu	HuD Neuronal nuclei
Opsoclonus-myoclonus	Breast	Anti-Ri	Neuronal nuclei
Cerebellar degeneration	Ovarian, breast	Anti-Yo	Purkinje cell
Lambert-Eaton syndrome	Small-cell lung	Anti-VGCC	Ca channel
Cancer-associated retinopathy	Small-cell lung	Anti-retinal	Photoreceptor

Anti-Hu antibody is a polyclonal, complement-fixing IgG that reacts strongly with the nuclei of virtually all neurons in the peripheral and central nervous system.

ANTIBODY TESTING IN NEUROMUSCULAR DISEASE

A positive anti-Hu antibody titer is seen in over 90% of patients with PSN or PEM/SN. A positive anti-Hu confirms the diagnosis of PSN (or PEM/PN) and should prompt an immediate search for cancer, since 90% of the time it is associated with small-cell lung cancer. If lung cancer is not detected by routine chest radiography, computed tomography should be obtained. If these are also negative, the search for a neoplasm should be broadened to consider other tumors. If this evaluation is also unrevealing, periodic screening for cancer is recommended. The prognosis for PSN patients is poor, but the tumor should be removed if possible, and plasmapheresis may be tried.

ANTI-SULFATIDE ANTIBODIES AND SENSORIMOTOR NEUROPATHY

Sulfatide is the major acidic glycosphingolipid in peripheral nerve myelin. The pathogenic role of sulfatide antibody to neuropathy is unknown.

A well-defined clinical syndrome has not been described associated with anti-sulfatide antibodies. Although most patients have predominantly sensory peripheral polyneuropathy, weakness is present in some individuals. The prevalence of anti-sulfatide neuropathy in the general population is also unclear. At this time, the available data does not justify the usefulness of routinely obtaining anti-sulfatide antibodies.

As for antibodies associated with disorders of neuromuscular junction as in myasthenia gravis or Lambert-Eaton myasthenic syndrome, see the discussions under Myasthenia Gravis and Lambert-Eaton Myasthenic Syndrome.

REFERENCES

Dalmau J et al: *Medicine* 71:59–72, 1992.
Kissel JT: *Semin Neurol* 18:83–94, 1998.
Van den Berg L et al: *Muscle Nerve* 19:637–643, 1996.
Yuki N et al: *Neurology* 43:414–417, 1993.

ANTIDEPRESSANTS

Antidepressants encompass several groups of compounds, including tricyclic and tetracyclic compounds, selective serotonin reuptake inhibitors (SSRI), and monoamine oxidase inhibitors. Table 4 summarizes the relative side effects of tricyclic antidepressants. Tricyclic antidepressants have notable anticholinergic side effects including blurred vision, dry mouth, constipation, urinary retention, memory dysfuncion, and exacerbation of narrow-angle glaucoma. Patients with dementia and concomitant depression may worsen as a result of anticholinergic effects, whereas patients with Parkinson's disease may improve. Patients with migraine or chronic pain may benefit from antidepressants with a relatively high affinity for serotonin receptors. Selective serotonin reuptake inhibitors (fluoxetine, sertraline, citalopram, and paroxetine) may cause headache. Choice of antidepressant must be based on assessment of the patient's clinical state, especially

TABLE 4
SIDE EFFECTS OF ANTIDEPRESSANT DRUGS*

Drug	Sedation	Insomnia	Anticholinergic Effects	Orthostatic Hypotension	Delay in Cardiac Conduction or Arrhythmia	Nausea
Tricyclic Drugs						
Amitriptyline	+++	0	+++	+++	Yes	0
Desipramine	+	+	+	+	Yes	0
Doxepin	+++	0	++	+++	Yes	0
Imipramine	++	0	++	++	Yes	0
Nortriptyline	++	0	+	+	Yes	0
Protriptyline	+	++	++	+	Yes	0
Monoamine Oxidase Inhibitors						
Phenelzine	+	+	0	+++	Very rare	0
Other SSRIs Agents						
Fluoxetine	0	++	0	0	Low	+
Trazodone	+++	0	0	0	Low	0
Alprazolam	+	0	0	High	None	0
Bupropion	0	High	0	0	Low	+
Sertraline	Very low	Moderate	0	0	0	+
Paroxetine	Low	Low	Low	0	0	+
Citalopram	Low	Low	0	0	0	Low

* Zero denotes no side effect, + a minor side effect, ++ a moderate side effect, and +++ a major side effect.
Adapted from Potter WZ et al: *N Engl J Med* 325:633–642, 1991.

A

ANTIDEPRESSANTS

cardiac conduction and ability to tolerate orthostatic hypotension, as well as the specific drug's side-effect profile. Suicide risk should be assessed in all depressed patients, since tricyclic antidepressant overdose is commonly fatal.

REFERENCES

Sadock BJ, Sadock VA, Kaplan HL: *Kaplan and Sadock's comprehensive textbook of psychiatry,* ed 7, Philadelphia, Lippincott Williams & Wilkins, 2000.

Stimmel GL: In Herfindal ET, Gourley DR, eds: *Textbook of therapeutics,* ed 7, Baltimore, Williams & Wilkins, 2000.

APHASIA

Aphasia is the acquired disorder of previously intact language ability. As such, it is not interchangeable with failure of language development. Aphasic patients have disturbances of speech, writing, and reading. The great majority of patients with aphasia have left hemisphere lesions, although occasional patients have language dominance in the right hemisphere.

Benson and Geschwind developed the most widely used classification of aphasia. In this classification three aspects of language are used to classify aphasias (see Tables 5 and 6).

1. Fluency refers to several features of spontaneous speech-rhythm, melody, articulation, and word production rate. Look for verbal (substitution of one word for another such as knife for spoon) and phonemic (substitution of incorrect sounds, such as "spork" for fork) paraphasic errors. Paraphasic errors (primarily in fluent aphasias) and naming abnormalities are the hallmark of aphasia.
2. Comprehension abilities vary from following midline commands (such as "stick out your tongue") to performing multistep requests (such as "take the paper in your left hand, fold it in half, and then put it on the floor"), to understanding relationships (as in "The lion was killed by the tiger. Which animal died?"), and to following more complex instructions.
3. Repetition of phrases may be impaired to various degrees; the most difficult phrases to repeat are those involving grammatical function or low frequency words (for instance, "The spy fled to Greece"). Additional testing of reading out loud, reading comprehension, and writing (to dictation or spontaneously) is useful.

Damage to the thalamus, caudate, putamen, and surrounding structures may produce aphasia (subcortical). Initial muteness improving to fluent or nonfluent hypophonic aphasia is common. Paraphasic errors in spontaneous speech, which disappear when the patient is asked to repeat phrases, and rapid resolution of deficits are hallmarks of these subcortical aphasias.

TABLE 5
APHASIAS WITH DISORDERED REPETITION*

	Type of Speech	Comprehension†	Other Signs	Emotional State	Localization
Broca's	Nonfluent	+	Right hemiparesis worse in arm	Depressed	Lower posterior frontal
Wernicke's	Fluent	–	Often none	Often euphoric and/or paranoid	Posterior superior temporal
Conduction	Fluent	+	Often none; cortical sensory loss in right arm	Depressed	Usually parietal operculum
Global	Nonfluent	–	Right hemiparesis worse in arm	Flat	Massive perisylvian lesion

From Geschwind N: Used by permission of the Continuing Professional Education Center, Princeton, NJ.
* Plus sign indicates relatively or fully intact; minus sign indicates definitely impaired.

A

APHASIA

APHASIAS WITH INTACT REPETITION

	Speech	Comprehension*	Localization
Transcortical motor	Nonfluent	+	Anterior to Broca's area or supplementary speech area
Transcortical sensory	Fluent	−	Surrounding Wernicke's area posteriorly
Transcortical mixed ("Isolation syndrome")	Nonfluent	−	Both of the above
Anomic	Fluent	+	Lesion of angular gyrus or second temporal gyrus

From Geschwind N: Used by permission of the Continuing Professional Education Center, Princeton, NJ.
* Plus sign indicates relatively or fully intact; − sign indicates definitely impaired.

Other syndromes related to aphasia but involving only a single language modality include *aphemia* or pure word dumbness (inferior frontal lobe dominant hemisphere lesions), pure word deafness (lesions of the dominant superior temporal lobe or bilateral middle portion of the superior temporal gyrus), *alexia without agraphia* (left occipital lesions, including posterior corpus callosum), and *sign language aphasia* (deaf signers can become aphasic in American Sign Language or other sign languages with left hemispheric damage).

Lesion of the right hemisphere cortices may lead to difficulties with "*utterances*," which refers to the automaticity of the speech, "*discourse*," which refers to the skill with which one can organize narrative, and impaired "prosody," which refers to inflection, stress, and melody of speech.

The classification of aphasia is based on patients with stable deficits; the acutely ill patient may not be easily classified. Spontaneous recovery often occurs in the first month after onset and may continue for many months. Speech therapy individualized for the form of aphasia may be helpful in recovery of language function.

REFERENCES

Benson DF: In Heilman KH, Valenstein E, eds: *Clinical neuropsychology*, ed 3, New York, Oxford University Press, 1993.
Mesulam MM: *Principal of behavioral and cognitive neurology*, New York, Oxford University Press, 2000.

APRAXIA

Apraxia is the inability to perform a previously learned skilled movement in the presence of intact motor, sensory, coordination, and comprehension systems. *Ideomotor apraxia* is the inability to voluntarily complete an act in response to a verbal command. However, the same act can be performed spontaneously. It may involve buccofacial, limb, or truncal musculature. It is often associated with lesion in the left hemisphere and often complicates Broca's aphasia. A lesion in the arcuate fasciculus may result in bilateral apraxia and conduction aphasia. *Callosal apraxia* results from a lesion in the anterior corpus callosum and manifests as left-sided apraxia with intact right-sided praxis. *Limb-kinetic apraxia* refers to loss of fine skilled movement following a premotor lesion. The patient is often clumsy and slow in executing motor tasks. *Ideational apraxia* (apraxia for object use) is the inability to perform sequential movements to use common objects in a proper manner despite the retained ability in performing the individual movements. *Constructional apraxia* occurs in two thirds of patients with right parietal lobe lesion. The patient is unable to copy or spontaneously draw figures and construct or mentally manipulate three-dimensional structures. *Oculomotor apraxia* occurs as part of Balint's syndrome (bilateral occipito-parietal lesions), *gait apraxia* is seen with frontal lesions and *dressing apraxia* with right parietal syndromes.

Testing for apraxia includes asking the patient to follow simple commands (such as "close your eyes" or "lick your lips"), to perform tasks with left and right extremities (for instance, comb hair, brush teeth, hammer a nail, or blow a kiss) and to use objects (as in lighting a match, or using the telephone). Patients with ideomotor apraxia are usually self sufficient because they can manipulate objects correctly on their own, whereas patients with ideational apraxia are often unable to care for themselves.

REFERENCE

Devinsky O: *Behavioral neurology: 100 maxims,* St Louis, Mosby, 1992.

ASTERIXIS

Asterixis is an abrupt, dysrhythmic loss of voluntary tone commonly elicited by extending the arms and dorsiflexing the wrists against gravity, although it may be present in any muscle group. Asterixis is preceded by a 50- to 110-millisecond period of EMG silence. In some cases, it may follow a sharp or biphasic EEG wave, indicating a possible cortical origin similar to cortical myoclonus.

Originally described in hepatic encephalopathy, asterixis may occur in any metabolic encephalopathy. Anticonvulsant-induced asterixis may occur in patients with elevated drug levels. Unilateral asterixis has been described contralateral to lesions in the midbrain, thalamus, internal capsule, and frontal or parietal lobe.

REFERENCE

Artieda J et al: *Mov Disord* 7(3):209–216, 1992.

ATAXIA

An abnormality of movement characterized by errors in rate, range, direction, timing, and force ("coordination") of motor activity. Elements of ataxia include:

1. Decomposition of movement into component parts.
2. Dysmetria-overshooting or undershooting a target.
3. Dysdiadochokinesia-impairment of rapid alternating movements.
4. Tremor.

Ataxia may involve limbs, trunk, eyes, or bulbar musculature and may be due to disease of the cerebellum, brainstem, spinal cord, or motor or sensory nerves. Cerebellar hemispheric disease commonly produces limb ataxia, whereas midline cerebellar disease manifests as truncal and gait ataxia. *Tremor* in cerebellar disease may be an action or intention tremor (disease of dentate nucleus or superior cerebellar peduncle) or more coarse ("rubral tremor"). *Titubation*, a nodding-head tremor, is seen with midline cerebellar disease and may involve the trunk. *Ataxic speech* has abnormal variability of volume, rate, and phonation and may be slow and slurred or have alternating loudness and quietness. Impaired proprioception resulting from tabes dorsalis, hereditary disease, or dorsal root ganglionopathies may lead to *sensory ataxia* with impaired gait and presence of Romberg sign. *Gait ataxia* may accompany vertigo in vestibular dysfunction.

ACUTE ONSET ATAXIA

Often results from cerebellar hemorrhage or infarction. Hemorrhage is usually associated with headache. Acute ataxia is also seen in basilar migraine. Viral cerebellitis causes an acute, reversible ataxia in children 2 to 10 years and is most common after chicken pox. Paraneoplastic syndromes in adults may be seen in association with bronchogenic or ovarian carcinoma.

SUBACUTE ATAXIA

Hydrocephalus, foramen magnum compression, posterior fossa tumor, abscess, or parasitic infection in any age group.

ATAXIA WITH EPISODIC COURSE

Multiple sclerosis, vertebrobasilar transient ischemic attacks, foramen magnum compression, intermittent obstruction of ventricular system due to colloid cyst and dominantly inherited periodic ataxia. In children metabolic causes including defects of the urea cycle, aminoaciduria, Leigh's disease and mitochondrial encephalomyopathies should be considered, also acetazolamide responsive episodic ataxia.

ATAXIA WITH CHRONIC PROGRESSIVE COURSE

Chronic alcoholism with progressive cerebellar degeneration but structural lesions such as posterior fossa tumors, foramen magnum compression, or hydrocephalus must be excluded first. Rarely, infectious agents such as chronic panencephalitis due to rubella in children or Creutzfeldt-Jakob disease can have chronic progressive course. Multiple sclerosis occasionally manifests as a chronic progressive cerebellar syndrome.

Spinocerebellar ataxias constitute a diverse group of genetic disorders that may present either in childhood or adulthood. All forms of inheritance have been described (see also Spinocerebellar Ataxias).

REFERENCE
Evidente VG et al: *Mayo Clin Proc* 75:475–490, 2000.

ATHETOSIS (see also Chorea)

Athetosis is an involuntary, slow, sinuous, irregular, writhing movement of any muscle group, usually most prominent in the distal extremities. It frequently coexists with other abnormal movements, particularly dystonia and chorea. Like those movements, athetosis is associated with lesions in the basal ganglia. EMG analysis reveals loss of reciprocation between agonists and antagonists. Common syndromes include posthemiplegic athetosis, generalized athetosis ("double athetosis" seen in cerebral palsy and post-kernicterus), and drug-induced athetosis (e.g., levodopa-induced dyskinesias). Athetosis may be seen in many inherited metabolic diseases such as Huntington's disease, Wilson's disease, Lesch-Nyhan syndrome, glutaric acidemia, glyceric acidemia, sulfite oxidase deficiency, Niemann-Pick disease, familial calcification of the basal ganglia, and Hallervorden-Spatz disease.

ATTENTION DEFICIT-HYPERACTIVITY DISORDER (ADHD)

ADHD is familial in 30% to 50% of cases, and is four to six times more common in boys. A *hypodopaminergic* state results in decreased activity of inhibitory areas of the prefrontal cortex, striatum, caudate, and thalamic nuclei leading to an inability of affected children to control their attention and/or impulses and motor activity. *Comorbid conditions* are frequent: 50% have obsessive-compulsive disorder (OCD), 30% to 50% have conduct disorders, 50% have oppositional defiant disorder, 15% to 20% have mood disorders, and 20% to 25% have anxiety disorders.

DSM-IV diagnostic criteria: (a) onset before age 7 years; (b) some impairment in two or more settings (e.g., school and home); (c) clinically significant impairment in social, academic, or occupational functioning; (d) absence of pervasive developmental or other mental disorder; (e) either six or more symptoms of inattention, or six or more symptoms of hyperactivity-impulsivity, for at least 6 months that is maladaptive and inconsistent with developmental level.

Inattention
1. Failure of close attention to details.
2. Has difficulty sustaining attention in tasks.
3. Often does not listen when spoken to directly.
4. Often does not follow through on instructions or fails to finish tasks.
5. Has difficulty organizing tasks or activities.
6. Often loses things necessary for tasks.
7. Is easily distracted by extraneous stimuli.
8. Is often forgetful in daily activities.

Hyperactivity
1. Often fidgets with limbs or squirms in seat.
2. Often leaves seat in classroom or other places where sitting is expected.
3. Often runs or climbs excessively.
4. Has difficulty playing quietly.
5. Is often "on the go" or often acts as if "driven by a motor."
6. Often talks excessively.

Impulsivity
1. Often blurts outs answers before questions are completed.
2. Often has difficulty awaiting turn.
3. Often interrupts or intrudes on others.

Management: A combination of behavior management at home and school, targeted educational assistance, and medication therapy. It requires a team of professionals that includes school officials, mental health professionals, and the physician working with the child and his/her family. Medications used most often include stimulants (methylphenidate, amphetamines, pemoline), antidepressants (nortriptyline, imipramine, desipramine, bupropion), α_2-adrenergic agents (clonidine, guanfacine), and mood stabilizers (lithium , carbamazepine, valproic acid). Stimulants are first-line drugs with a 70% to 90% response rate. *Methyphenidate increases levels of norepinephrine and dopamine in synaptic clefts.* Side effects include insomnia, anorexia, irritability, rebound phenomena, growth suppression, cardiovascular effects, potential for drug addiction, and an increase in seizure frequency. *Children with strong family history of tics or Tourette's disorder should be referred to a specialist prior to initiating therapy as both conditions may be precipitated prematurely by stimulant use.* Pemoline can be used with substance-abusing patients but is associated with acute liver failure. Nonstimulants are used in children who fail to respond to or cannot tolerate the stimulants and in those with significant comorbid conditions such as anxiety, depression, tics, aggression, or substance abuse.

Prognosis: Thirty percent will outgrow their symptoms, 40% will continue to display significant symptoms often accompanied by depression and anxiety, and 30% will decline with development of additional psychopathology such as alcoholism, substance abuse, or antisocial personality disorders. About 60% will continue with symptoms into adulthood where it may impact social or occupational functioning.

REFERENCE

Taylor MA: *Comp Ther* 25:313–325, 1999.

AUTISM

Clinical features: Normal early milestones followed by regression at age 1 to 3 years; characterized by abnormal language (parrotlike and echolalic), social dysfunction (aloof, passive, or odd), and restricted range of behaviors, interests, or activities (repetitive, stereotyped movements or idiot savant). One third of patients with autism develop epilepsy. *Diagnostic evaluation* should include formal audiologic assessment and EEG. Imaging is rarely indicated. *Treatment* consists of special education and behavior modification programs and medications targeted at specific behaviors.

I. Autistic spectrum
    A. *Asperger syndrome:* flat affect, insensitive to social cues, obsessively indulged special interests, need for sameness, unable to communicate effectively, though language skills develop normally.
    B. *Pervasive developmental disorder:* onset after 30 months of age; impaired social skills, anxious, resistant to change, odd mannerisms and speech, and occasionally self-mutilation
II. Syndromes with prominent autistic features
    A. *Fragile X syndrome:* most common cause of mental retardation; dysmorphic faces, macro-orchidism after puberty, hyperactive; one third of female heterozygotes are mildly retarded.
    B. *Angelman's syndrome* ("Happy puppet" syndrome): maternal 15q deletion; infantile feeding problems, severe retardation, microcephaly, autism, jerky puppetlike ataxia, paroxysmal laughter, protruding tongue. By contrast, *Prader-Willi syndrome* (paternal 15q deletion) presents with hypotonia at birth; dysmorphism, mental retardation; later, hyperphagia, hypogonadism, Pickwinian syndrome.
    C. *Rett's syndrome:* girls develop normally until 6 to 12 months of age; thereafter, regression with acquired microcephaly, ataxia, and autistic-like behavior; repetitive hand-wringing or hand-wetting movements; irregular breathing.
    D. *Others:* tuberous sclerosis; hypomelanosis of Ito.

REFERENCES

Gillberg C: *Curr Opin Neurol* 11:109–114, 1998.
Menkes JH: *Textbook of child neurology*, Baltimore, Williams & Wilkins, 1995.

AUTONOMIC DYSFUNCTION

Classification: Disorders marked by autonomic dysfunction are given in Table 7. Progressive autonomic failure can occur either as an isolated

TABLE 7

CLASSIFICATION OF AUTONOMIC DISORDERS

I.   Diseases affecting the central nervous system
    A. Progressive autonomic failure ([PAF], idiopathic orthostatic hypotension)
        1. Pure PAF
        2. PAF with multiple-system atrophy (Shy-Drager syndrome)
            a. With parkinsonian features
            b. With spinocerebellar degeneration
    B. Parkinson's disease
    C. Spinal cord lesions
    D. Wernicke's encephalopathy
    E. Miscellaneous diseases
        1. Cerebrovascular disease
        2. Brainstem tumors
        3. Multiple sclerosis
        4. Adie's syndrome
        5. Tabes dorsalis
II. Diseases affecting the peripheral autonomic nervous system
    A. Disorders with no associated sensory-motor peripheral neuropathy
        1. Acute and subacute autonomic neuropathy
            a. Pandysautonomia
            b. Cholinergic dysautonomia
        2. Botulism
    B. Diseases associated with sensory-motor peripheral neuropathy in which autonomic dysfunction is clinically important
        1. Diabetes
        2. Amyloidosis
        3. Guillain Barré syndrome
        4. Acute intermittent porphyria
        5. Familial dysautonomia (Riley-Day syndrome: HMSN III [Hereditary Motor-Sensory Neuropathy])
        6. Chronic sensory and autonomic neuropathy
    C. Disorders in which autonomic dysfunction is usually clinically unimportant
        1. Alcohol-induced neuropathy
        2. Toxic neuropathies (caused by vincristine sulfate, acrylamide, heavy metals, perhexiline maleate, or organic solvents)
        3. HMSNs I, II and V
        4. Malignancy
        5. Vitamin B_{12} deficiency
        6. Rheumatoid arthritis
        7. Chronic renal failure
        8. Systemic lupus erythematosus
        9. Mixed connective tissue disease
      10. Fabry's disease
      11. Chronic inflammatory neuropathy

Adapted from McLeod JG, Tuck RR: *Ann Neurol* 21:419–430, 1987.

syndrome of orthostatic hypotension or in association with spinocerebellar and/or Parkinsonian features in the syndromes collectively referred to as multiple-system atrophy. Autonomic dysreflexia occurs in the context of spinal cord lesions above the T6 level. This is mediated by an interruption in the brain's ability to dilate the splanchnic vascular bed and manifests as a marked rise in blood pressure along with headache, goose flesh, diaphoresis, flushing, or chills; it affects half to three quarters of this population. Acute pandysautonomia may occur as a variant of Guillain-Barré syndrome or may complicate more typical cases of Guillain-Barré syndrome. A number of hereditary acquired or peripheral small fiber neuropathies can have autonomic features.

Diagnosis: Autonomic dysfunction is suspected in the presence of orthostatic hypotension or other derangement of cardiovascular regulation, loss of sweating, bladder or bowel dysfunction, impotence, or pupillary abnormalities. The following screening tests can be performed at the bedside: (1) Orthostatic blood pressure and heart rate. An estimate is made of the time typically required to produce symptoms on standing. After 20 minutes of inactivity, baseline supine heart rate and blood pressure are recorded. The standing measurements are taken at 3 minutes or after the estimated time interval that takes the patient to become symptomatic. The cuff on the arm is kept at the level of the heart at all times. Orthostatic hypotension is defined as a reduction in SBP of at least 20 mmHg or in DBP of at least 10 mmHg within 3 minutes of standing. Heart rate normally increases by 11 to 29 beats per minute immediately on standing. If the patient has had electrocardiogram (ECG) leads placed prior to testing, the ratio between the longest R-R interval (slowest rate), which occurs about 30 beats after standing, divided by the shortest R-R interval, which occurs at about 15 beats, is called the 30:15 ratio. Normal 30:15 ratio is >1.04 with slight age-related variation. Orthostatic BP assesses sympathetic adrenergic efferents, while the heart rate tests assess parasympathetic cholinergic (cardiovagal) efferents; both assess baroreceptor and CN IX and X integrity. (2) *Respiratory heart rate variation.* The patient breathes deeply at six breaths per minute while ECG is recording, and the times of inspiration and expiration are noted on the ECG tracing. A difference in heart rate between inspiration and expiration of less than 10 beats per minute or an expiration-to-inspiration ratio of R-R intervals of less than 1:2 is abnormal in individuals under age 40. Normally the heart rate increases during inspiration (respiratory sinus arrhythmia) as a result of decreased cardiovagal activity. This is the single best cardiovagal test, though the effect decreases with advancing age. (3) *Tests of pupillary function.* Installation of dilute 0.1% epinephrine into the conjunctival sac has no effect on a normal pupil but dilates a pupil with a lesion in the postganglionic sympathetic innervation because of denervation supersensitivity. Likewise, dilute 0.125% pilocarpine causes little or no constriction in normal pupils but causes miosis in the presence of abnormal parasympathetic innervation. All pharmacologic tests of pupillary function are distorted by corneal trauma (e.g., contact lenses, corneal reflex testing) within 24 hours of the eye drops.

A

AUTONOMIC DYSFUNCTION

Other tests. More extensive autonomic testing includes measurement of plasma norepinephrine levels and determination of denervation supersensitivity, Valsalva maneuver and tilt-table testing, baroreflex sensitivity testing, thermal sweat testing, and skin blood-flow measurements.

Treatment: Management of orthostatic hypotension begins with supportive measures:

1. Avoiding or optimizing drugs that may lead to orthostasis, including diuretics, antihypertensives, and psychotropic agents.
2. Avoid sudden standing, straining during urination or defecation, excessive heat, large meals, and alcohol. Elevation of the head of the bed reduces nocturnal volume loss and is generally recommended, as is increased salt intake unless there is associated congestive heart failure.
3. Waist-high elastic garments may be helpful but are cumbersome.
4. Drinking coffee after large meals may help reduce postprandial hypotension.

Pharmacologic therapy:

1. Fludrocortisone—a starting dose of 0.1 mg per day is increased by 0.1 mg every 3 to 4 days until symptoms are controlled or until a maximum dosage of 1 mg per day is reached. Complications include supine hypertension, peripheral edema, hypokalemia, and congestive heart failure.
2. Midodrine—starting at 10 mg three times a day.
3. Pseudophedrine—30 mg four times a day.

REFERENCES

Grubb BP: *Am J Cardiol* 84(8A):3Q–9Q, 1999.
Ravits JM: *Muscle Nerve* 20(8):919–937, 1997.

B

BENZODIAZEPINES

Benzodiazepines are used in the treatment of anxiety, insomnia, epilepsy, vertigo, and certain movement disorders. They are also used in the management of ethanol withdrawal. Prolonged use of any drug in this class may cause physical dependence, particularly in patients with a history of alcohol or substance abuse. Therefore only the lowest effective doses should be used for the shortest possible period. Side effects include sedation, suppression of REM sleep, amnesia, agitation, and gait disorder. Withdrawal symptoms may occur after 4 to 6 weeks of use and include flulike symptoms, insomnia, irritability, seizures, nausea, headache, tremor, and muscle cramps. In those at risk for withdrawal, the dose should be tapered over several weeks. Acute intoxication with depressed mental status may be reversed with the benzodiazepine receptor antagonist flumazenil, starting at 0.2 mg IV over 30 seconds. Failure to respond to a total dose of 5 mg makes it unlikely that sedation is due to benzodiazepines.

BLADDER

Normal bladder function is controlled by bladder stretch receptors (generating sympathetic input to spinal cord), the bladder wall detrusor muscle (activated by parasympathetic outflow), the internal sphincter (smooth muscle), and the external sphincter (striated muscle under voluntary control). Neural control is mediated by cerebral hemispheric centers, the pontine micturition center, the sacral micturition center, and the hypogastric, pelvic, and pudendal nerves (Figure 4). These centers and nerves work together to achieve (1) storage of urine without leaking; (2) adequate perception of increased intravesical pressure; (3) release of cortical inhibition of emptying in appropriate circumstances; (4) proper synergy of urinary tract muscular structures; and (5) complete bladder emptying. Thus disorders of bladder control can be caused by local factors (such as previous childbirth, pelvic surgery, or urinary tract infection) or disorders of the upper or lower motor neuron (see Table 8).

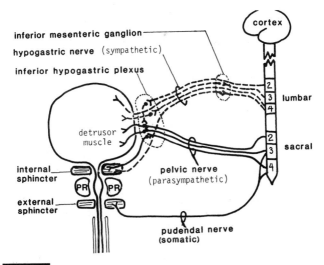

FIGURE 4

Neuroanatomy of bladder control.

TABLE 8

BLADDER DYSFUNCTION

Upper Motor Neuron	Lower Motor Neuron
Characteristic Feature	
Decreased capacity for storage	Decreased emptying ability
Cause	
Hemisphere or cord injury above T12 (trauma, multiple sclerosis, stroke, tumor)	1. Sensory: diabetes mellitus, tabes dorsalis 2. Motor: amyotrophic lateral sclerosis 3. Mixed sensory and motor: spinal dysraphism (meningomyelocele), tumor or trauma of lower cord, conus, or cauda
History	
Urge incontinence with dry intervals Wet at night	Overflow incontinence Urinary retention Straining to void Wet or dry at night
Bulbocavernous Reflex	
Present	Absent
Cystometrogram	
"Hyperreflexic bladder" Small bladder capacity Small residual volumes Vesicoureteral reflux (and upper urinary tract damage) may occur at peak pressures.	"Flaccid bladder" Large bladder capacity Large residual volumes Vesicoureteral reflux and upper urinary tract damage can occur with persisting urinary retention.

Detrusor hyperreflexia resulting from *cerebral cortical dysfunction* is a deficit of normal inhibitory mechanisms in which the micturition reflex itself is intact, since the lesion is above the pontine micturition center. Symptoms include frequency, urgency, and urge incontinence. Common neurologic disorders leading to uninhibited bladder contraction include stroke, mass lesion, and hydrocephalus. *Bladder dyssynergia* due to *suprasacral spinal cord lesions* leads to loss of detrusor-sphincter coordination. Simultaneous contraction of detrusor and sphincter can lead to increased intravesical pressures and upper urinary tract damage. Multiple sclerosis, spinal cord tumor or trauma, vascular malformation, and herniated intervertebral disk are common causes.

Table 9 includes agents traditionally used in the pharmacologic management of upper and lower motor neuron bladder dysfunction. Tolterodine (Detrol) is a new agent recently approved for detrusor hyperreflexia (symptoms of frequency, urgency, urge incontinence) that acts as a non-subtype selective antimuscarinic agent. Its efficacy is equivalent to oxybutynin, and it offers the advantages of twice daily dosing and fewer anticholinergic side

---

TABLE 9

TREATMENT OF BLADDER DYSFUNCTION

Upper Motor Neuron	Lower Motor Neuron
Treatment goal	
Increase storage capacity	Increase bladder tone; avoid storage of large urinary volumes; promote bladder emptying
Treatment	
Oxybutynin (Ditropan) anticholinergic	Bethanechol (Urecholine) cholinergic
Dose:	Dose:
Child: 2.5 mg PO bid–tid	Child: 5 mg/day, increase as below for adult
Adult: 5 mg PO tid–qid	Adult: 2.5–10 mg SC tid–qid, or 5–50 mg PO tid–qid
Side effects: dry mouth, blurred vision	Contraindicated asthma, hyperthyroidism, coronary artery disease, ulcer disease
Propantheline bromide (Pro-Banthine) anticholinergic	Phenoxybenzamine (Dibenzyline) antiadrenergic
Dose:	Dose:
Child: not currently approved for use (USA)	Child: 0.3–0.5 mg/kg/day
Adult: 15–30 mg PO tid–qid	Adult: 10–30 mg/day
	Side effects: retrograde ejaculation, drowsiness, orthostatic hypotension
Side effects: dry mouth, blurred vision	
Imipramine (Tofranil) mixed anticholinergic and adrenergic	
Dose:	
Child: 1.5–2 mg/kg qid	
Adult: 25 mg PO qid	
Side effects: dry mouth, blurred vision, constipation, tachycardia, sweating, fatigue, tremor	
Intermittent self-catheterization	Intermittent self-catheterization or Crédé maneuver

effects. However, at present its expense may reserve its use for those patients who are intolerant of or fail oxybutynin.

Detrusor areflexia is due to lesions of the *sacral micturition center* or its connections to the bladder. Sphincter function is preserved but detrusor contraction is not activated, commonly resulting in overflow incontinence. Causes include myelopathy resulting from herniated disk or tumor and interruption of the reflex arc as a result of pelvic or pudendal nerve injury following trauma or operation.

Autonomic dysreflexia occurs after spinal cord lesions above the region of major sympathetic outflow (T5 to L2). Splanchnic sympathetic outflow is no longer moderated by supraspinal centers, and bladder distention, catheterization, or other manipulation causes an acute syndrome of severe hypertension, anxiety, sweating headache, and bradycardia. Prompt recognition and treatment (blood pressure control and treatment of local bladder problems) are essential.

REFERENCES

Fowler CJ: *Brain* 122(Pt 7):1213–1231, 1999.
Guay DRP: *Pharmacotherapy* 19(3):267–280, 1999.
Madersbacher HG: *Curr Opin Urol* 9(4):303–307, 1999.

BRACHIAL PLEXUS

The brachial plexus (Figure 5) comprises the anastomoses derived from the anterior primary rami of vertebral segments C5 to T1. Trauma (penetrating, traction, avulsion, compression, or stretch) is the most common cause of damage. Other causes include radiation, neoplastic infiltration, and infections, damage also may be vaccine induced.

Upper plexus lesions (C5–6, upper trunk, *Duchenne-Erb palsy*) are the most common; they usually result from forceful separation of the head and shoulder but may be seen with chronic pressure on the shoulder (*knap-*

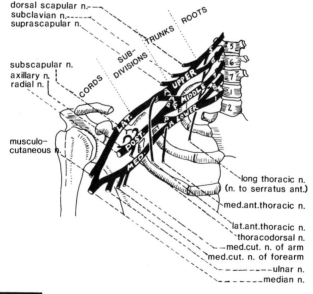

FIGURE 5

Brachial plexus. (From Haymaker W, Woodhall B: *Peripheral nerve injuries: Principles of diagnosis,* Philadelphia, WB Saunders, 1953.)

sack paralysis). The lesions are characterized by weakness of shoulder abduction, external rotation, elbow flexion, and forearm supination as well as variable amounts of triceps weakness. Sensory loss is variable and may involve the deltoid region, the external aspect of the upper arm, and the radial side of the forearm.

Lower plexus lesions (C8–T1, *Dejerine-Klumpke palsy*) are usually due to traction of an already abducted arm or to infiltration or compression resulting from tumors of the lung apex (*Pancoast's syndrome*). The lesions are characterized by weakness of intrinsic hand muscles, longer finger flexors, and extensors. Sensory loss may involve the medial arm and forearm and the ulnar aspect of the hand. The cords of the brachial plexus are usually injured in variable combinations as a result of humeral head dislocation, direct axillary trauma, and supraclavicular compression.

Radiation brachial plexopathy occurs between 5 months and many years after radiation. In contrast to plexopathy due to tumor infiltration, the upper trunk or entire plexus is affected, pain is less common, lymphedema is frequent, and Horner's syndrome is rare.

Idiopathic brachial plexus neuritis (*Parsonage-Turner syndrome, neuralgic amyotrophy*) develops suddenly; shoulder pain is exacerbated by shoulder or arm movement but not by neck movement or Valsalva maneuver. Pain persists for several weeks, followed by weakness and atrophy. Onset may be preceded by a viral illness or immunization. In one-third of cases the neuritis is bilateral. Prognosis is usually good, and treatment should include range-of-motion exercises to prevent shoulder arthropathy.

REFERENCE

Dyck PJ, Thomas PK: *Peripheral neuropathy*, ed 3, Philadelphia, WB Saunders, 1993.

BRAIN DEATH

An irreversible loss of all recognizable brain function (incompatible with continued cardiopulmonary function off mechanical support). Legal criteria for death vary by state. Each institution may also set policy defining more specific requirements for brain death or discontinuation of life-sustaining measures. An interdisciplinary task force developed the following commonly accepted guidelines for the diagnosis of brain death in adults. There are also specific criteria for establishment of brain death in children; a pediatric neurologist should be consulted.

I. Clinical criteria (*all* are mandatory).
    A. Preceding coma of known cause due to an irreversible cerebral process. Must not be due to CNS depressant or neuromuscular-blocking drugs, shock, hypothermia (<32°C/90°F), metabolic or endocrine disturbances.
    B. No cerebral function. No behavioral or reflex responses involving structures above the cervical spinal cord can be elicited by stimuli to any part of the body. No spontaneous movement or posturing to

deep pain. Spinal reflex withdrawal is allowable. Deep tendon (spinal) reflexes may be present if all other criteria are met.
  C. No brainstem function (including reflexes).
    1. Pupils unreactive to light (midposition or dilated).
    2. Corneal reflexes absent.
    3. Vestibular-ocular reflexes absent. No response to oculocephalic maneuvers and 50-ml ice water caloric stimuli in each ear.
    4. Gag reflex absent (move endotracheal tube to elicit).
    5. No other brainstem reflexes (e.g., blink, ciliospinal, cough, snout).
  D. Criteria should be present for 6 hours (minimum).
II. Laboratory criteria (confirmatory).
  A. Negative toxicology screen or specific drug levels.
  B. Isoelectric EEG. Technical standards published by the American Electroencephalographic Society (Guidelines in EEG, Pts. 1–7, *J Clin Neurophysiol* 3:131–168, 1986).
  C. Brainstem auditory and somatosensory-evoked potentials can provide additional evidence of absent brainstem functions.
  D. Absence of cerebral circulation *may* be demonstrated by cerebral arteriography, transcranial Doppler, bolus radioisotope angiography, or intracranial pressure (by ICP monitor) exceeding mean systolic pressure for ≥ 1 hour.
  E. No spontaneous respiration of respiratory effort during apneic oxygenation for 10 minutes or with a Pco_2 >60 (caution in using Pco_2 with chronic lung disease patients). Patients are ventilated for 10 to 30 minutes with 100% O_2 (maintain baseline, Pco_2) and then disconnected from the ventilator while 100% O_2 is supplied by tracheal catheter at ≥ 6 L/minute. Blood gas levels are measured before the ventilator is disconnected and 5 to 10 minutes after disconnecting the ventilator.

REFERENCES

Farnell MM, Levin DL: *Crit Care Med* 21(12):1951–1965, 1993.
Manks SJ, Zisfein J: *Arch Neurol* 47:1066–1068, 1990.
Quality Standards Subcommittee of the American Academy of Neurology: *Neurology* 45(5):1012–1014, 1995.
Wijdicks EF: *N Engl J Med* 344(16):1215–1221, 2001.

BULBAR PALSY

A syndrome of weakness or paralysis of muscles supplied by cranial nerves IX, X, XI, and XII, due to lesions of the nuclei or nerves (see Pseudobulbar Palsy for lesions of the supranuclear pathways). Involved muscles include those of the pharynx, larynx, sternocleidomastoid, upper trapezius, and tongue. Patients may present clinically with dysarthria, dysphagia, hoarseness, nasal voice, palatal deviation, diminished gag reflex, or weakness of the sternocleidomastoid, upper trapezius, or tongue (may have atrophy and fasciculations). Etiologies include motor neuron disease ("progressive bulbar palsy" is one form), cerebrovascular lesions of the brainstem, intra- and extramedullary posterior fossa tumors, syringobulbia (may be associated with syringomyelia), meningitis, encephalitis, herpes zoster, poliomyelitis, diphtheria, aneurysms (uncommon), granulomatous disease, Brown-Vialetto-van Laere syndrome (also known as *pontobulbar palsy with deafness* a very rare disorder characterized by bilateral nerve deafness, a variety of cranial nerve disorders usually involving the motor components of the 7th and 9th to 12th cranial nerves, and less commonly an involvement of spinal motor nerves and upper motor neurons), bone lesions (platybasia, Paget's, foraminal syndromes), and radiation induced. Peripheral nervous system lesions as seen in Guillain-Barré syndrome, myasthenia gravis, and other neuromuscular disorders affecting bulbar innervated muscles must also be considered.

REFERENCE

Belsh JM: *Neurology* 53:S26–S30, 1999.

C

CALCIFICATION, CEREBRAL

Calcification may be physiologic or pathologic. Physiologic calcification is rare under 10 years of age. Basal ganglia calcification is most often idiopathic (especially in the elderly), as is calcification in the pineal gland, choroid plexus, falx, tentorium, habenula, dentate nucleus, dura and large vessels.

Causes of pathological calcification include the following.

A. Congenital/developmental: tuberous sclerosis, Sturge-Weber, Fahr's disease, familial idiopathic (autosomal dominant with basal ganglia and dentate calcifications), Gorlin's syndrome (basal cell nevus), neurofibromatosis, Cockayne's syndrome, Down's syndrome.

B. Inflammatory/infectious: "TORCH" (toxoplasmosis, syphilis, rubella, cytomegalovirus, herpes), bacterial, tuberculosis, HIV, parasitic (cysticerosis, coccidiomycosis, echinococcosis, granuloma.

C. Metabolic/endocrine: hyper- and hypoparathyroidism, pseudohyperparathyroidism, celiac disease with low serum folate.

D. Vascular: cavernous angiomas (50%), AVM's (25%), aneurysms (5%), infarcts (rare).

E. Trauma: chronic subdurals and other hematomas (rare).

F. Toxic: post-radiotherapy (especially combined with methotrexate), carbon monoxide, lead encephalopathy, birth anoxia.

G. Neoplastic: virtually all types of neoplasms can calcify. Most common are low grade astrocytoma (10%), oligodendroglioma *(50%)*, medulloblastoma (5%), ependymoma (33% to 66%), craniopharyngioma

(70% to 80%), meningioma (10% to 20%, with adjacent bony sclerosis), dermoid, and teratoma. Metastases may rarely calcify.

REFERENCE

Osborn AG: *Diagnostic neuroradiology*, St. Louis, Mosby, 1994.

CALORICS

Water that is colder or warmer than body temperature, when applied to the tympanic membrane, changes the firing rate of the ipsilateral vestibular nerve, causing ocular deviation and nystagmus. Cold water normally induces a slow ipsilateral deviation with contralateral "corrective" fast phases. Warm water induces a slow contralateral deviation and ipsilateral fast phases. Since the direction of nystagmus is conventionally described as that of the fast phase, the mnemonic COWS ("cold opposite, warm same") indicates the direction of caloric nystagmus for cold and warm stimuli. Bilateral irrigation induces vertical nystagmus; the mnemonic CUWD ("cold up, warm down") refers to the fast phases.

Caloric testing may be done at the bedside or quantitatively in a laboratory. Quantitative caloric testing is used to evaluate vestibular function. Bedside caloric testing is used (1) to establish the integrity of the ocular motor system in patients with an apparent gaze paresis and (2) to evaluate altered states of consciousness. Caloric stimulation may be used to elicit vestibular eye movements if oculocephalic maneuvers (see Vestibulo-Ocular Reflex) have negative results or when a cervical injury is suspected.

Bedside caloric testing is performed after the external auditory canal has been examined, the impacted cerumen removed, and the tympanic membrane established to be intact. The head is elevated 30 degrees from horizontal, aligning the horizontal semicircular canal in the vertical plane and maximizing lateral horizontal nystagmus. Water is gently injected with a syringe through a soft catheter inserted in the external auditory canal. Usually 1 ml of ice water is sufficient in alert patients and minimizes discomfort. Up to 100 ml of ice water can be used in unresponsive patients, and several minutes should be allowed for a response. Irrigation is repeated in the opposite ear after waiting at least 5 minutes for vestibular equilibration. Warm water (44° C) may also be used. Because of the risk of thermal injury, hot water should never be used.

Eye movements elicited by vestibular stimuli, whether passive head rotation or caloric, may allow localization within the ocular motor system. Impaired movement of both eyes to one side occurs with lesions of the ipsilateral paramedian pontine reticular formation. Impaired abduction in one eye suggests a palsy of cranial nerve VI. Impaired adduction is seen in third-nerve palsies and in the eye ipsilateral to a medial longitudinal fasciculus lesion (internuclear ophthalmoplegia). Bilateral internuclear ophthalmoplegias cause, in addition to bilateral adduction weakness, impaired vertical vestibular eye movements. Eye deviation may occur in aberrant directions in patients with drug intoxication or structural disease of central vestibular connections.

As consciousness declines, the caloric stimulus-induced eye movements relate to the integrity of brainstem structures. Tonic eye deviation indicates integrity of brainstem function. Asymmetric horizontal responses are interpreted as previously described and may give localizing information. Lack of any response may result from lesions of vestibulo-ocular reflex pathways in the medulla or pons, the eighth cranial nerve, labyrinth or drug intoxications, such as those resulting from vestibular suppressants (barbiturates, phenytoin, tricyclic antidepressants, or major transquilizers), and neuromuscular blockers. The presence of caloric-induced nystagmus in an acutely unresponsive patient suggests a psychogenic cause of unresponsiveness.

REFERENCE

Plum F, Posner JB: *The diagnosis of stupor and coma*, ed 3, Philadelphia, FA Davis, 1982.

CARDIOPULMONARY ARREST (see also Brain Death, Coma)

Prediction of neurologic outcome following cardiopulmonary arrest requires serial evaluations and is not completely accurate. Most patients with good outcome (independent self-care) emerge from coma within 24 to 48 hours. Conversely, coma duration greater than 48 hours has high likelihood of mortality or permanent neurologic deficit. Deterioration in level of consciousness is indicative of poor prognosis. Absence of pupillary light reflex at initial exam, absence of motor responses at 1 day, and failure to follow commands at 1 week are all strong predictors of poor neurologic outcome.

Pre-arrest morbidity affects survival. Preexisting pneumonia, hypotension, renal failure, cancer, or home-bound lifestyle are predictive of poor prognosis. Arrest for longer than 15 minutes is associated with an in-hospital mortality rate of 95%.

REFERENCES

Bedell SE et al: *N Engl J Med* 309:569–576, 1983.
Levy DE et al: *JAMA* 253:1420–1426, 1985.
Longstreth WT, Diehr P, Inui TS: *N Engl J Med* 308:1378–1382, 1983.

CARPAL TUNNEL SYNDROME

Carpal tunnel syndrome (CTS) occurs as a result of compression of the median nerve as it courses beneath the transverse carpal ligament. Incidence is 1/1,000 population. Eighty-two percent of patients are over

40 years old, and 65% to 75% are women. Approximately half of the patients have bilateral symptoms. Acute CTS is commonly related to distal radius fracture; other causes include hemorrhage into the carpal tunnel (due to trauma or coagulopathy), burn, infections, and injection injuries. Chronic CTS is usually idiopathic or may be related to repetitive motion injury; other causes are anatomic (ganglion, neuroma, lipoma, and myeloma), neuropathic (diabetes, alcoholism, amyloidosis, and mucopolysaccharidoses), inflammatory (tenosynovitis, hypertrophic synovium, rheumatoid arthritis, gout, dermatomyositis, scleroderma, systemic lupus erythematosus [SLE]), infection (TB), alteration of fluid balance (pregnancy, myxedema, obesity, long-term hemodialysis, congestive heart failure), acromegaly, and Paget's disease.

Patients characteristically complain of nocturnal numbness and paresthesia or burning pain in the median distribution (but may radiate to the forearm, elbow, or shoulder). Weakness and atrophy of the opponens pollicus, abductor pollicis brevis, and first two lumbricals and loss of two-point discrimination are late signs of long-term involvement. The symptoms are reproduced by tapping over the medial nerve at the carpal tunnel (*Tinel's sign*) or by maximum flexion of the wrist for 60 seconds (*Phalen's sign*), which has 75% to 88% sensitivity and 100% specificity. Also, inflating a sphygmomanometer to 150 mmHg at the wrist for 30 seconds has a 100% specificity and 97% sensitivity. Electromyogram (EMG) studies show prolongation of distal median motor and sensory (more sensitive) latencies and a difference between the distal median and ulnar motor latencies. Fibrillation potentials are infrequent. Bilateral EMG and nerve conduction abnormalities are common, even in asymptomatic patients. Recently, sonography and MRI have been shown to help in establishing the diagnosis.

Differential diagnosis includes C6 or C7 radiculopathy, thoracic outlet syndrome, brachial plexopathy, peripheral polyneuropathy, sensory stroke, syringomyelia, and more proximal median neuropathies.

Treatment consists of avoiding activities that precipitate symptoms and wearing a wrist extension splint at night. Local steroid with or without lidocaine injections may provide limited relief. Indications for surgery are weakness, atrophy, or EMG evidence of denervation. Surgical treatment, which can be done by either open or endoscopic approach, is usually not necessary during pregnancy as symptoms resolve spontaneously.

REFERENCE

Sternbach G: *J Emerg Med* 17:519–523, 1999.

CAUDA EQUINA AND CONUS MEDULLARIS

Clinical features of cauda equina and conus medullaris syndromes are summarized in Table 10.

TABLE 10

CLINICAL DIFFERENTIATION OF CAUDA EQUINA AND CONUS MEDULLARIS SYNDROMES

Conus Medullaris (Lower Sacral Cord)	Cauda Equina (Lumbosacral Roots)
Sensory Deficit	
Saddle distribution	Saddle distribution
Bilateral, symmetric	Asymmetric
Sensory dissociation present	Sensory dissociation absent
Presents early	Presents relatively later
Pain	
Uncommon	Prominent, early
Relatively mild	Severe
Bilateral, symmetric	Asymmetric
Perineum and thighs	Radicular
Motor Deficit	
Symmetric	Asymmetric
Mild	Moderate to severe
Atrophy absent	Atrophy more prominent
Reflexes	
Achilles reflex absent	Reflexes variably involved
Patellar reflex normal	
Sphincter Dysfunction	
Early, severe	Late, less severe
Absent anal and bulbo cavernosus reflex	Reflex abnormalities less common
Sexual Dysfunction	
Erection and ejaculation impaired	Less common

Modified from DeJong RN: *The neurologic examination*, ed 4, New York, Harper & Row, 1979.

C

CEREBELLUM

CEREBELLUM

The cerebellum is derived from ectodermal thickenings known as rhombic lip. It constitutes 10% of brain volume, yet it contains more than half of all the neurons.

It is composed of an outer gray mantle (cerebellar cortex), internal white matter, and three pairs of deep nuclei, which project out of the cerebellum. From medial to lateral, the nuclei pairs are the fastigial, the interposed (two nuclei, the globose posteriorly and the emboliform anteriorly), and the dentate nuclei. The primary fissure, located on the upper surface, divides the cerebellum into anterior and posterior lobes. The posterolateral fissure on the underside of the cerebellum separates the large posterior lobe from the small flocculonodular lobe. Shallower fissures subdivide the anterior and posterior lobes into several lobules from anterior to posterior: Lingula, central, culmen, declive, folium, tuber, pyramis, uvula, tonsil, nodulus, and flocculus. Two longitudinal furrows, most prominent on the undersurface of the cerebellum's posterior lobe, separate three areas: a thin midline longitudinal strip, the Vermis, and left and right cerebellar hemispheres (see Figure 6).

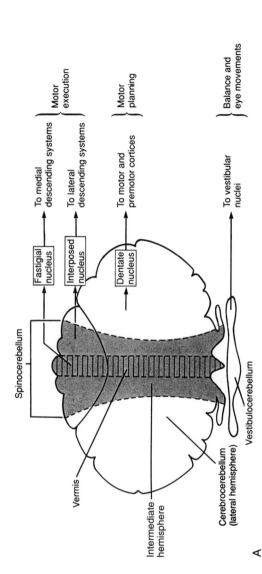

FIGURE 6

The cerebellum has three functional components with different outputs (A) and inputs (B).

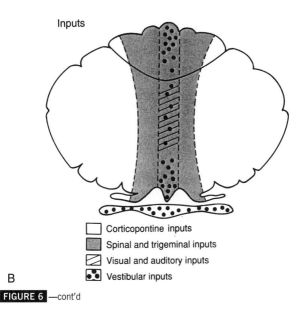

Inputs

☐ Corticopontine inputs
▨ Spinal and trigeminal inputs
◪ Visual and auditory inputs
⬤⬤ Vestibular inputs

B

FIGURE 6 —cont'd

    These parts represent distinct functional subdivisions that have distinct connections. The vermis projects by way of the fastigial nucleus to give rise to the medial descending systems, controlling proximal muscles. The intermediate zone projects via the interposed nucleus to give rise to the lateral descending systems, through which distal limb muscles are controlled. The lateral zone projects to the dentate nucleus, which connects primarily with motor and premotor regions of the cerebral cortex; these regions are involved in the planning of voluntary movements.

    The input and output connections of the cerebellum run through three symmetrical pairs of tracts that connect to the brainstem. These tracts, called the cerebellar peduncles, consist of the inferior, middle, and superior cerebellar peduncles (restiform body and brachium pontis and conjunctivum, respectively) (see Table 11).

CELLULAR ORGANIZATION OF THE CEREBELLUM

The molecular layer is the outermost and is composed primarily of the axons of granular cells, known as parallel fibers, that run parallel to the long axis of a folium. It also contains scattered stellate and basket cells, which function as interneurons.

    The Purkinje cell layer is beneath the molecular layer and contains the large cell bodies of the Purkinje neurons that are arranged side by side in a single layer. The Purkinje neurons have extensive dendritic trees that extend up into the molecular layer in a single plain perpendicular to the

TABLE 11

PRINCIPAL INPUT AND OUTPUT PATHWAYS OF CEREBELLUM

Functional Region	Anatomical Region	Principal Input	Deep Nucleus	Principal Destination	Functions
Vestibulocerebellum	Flocculonodular lobe	Vestibular labyrinth	Lateral vestibular	Medial systems: axial motor neurons	Axial control and vestibular reflexes
Spinocerebellum	Vermis	Vestibular labyrinth, proximal body parts, facial, visual, and auditory inputs to posterior lobe only	Fastigial	Medial systems: vestibular nucleus, reticular formation, and motor cortex	Axial and proximal motor control, ongoing execution of movement
Spinocerebellum	Intermediate part of hemisphere	Spinal afferents, distal body parts	Interposed	Lateral systems: red nucleus and distal motor cortex areas	Distal motor control, ongoing execution
Cerebrocerebellum	Lateral part of hemisphere	Cortical afferents	Dentate	Integration areas: red nucleus (parvocellular part) and premotor cortex (area 6)	Initiation, planning, and timing

main axis of a folium and their axons extend down into the underlying white matter. They are the sole output of the cerebellar cortex. All Purkinje neurons are inhibitory and utilize gamma-aminobutyric acid (GABA) as their neurotransmitter.

The granular layer is the innermost and contains a vast number of densely packed small neurons, mostly small granule cells. The granular layer contains small clear spaces called cerebellar glomeruli, where cells in the granular layer form complex synaptic contacts with the bulbous expansions of afferent (mossy) fibers.

CORTICAL INPUT (see Table 11)

Within the cerebellar cortex afferent fibers lose their myelin sheath and end either as mossy fibers or climbing fibers. Both send collateral axon branches to the deep cerebellar nuclei. These collateral pathways, given off by the mossy and climbing fibers to activate neurons in deep nuclei, form the primary cerebellar circuit. This primary circuit is then modulated by inhibitory action of the cerebellar cortex (mediated by the Purkinje neurons), which is driven by the same inputs.

Mossy fibers originate from a variety of brainstem nuclei and from neurons in the spinal cord that give rise to the spinocerebellar tracts. Mossy fibers influence Purkinje cells indirectly through synapses with the granule cells, which are excitatory interneurons in cerebellar glomeruli. The mossy fiber pathway activated by peripheral stimuli typically activates local clusters of granule cells. Granule cell axons ascend into the molecular layer and along the way make excitatory connections with nearby Purkinje cells. In the molecular layer, the axons bifurcate and give rise to parallel fibers. The parallel fibers intersect the dendrites of a row of Purkinje cells, all of which are oriented perpendicular to the parallel fibers.

The climbing fibers originate in the inferior olivary nucleus. Climbing fibers are so named because of the morphology of their terminations on the Purkinje cells (see Figure 6). The climbing fiber contacts only 1 to 10 Purkinje cells, and each Purkinje cell receives synaptic input from only a single climbing fiber. A single action potential in a climbing fiber elicits very large excitatory postsynaptic potentials in both the soma and dendrites of the Purkinje cells that trigger a large action potential followed by a high frequency burst of smaller action potentials. This characteristic grouping is called a complex spike and is associated with a large Ca^{2+} influx into a Purkinje cell.

The neurons giving rise to the mossy fibers and the granule cells both fire spontaneously at high rates, producing 50 to 100 spikes per second in Purkinje cells. Sensory stimuli or voluntary movements acting through mossy fibers can modulate this firing and control the moment-to-moment firing rate of Purkinje cells. In contrast, the neurons in the inferior olivary nucleus, which gives rise to the climbing fibers, fire spontaneously at low rates, producing on average one complex spike per second in the Purkinje cell. Sensory stimuli or movement elicit only one or two complex spikes.

However, climbing fiber input to the Purkinje cells is important in modulating the effect of mossy fibers upon Purkinje cells by transiently enhancing the effect of mossy fiber inputs on Purkinje cells. The climbing fibers also can produce a long-lasting depression of the efficacy of selected mossy fiber inputs through a heterosynaptic action responsible for some forms of motor learning.

The projection from the raphe nuclei to the cerebellar cortex is serotonergic and terminates in both the granular and the molecular layers. The projection from the locus ceruleus is noradrenergic and terminates as a plexus in all three layers of the cerebellar cortex.

INHIBITORY INTERNEURONES

Stellate and basket cells are interneurons; they receive excitatory connections from the parallel fibers. Stellate cells have short axons that contact nearby dendrites of Purkinje cells in the molecular layer, while basket cell axons run perpendicular to the parallel fibers and contact the cell bodies of more distant Purkinje cells. As a result, when a group of parallel fibers excites a row of Purkinje cells and neighboring basket cells, the excited basket cells inhibit the Purkinje cells outside the beam of excitation. This results in a field of activity that resembles the center-surround antagonism that we have encountered in sensory neurons. The third inhibitory interneuron, the Golgi cell located in the granular layer, has an elaborate dendritic tree in the molecular layer, where it receives its principal input (excitatory) from the parallel fibers. In the granular layer, the terminals of Golgi cells are distributed to the granule cells as an axodendritic synapses within the glomeruli. Thus, the Golgi neurons suppress the excitation of the granule cells to mossy fiber input and curtail the duration of the excitation, ultimately reaching the Purkinje cell through the parallel fibers. GABA appears to be the neurotransmitter used by Golgi neurons.

FUNCTIONAL DIVISION OF THE CEREBELLUM

The vestibulocerebellum, the spinocerebellum, and the cerebrocerebellum correspond roughly to anatomical subdivisions.

THE VESTIBULOCEREBELLUM

The vestibulocerebellum, also called the archicerebellum, is phylogenetically the oldest part and corresponds to the flocculonodular lobe. It receives its input from the vestibular nuclei in the medulla and projects back to them. The dominant afferent inputs come from two sources: semicircular canals (changes in head position) and otolith organs (orientation of the head with respect to gravity).

These two types of primary vestibular afferents are the only afferents that reach the cerebellar cortex directly from ganglion cells in the periphery. Secondary afferents arise from the vestibular nuclei. The vestibulocerebellum receives visual information from the lateral geniculate nucleus, superior colliculi, and striate cortex. The output of the vestibulocerebellum is projected back to the vestibular nuclei. The vestibulocerebellum governs balance and eye movements (and coordinates them with head movement) and body equilibrium during stance and gait. Diseases of the flocculonodular lobe cause disturbances of equilibrium, including ataxic gait, a compensatory wide-based standing position, and nystagmus. Patients with diseases of the flocculonodular lobe lack the ability to use vestibular information to coordinate movements of either the body or eyes. However, when the patient moves while lying down, no deficits are seen.

THE SPINOCEREBELLUM

The spinocerebellum, also called the paleocerebellum, extends rostrocaudally through the central part of both the anterior and posterior lobes and includes the vermis and the intermediate part of the hemispheres. Fastigial nuclei receive somatotopically organized projections from the vermis in the anterior and posterior lobes and project bilaterally to the brainstem reticular formation and to the lateral vestibular nuclei, which give rise to fibers that descend to the spinal cord. The fastigial nuclei also have crossed ascending projections that reach the ventrolateral nucleus of thalamus, where information is relayed to the primary motor cortex. These connections are involved in the control of the proximal and axial muscles. The intermediate part of the cerebellar hemisphere projects to the interposed nuclei. The interposed nuclei project to the contralateral magnocellular portion of the red nucleus in the brainstem via the superior cerebellar peduncle. Many of these fibers continue to the ventral lateral nucleus of the thalamus, where they end on neurons projecting to the limb areas of the motor cortex, mainly the distal muscles. The principal input is somatosensory information from the spinal cord through the topographically arranged spinocerebellar tracts. The body map in the anterior lobe has the feet oriented forward while the face extends backward into the first lobule of the posterior lobe. The body map in the posterior lobe is oriented head forward and is located in the vermis and the intermediate part of the hemisphere. The spinocerebellum also receives information from the auditory, visual, and vestibular systems, and topographically organized projections from the primary motor and somatic sensory cortex. The spinocerebellum controls the execution of movement and regulates muscle tone. Lesions in the spinocerebellum will lead to appendicular ataxia and hypotonia ipsilateral to the lesion due to the double crossing (one in the cerebellocortical projection and the second during the corticospinal projection).

THE NEOCEREBELLUM

The neocerebellum, also called the cerebrocerebellum, is the largest and phylogenetically newest part of the cerebellum. It is the lateral part of the cerebellar hemisphere and forms a third sagittal region in the main body of the cerebellum. Its input originates exclusively in pontine nuclei that relay information from the premotor, motor, and sensory cortices to the contralateral cerebellar hemisphere through the middle cerebellar peduncle. The output is conveyed from the dentate nucleus via the superior cerebellar peduncle to the ventrolateral thalmus and from there to the motor and premotor cortices. The dentate nucleus also projects to the parvocellular component of the red nucleus, which is part of a complex feedback circuit that sends information back to the cerebellum, primarily through the ipsilateral inferior olivary nucleus. The neocerebellum coordinates the planning and initiation of limb movements. It is the center of a complex feedback circuit that modulates cortical motor commands. The lateral parts of the cerebellar hemispheres are largely devoted to achieving precision in the control of rapid limb movements and in tasks requiring fine dexterity.

Lesions of the dentate nuclei or the overlying cortex produce four kinds of disturbances:

1. Delay in initiating and terminating movement.
2. Terminal tremor at the end of movement.
3. Disorders in the temporal coordination of movements involving multiple joints.
4. Disorders in the spatial coordination of hands and finger muscles.

SIGNS AND SYMPTOMS OF CEREBELLAR DISEASE
Hypotonia
Hypotonia accompanies acute hemispheric lesions more than chronic lesions. It is usually more noticeable in the proximal upper limbs. Hypotonic extremities often exhibit pendular reflexes. It is due to diminished resistance and delay in the response to passive and rapid imposed movements, also called lack of check, and reflects the patient's inability to stop the limb rapidly so that the limb overshoots and may rebound excessively.

Ataxia
Ataxia refers to a disturbance in the smooth performance of voluntary motor acts. It results from defective timing of sequential contractions of agonist and antagonist muscles. Errors in movements occur in rate, force, and duration. Ataxia may affect limbs, the trunk, or gait and may be acute, episodic, or progressive. Ataxia secondary to cerebellar injury characteristically persists despite visual cues. The term ataxia includes other abnormalities of voluntary movement control, such as asynergia (movements are broken up into isolated successive parts—decomposition of movement due to lack of synergy), dysmetria (abnormal excursions in movement), dysdiadochokinesia (impaired performance of rapidly alternating movements), and past-pointing. Also associated is an impaired checking response and an excessive rebound phenomenon, when an opposed-force is suddenly released. Typically patients with cerebellar disease have a wide-based stance and a gait characterized by staggering and impaired tandem walking. Truncal instability may be manifested by falls in any direction. Truncal ataxia and titubations suggest a midline cerebellar lesion.

Tremor

Cerebellar type tremor may be an action tremor or intention tremor, although it is the act of moving rather than the intention to move that causes the tremor. Characteristically it becomes most marked at the end of movement.

Cerebellar Dysarthria

Cerebellar dysarthria is characterized by abnormalities in articulation and prosody together or independently. The speech has been described as scanning, slurring, staccato, explosive, hesitant, slow altered accent, and garbled.

Ocular Dysmotility

Gaze-evoked nystagmus, upbeat nystagmus, rebound nystagmus, and optokinetic nystagmus may be seen with midline cerebellar lesions and may also occur with hemispheric disorders. Positional nystagmus, mimicking positional nystagmus of the benign paroxysmal type, may occur with posterior fossa tumors. Ocular dysmetria—a conjugate overshoot and undershoot of a target with voluntary saccades—may occur with midline or lateral cerebellar lesions.

VASCULAR BLOOD SUPPLY OF CEREBELLUM

Posterior Inferior Cerebellar Artery (PICA)

The PICA is a branch of the vertebral artery or basilar artery, curves upwards on the inferior surface of the cerebellum, and supplies the inferior cerebellar peduncle, ipsilateral portion of the inferior vermis (uvula and nodulus), cerebellar tonsil, and the inferior surface of the cerebellar hemisphere. The medial branch of PICA supplies the medial cerebellum, and the lateral branch supplies the inferoposterolateral aspect of the cerebellum. Medial branches also supply parts of the choroid plexus of the fourth ventricle.

Anterior Inferior Cerebellar Artery (AICA)

The AICA arises from the basilar artery. It lies on the inferior surface of the cerebellum. Its branches supply the pyramids, tuber, flocculus, and parts of the inferior surface of the cerebellar hemisphere and the lower portion of the middle cerebellar peduncle. Penetrating branches supply portions of the dentate nucleus and the surrounding white matter; smaller branches also contribute to the blood supply of the choroid plexus of the fourth ventricle.

Superior Cerebellar Artery (SCA)

The SCA arises near the distal segment of the basilar artery just below the terminal bifurcation into paired posterior cerebral arteries and lies on the superior surface of the cerebellum. It divides into medial and lateral branches. It supplies the superior surface of the cerebellar hemisphere, the ipsilateral portion of the superior vermis, most of the dentate nucleus, the upper portion of middle cerebellar peduncle, and the superior cerebellar peduncle. Some branches contribute to the choroid plexus of the fourth ventricle.

CEREBELLAR SYNDROMES

The Rostral Vermis Syndrome (Anterior Lobe)

The clinical features of this syndrome may include the following: wide-based stance and gait, and gait ataxia, with proportionally little ataxia on the heel-to-shin maneuver; normal or only slightly impaired arm coordination; and infrequent presence of hypotonia, nystagmus, and dysarthria. This syndrome is seen in the restricted form of cerebellar cortical degeneration that occurs in alcoholic patients. The pathologic changes in this condition affect the anterior and superior vermis.

The Caudal Vermis Syndrome (Flocculonodular and Posterior Lobe)

The clinical features of this syndrome include the following: axial disequilibrium and staggering gait, little or no limb ataxia, and sometimes spontaneous nystagmus and rotated postures of the head. This syndrome is typically seen with damage to the flocculonodular lobe, especially medulloblastoma in children early on.

The Hemispheric Syndrome (Posterior Lobe, Variably Anterior Lobe)

Patients with this syndrome show ipsilateral appendicular incoordination. Thus this coordination affects mainly muscles that are closely controlled by the precentral cortex, such as those involved in speech and finger movements. The most likely etiologies include infarcts, neoplasms, and abscesses.

The Pancerebellar Syndrome (All Lobes)

This syndrome is a combination of all the other cerebellar syndromes and is characterized by bilateral signs of cerebellar dysfunction affecting the trunk, limbs, and cranial musculature. It is seen with infectious and parainfectious processes, hypoglycemia, hyperthermia, paraneoplastic disorders, and other toxic-metabolic disorders.

SYNDROMES OF CEREBELLAR INFARCTION

These account for 2% of all acute ischemic stroke and in order of frequency are posterior inferior cerebellar artery (40%), superior cerebellar artery (35%), border zone infarcts (20%) and anterior inferior cerebellar artery (5%). SCA infarcts are more likely to produce mass effect and herniation; other types may also be accompanied with mass effect depending on the size of the infarction.

REFERENCES

Belden JR, Caplan LR et al: *Neurology* 53:1312–1318, 1999.

Brazis PW, Masdeu JC, Biller J, eds: *Localization in clinical neurology*, ed 3, Boston, Little Brown, 1996.

Carpenter MB: *Core text of neuroanatomy*, ed 4, Baltimore, Williams & Wilkins, 1991.

Kandel ER, Schwartz JH, Jessel TM: *Principles of neural science*, ed 3, Norwalk, CT, Appleton & Lange, 1991.

CEREBRAL CORTEX

The cerebral cortex is divided into discrete areas, originally mapped by Brodmann, based on cytoarchitectonics. Figure 7 shows Brodmann's areas in lateral and medial views.

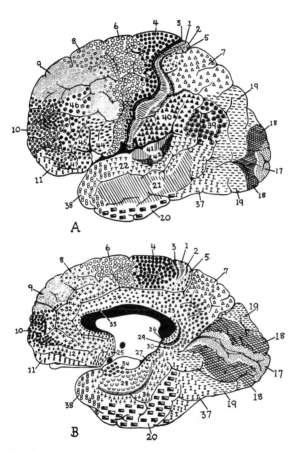

FIGURE 7

Brodmann's cytoarchitectural map of cerebral cortex, indicating major functional areas. *4*, Primary motor strip; *3*, *1*, and *2*, sensory strip; *17*, primary visual cortex; *18* and *19*, visual association cortex; *8*, frontal eye fields; *6*, premotor cortex; *41* and *42*, auditory cortex; *5* and *7*, somaesthetic association cortex. Areas *13* to *16* (not shown) make up the insula. Labeling is from anterior to posterior. (From Carpenter MB: *Core text of neuroanatomy*, ed 4, Baltimore, 1991, Williams & Wilkins.)

CEREBRAL HEMORRHAGE

Primary intraparenchymal (intracerebral) hemorrhage accounts for 10% of all strokes. Hypertension is the predominant risk factor. Chronic hypertension causes lipohyalinosis of the small intraparenchymal arteries, resulting in arteriolar wall weakness and subsequent rupture. Location of hemorrhage in order of frequency is as follows: putaminal (35% to 50%), subcortical white matter (30%), cerebellar (15%), thalamic (10% to 15%), and pontine (5% to 12%). The duration of active bleeding usually lasts only a short time, and later clinical deterioration is most often ascribed to surrounding edema and ischemia, rather than continued hemorrhage.

The signs and symptoms of cerebral hemorrhage correlate with anatomic location, size, and degree of associated mass effect. Headache is a frequent accompanying symptom.

Putamenal hemorrhage is associated with contralateral hemiparesis, hemianesthesia, and homonymous hemianopsia with aphasia or neglect (depending on which hemisphere is involved). There is also decreased level of consciousness (disproportionate to the weakness), ipsilateral eye deviation, and normal pupils.

Thalamic hemorrhage produces contralateral hemisensory loss with variable hemiparesis, contralateral homonymous hemianopsia, vertical or lateral-gaze palsies (including "wrong way" deviation) and, occasionally, nystagmus.

Cerebellar hemorrhage is associated with severe occipital headache, sudden nausea and vomiting, and truncal ataxia. It is a potential neurosurgical emergency when brainstem compression is imminent.

Pontine hemorrhage causes coma, pinpoint pupils (reactive to light), bilateral extensor posturing, impaired ocular motility, and caloric testing.

Acute mortality in intracerebral hemorrhage is usually due to mass effect with herniation or brainstem compression. Mortality may be high, especially in posterior fossa hemorrhage. The long-term prognosis for recovery of function may be better than in infarction, since there is usually displacement of tissue instead of primary tissue damage and necrosis.

Diagnosis is made by CT; blood appears as a hyperdensity acutely. The size is estimated based on the CT findings using the simple formula A B C/2 (A=width, B=length, C=number of cuts). Angiography may be necessary to exclude underlying vascular malformation or tumor.

Management may require an intensive care setting with frequent neurologic evaluation, and tight blood pressure control. Maintain adequate ventilation, pulmonary/pharyngeal toilet, adequate fluid, and electrolyte balance. Antiedemic agents (steroids, osmotic diuretics) may be used, but their efficacy is uncertain. Hyperventilation with induction of hypocapnia to keep Pco_2 between 28 and 32 can also be used to decrease intracranial pressure (ICP). This is a temporary measure before the ultimate therapy to control ICP is used, because maintaining Pco_2 below 30 for long periods risk compounding any concurrent ischemia by decreasing intracranial blood flow.

Blood pressure management is controversial; injudicious lowering of the pressure is contraindicated. Neurosurgical evaluation should be obtained for superficially located cerebral hemorrhages and all cerebellar hemorrhages.

Other causes of intraparenchymal hemorrhage:

1. Trauma accounts for up to 50% of nonhypertensive cerebral hemorrhage.
2. Ruptured AVM.
3. Ruptured aneurysm with parenchymal extension.
4. Metastatic carcinoma, especially lung, choriocarcinoma, melanoma, and renal adenocarcinoma.
5. Primary neoplasms (glioblastoma multiforme, pituitary adenoma).
6. Embolic infarction with secondary hemorrhage (up to one third of embolic infarcts).
7. Hematologic disorders, including leukemia, lymphoma, thrombocytopenic purpura, aplastic anemia, sickle cell anemia, hemophilia, hypoprothrombinemia, afibrinogenemia, and Waldenström's macroglobulinemia.
8. Anticoagulant therapy.
9. Cerebral amyloid angiopathy. This usually presents as multiple, recurrent hemorrhages in the white matter or cortex, sparing deep gray matter (as opposed to hypertensive hemorrhages). Amyloid angiopathy may be the cause in 5% to 10% of sporadic intracerebral hemorrhage. It is associated with dementia in about 30% of cases; familial cases are associated with mutations in the amyloid precursor protein on chromosome 21 (Dutch and Icelandic forms). Attempts at surgical evacuation are usually futile, since the vessels are very fragile, bleeding is very difficult to control, and there is a high incidence of recurrent hemorrhages.
10. Vasculopathies such as lupus, polyarteritis nodosa, and granulomatous arteritis.
11. Cortical vein thrombosis with secondary hemorrhage.
12. Drugs, including methamphetamine, amphetamine, pseudoephedrine, phenylpropanolamine, and cocaine.

Subarachnoid hemorrhage occurs with an incidence of 15/100,000 with peak incidence at 55 to 60 years of age. The majority of cases are due to rupture of cerebral aneurysm or trauma (see Aneurysm for further discussion).

Subdural hemorrhage (SDH) may be acute or chronic. Acute SDH is usually due to trauma with tearing of bridging veins. There may be an initial loss of consciousness with regaining of consciousness (lucid interval) followed in several hours by progressive deterioration of mental status and headache. Lateralizing signs may be present. Diagnosis is based on clinical course, emergency CT (appears as hyperdensity over cortex), and, if necessary, angiography. Treatment consists of neurosurgical evacuation. Dialysis patients and alcoholics are particularly prone to develop SDH.

Chronic SDH is less clearly related to trauma and may follow minor head trauma in the elderly and in patients on anticoagulants. Symptoms and signs resemble those in acute SDH but develop gradually over several days to months. Lateralizing signs are common. Mental status changes may suggest dementia. Diagnosis is as for acute SDH, although the lesion on CT is usually hypo or isodense. Treatment is neurosurgical evacuation.

The prognosis for survival and recovery in surgically treated patients is generally good but recurrence may occur.

Acute epidural hemorrhage results from skull fracture with laceration of the middle meningeal artery and vein. The clinical course is similar to acute SDH but is more rapidly progressive. Rapid herniation, respiratory depression, and death may ensue. The diagnosis is established emergently as for acute SDH. The CT appearance is a lens-shaped hyperdensity. This is a neurosurgical emergency and treated by immediate evacuation.

REFERENCE

Selman WR, Ratcheson RA: In Bradley WG, Daroff RB, Fenichel GM, Marsden CD, eds: *Neurology in clinical practice*, Boston, ed 3, Butterworth-Heinemann, 2000.

CEREBRAL PALSY (CP)

Static encephalopathy or CP refers to a group of an early-onset nonprogressive disorders of the CNS manifested by aberrant control of movement, tone, or posture.

Risk factors for development of CP:

1. Gestational age (prematurity and low birth weight).
2. Multiple gestation and transient hypothyroxinemia in premature infants.
3. Intrauterine exposure to infection or inflammation (nine-fold increased risk for CP).
4. Disorders of coagulation.
5. Asphyxia (contributes 6% of spastic CP).
6. Placental abnormalities leading to embolization to the fetal circulation, reaching cerebral circulation via the patent foramen ovale.
7. Maternal mental retardation. Interestingly, antenatal exposure to steroids may be protective and premature babies born to preeclamptic mothers have a lower risk of CP than babies born similarly premature for other indications.

Neurologic manifestations may include cognitive impairment, seizures, or impairments in vision (optic atrophy), hearing, or speech (pseudobulbar signs) in addition to the motor disability. The main categories are:

1. *spastic* form, which includes spastic *quadriplegia*, *diplegia*, or *hemi-paresis* with unilateral hemispheric atrophy and thickening of the skull on the same side (*Davidoff-Dyke-Masson syndrome*).
2. *dyskinetic* type consisting of chorea, choreoathetosis, or dystonia.
3. *ataxic* form.
4. *hyptonic* or atonic variant.
5. *mixed* form.

Diagnosis is usually made by exclusion. Imaging may be necessary to exclude remediable causes such as hydrocephalus.

Treatment includes the use of supportive care with physical therapy and orthosis. Surgical treatment for tendon release and transfer. Medical treatment for the spastic type may be tried with dantrolene sodium or baclofen, for the ataxic type with gabapentin, and for the dyskinetic type with dopaminergic medications. Botulinum toxin may be used to treat dynamic equinus foot deformity due to spasticity in ambulant pediatric CP patients, 2 years of age or older.

Prognosis depends on the severity of the disease; most of the hemi-paretic patients tend to do well. Patients with seizure, mental retardation, or dyskinetic and ataxic types have less favorable outcomes.

REFERENCES

Carr LJ et al: *Arch Dis Child* 79:271–273, 1998.
Grice J: *Arch Dis Child* 80:300, 1999.
Nelson KB, Grether JK: *Curr Opin Pediatr* 11:487–491, 1999.

CEREBROSPINAL FLUID

FORMATION

Cerebrospinal fluid (CSF) is produced mainly by the choroid plexuses (95%) but also in the interstitial space and ependyma (5%). The rate of CSF formation is about 500 ml per day, and total CSF volume is 150 ml (50% intracranial, 50% spinal). Secretion is an energy-requiring process related to ion-exchange (Na/K). Production is also dependent on the cytosolic enzyme carbonic anhydrase. Therefore, carbonic anhydrase inhibitors (e.g., acetazolamide) substantially reduce CSF formation. CSF is absorbed primarily by arachnoid villi extending into the dural venous sinuses. Normal CSF opening pressure during lumbar puncture (LP) should be less than 20 mm H_2O (see Table 12).

APPEARANCE

Normal CSF is clear and colorless (s.g. 1.007, pH 7.33 to 7.35); when cell counts reach approximately 200 WBC/mm^3 or 400 RBC/mm^3, it may become cloudy. Lower cell counts can be detected by observing for *Tyndall's effect*. This phenomenon refers to a sparkling quality of CSF when viewed in direct light and results from suspended particles scattering ambient light.

C

CEREBROSPINAL FLUID

TABLE 12

NORMAL VALUES FOR LUMBAR FLUID

Age	Protein mg/dl	Glucose mg/dl	Cell Count/mm³	Lymph/PMN Ratio	Opening Pressure (mm CSF)
Preterm	115	50	9	40/60	
Term	90	52	8	40/60	80–100
Child	5–40	40–80	0–5		60–200
Adult	20–40	50–70	0–5	100/0	60–200
Ventricular	6–15				
Cervical	20–30				

IgG/albumin ratio (CSF IgG/Alb) upper limit: 0.27
IgG/albumin index (CSF IgG/Alb)/(serum IgG/Alb) upper limit: 0.60
Myelin basic protein upper limit: 4 ng/ml
Corrections
  WBC: Reduce WBC by one cell for every 700 RBC (if hematocrit is normal)
                     OR
  WBC (corr) = WBC(csf) − WBC(blood) × RBC(csf)/RBC(blood)
  Protein: Subtract 1 mg/ml for every 1000 RBC

Viscous CSF can result from large numbers of cryptococci within the CSF, secondary to their polysaccharide capsules. Clot or pellicle formation occurs with elevated proteins. *Froin's syndrome* refers to clot formation in the setting of complete spinal block and very high protein. CSF is perceived as grossly bloody with cell counts greater than 6000 RBC/mm³ and, at cell counts of more than 500, *xanthochromia* appears. Xanthochromia refers to the yellow, pink, or orange coloration of the CSF corresponding to the breakdown products of RBCs. Oxyhemoglobin released from RBCs can be detected within the supernatant fluid within 2 to 4 hours after the release of blood into the subarachnoid space; it reaches a maximum at about 36 hours and disappears in about 7 to 10 days. Supernatant fluid may, however, remain clear for up to 12 hours after a subarachnoid bleed. Differential diagnosis of xanthochromia includes hyperbilirubinemia, hyperproteinemia, hypercarotenemia, and drugs (rifampin).

CYTOLOGY

Cytological analysis should be done soon after lumbar puncture. Prompt refrigeration is necessary. Lymphocytes are the predominant leukocyte forms in normal CSF. An occasional granulocyte is seen in normal fluid and is not necessarily pathological if the total white count is normal (0 to 3 cells/mm³). A few or moderate numbers of granulocytes may occur following spinal anesthesia, myelography, or other intrathecal injections or with trauma, hemorrhage, or infarct in the absence of infection. No RBCs should be present in normal CSF. In a traumatic tap, it is important to differentiate whether the WBCs are truly elevated or whether they are present in the same WBC/RBC ratio as in the peripheral blood. In a non-anemic patient as an approximation, subtract 1 WBC for every 700 RBCs.

Fishman's formula can be used for correction of WBC counts in the presence of significant anemia or peripheral leukocytosis. It estimates the WBC count in the CSF before the LP (actual $WBC_{CSF} = WBC_{CSF} \times RBC_{CSF} / RBC_{BLOOD}$). Detection of tumor cells is enhanced by collection of large volumes of CSF (20 ml), repeated CSF examination, and/or cisternal taps.

PROTEIN

Protein is a nonspecific indicator of disease. Normally, the blood-brain barrier keeps serum proteins out of the CSF (normal adult 15 to 45 mg%). Many CNS diseases disrupt the barrier, allowing entrance of serum protein and consequently elevation of CSF protein (see Table 13). Increases greater than 500 mg/dl are rare, and occur mainly in spinal block, meningitis, arachnoiditis, and subarachnoid hemorrhage (SAH). Metabolic conditions such as myxedema and diabetic neuropathy may cause an increase in protein levels. The major immunoglobulin in normal CSF is IgG. The IgG index and synthesis rate correct for serum IgG. Elevated levels may result from production within the CNS in various immune response disorders. Oligoclonal bands indicate the presence of an immune-mediated pathologic process such as multiple sclerosis and subacute sclerosing panencephalitis. Oligoclonal bands occur in 80 to 90% of patients with clinically definite MS. Myelin basic protein, a product of oligodendroglia, may be increased by any processes that result in myelin breakdown, such as stroke or anoxia; elevated levels are not a specific marker of demyelinating disease. Low CSF protein may occur with dural leaks and in benign intracranial hypertension. Protein in cisternal CSF is 50% of the lumbar value and is even lower (25%) within the lateral ventricles.

GLUCOSE

Glucose is derived from serum and is a reflection of the previous 4 hours of systemic glucose levels. Normal CSF to blood ratio is 0.6 with a usual value of 40 to 80 mg%. Simultaneous serum glucose level should be done. Hypoglycorrhachia occurs in bacterial, fungal, or TB meningitis, and inflammatory processes such as sarcoidosis, carcinomatous meningitis, and SAH. The mechanism of hypoglycorrhachia in meningeal disorders is related to an increase in anaerobic glycolysis in brain and spinal cord and, to a variable degree, PMNs as well as an inhibition of glucose entry from altered glucose membrane transport.

COMPLICATIONS OF LUMBAR PUNCTURE
Headache

Results from persistent dural CSF leak. Incidence 10%. Onset is 5 minutes to 4 days after LP. Pain is positional. Post-LP headache usually resolves spontaneously, the majority within 1 week, but may persist up to several months. These headaches are more common in women and younger patients. The risk factors are related to needle size, the amount of CSF obtained, and placing the stylet back before removing the needle. Preventive

TABLE 13

CSF PROFILES IN VARIOUS DISEASES

	Pressure	Cell Count/mm³	Protein	Glucose
Purulent meningitis	Increased (inc) in 90% 200–1500 mm H_2O	100–10,000 90%–95% PMN	Nl–2200	Decreased (dec)
Aseptic meningitis	May be inc	10–1000 L + M (PMN early)	Nl to 400	Nl
Fungal meningitis	Nl	Inc PMN + L + M Need to check india ink and cryptococcal antigen.	Nl or inc	Dec
Tuberculous meningitis	Inc	50–500	100–1000	Dec
Sarcoidosis	Nl or inc	10–100 L + M	50–200	Nl or dec
Neoplastic meningitis	Nl or inc	0–500 PMN + L + M Cytology may show atypical cells, and cell surface markers may be helpful.	Nl or inc	Nl or dec
Subarachnoid hemorrhage	Inc	Nl or inc Lysis of RBC begins after 2 to 4 hours. Xanthochromia is visible after 8 to 10 hours and may persist for weeks.	Nl or inc	Nl or dec
Herpes encephalitis	Nl	50–100 L + M RBC and xanthochromia are often present (which distinguishes this disease from other viral meningitides).	Nl	Nl
SSPE	Nl	Nl Gammaglobulins are markedly inc and may account for 50% of the total protein. Oligoclonal bands are present.	Nl or inc	Nl
Guillain-Barré	Nl	0–25 L + M Protein values peak between day 4 and day 18. Oligoclonal bands are often present.	Nl or inc	Nl
Migraine	Nl or inc	5–15 L + M A migrainous syndrome with white blood cell counts greater than 200/mm³ has been described.	Nl	Nl
Optic neuritis	Nl	Nl or inc Less than 25 L + M	Nl or inc	Nl
Multiple sclerosis	Nl	Nl or inc Less than 25 L + M Oligoclonal bands, IgG/albumin index and ratio elevated, indicating intra-CNS antibody production. Myelin basic protein may increase with an exacerbation.	Nl or inc	Nl
Acute disseminated encephalomyelitis	Nl or inc	5–150 L + M + PMN	Nl or inc	Nl

continued

TABLE 13 —cont'd
CSF PROFILES IN VARIOUS DISEASES

	Pressure	Cell Count/mm³	Protein	Glucose
Spinal block	Dec	Nl or inc	Markedly increased	Nl
	Clotting (Froin's syndrome) occurs when the protein value is greater than 1000.			
Seizure	Nl	Nl or inc Up to 25 L + M rarely PMN	Nl or Inc	Nl
	Pleocytosis is usually associated with prolonged or frequent seizures.			
CNS Lyme disease	Nl or inc	Inc L + M Up to 20% plasma cells	Inc	Nl or dec
	Oligoclonal bands, IgG/albumin index and ratio may be elevated, indicating intrathecal anti-*Borrelia* antibody production.			
HIV and AIDS				
Encephalopathy	Nl	Nl	Nl or inc	Nl
Toxoplasmosis	Nl or increased	Inc Positive Toxo. antibody	Inc	Nl
Cryptococcosis	Nl or inc	Nl or inc Positive cryptococcal antigen	Nl or inc	Nl or dec
Polyneuropathy				
Distal, symmetric	Nl	Nl	Nl or inc	Nl
Chronic inflammatory	Nl or inc	Inc	Inc	Nl

C

CEREBROSPINAL FLUID

measures include use of the smallest gauge needle, insertion of the needle bevel parallel to the dural fibers of the posterior longitudinal ligament, and the use of short bevel needles. Treatment of an established post-LP headache involves bed rest, adequate hydration (particularly if nausea and vomiting occur), and analgesics. Caffeine 300 to 500 mg PO and theophylline may be used. Intractable cases may be treated with epidural blood patching by injection of 10 ml of the patient's freshly drawn blood into the epidural space, where it can clot. It is curative in the majority of cases.

Brain Herniation
May occur immediately or up to 12 hours after an LP. Occurs in patients with supratentorial mass lesions and midline shift or obstructing posterior fossa tumors.

Bleeding
Spinal subdural, epidural, and subarachnoid hemorrhage may occur in patients treated with anticoagulants or those with thrombocytopenia or bleeding diathesis.

Diplopia
Rare transient unilateral or bilateral abducens palsy.

Others
Radicular irritation, meningitis, implantation of epidermoid tumor.

LP contraindications
Infection over the site of entry, coagulopathy, presence of a known or suspected intracranial mass especially with midline shift and noncommunicating hydrocephalus (always try to obtain CT before procedure). Elevated ICP as reflected by papilledema by itself is not an absolute contraindication to spinal tap because LP is actually used as a treatment in pseudotumor cerebri.

REFERENCES

Fishman RA: *Cerebrospinal fluid in diseases of the nervous system*, Philadelphia, WB Saunders, 1992.
Zaidat OO, Suarez JI: *JAMA* 283:1004, 2000.

CHEMOTHERAPY, NEUROLOGIC COMPLICATIONS

NEUROTOXIC SIGNS CAUSED BY AGENTS COMMONLY USED IN PATIENTS WITH CANCER

Acute Encephalopathy
Corticosteroids, methotrexate (MTX) (see Table 14), cis-platinum, vincristine, aspariginase, procarbazine, 5-FU, ara-C, nitrosoureas, cyclosporine, interleukin 2, ifosfamide/mesna, interferons, tamoxifen, VP-16 (high-dose), PALA.

Chronic Encephalopathy
MTX, BCNU, ara-C, Carmofur, fludarabine.

Stroke/Stroke-like/TIA
MTX, L-aspariginase, cisplatin, interleukin 2.

Visual Loss/Other Cranial Neuropathy
Tamoxifen, gallium nitrate, nitrosoureas (intra-arterial), cis-platinum, vincristine.

Cerebellar Dysfunction/Ataxia
5-FU, ara-C, procarbazine, hexamethylmelamine, vincristine, cyclosporine A.

Aseptic Meningitis
IVI, levamisole, monoclonal antibodies, metrizamide, OTK3, ara-C, MTX.

Seizures
MTX, VP-16 (high dose), OTK3 antibody, cis-platinum, vincristine, aspariginase, nitrogen mustard, BCNU, dacarbazine, PALA, mAmsa, busulfan (high dose), cyclosporine.

Myelopathy
MTX (IT), ara-C (IT), thiotepa (IT), cyclosporine.

TABLE 14
HIGH-DOSE METHOTREXATE NEUROTOXICITY

Characteristics	Acute Encephalopathy	Subacute Encephalopathy	Chronic Leukoencephalopathy
Onset	<48 hr	3–10 days	≥ 3 mo
Symptoms	Confusion, lethargy, headaches, seizures	Multifocal deficits	Spasticity, dementia, seizures
Abnormal CT	No	Rarely	White-matter hypodensity, calcifications
Clinical outcome	Full recovery	Usually full recovery	Persistent neurologic deficits, death

Adapted from Posner JB: *Neurologic complications of cancer*, ed 2, Philadelphia, FA Davis, 1995, 297.

Peripheral Neuropathy
Vinca alkaloids, cis-platinum, hexamethylmelamine, procarbazine, 5-azacytidine, VP-16, VM-26, methyl-G, ara-C, taxol, suramin, mitotane, vincristine (subacute to chronic; almost 100%), cyclosporine, interferon-alpha.

Myopathy
Vincristine (subacute), cyclosporine, corticosteroids.

Adapted from Posner JB: *Neurologic complications of cancer*, ed 2, Philadelphia, FA Davis, 1995, 284.

REFERENCES
Posner JB: *Neurologic complications of cancer*, ed 2, Philadelphia, FA Davis, 1995, 282–310.
MacDonald DR: *Neurol Clin* 9(4):955–967, 1991.

CHILD NEUROLOGY

I. History: Pregnancy, labor, delivery (drugs, illnesses, complications, etc.) and mode of delivery; weeks of gestation, Apgar scores, complications of delivery; birth weight; length of neonate's hospital stay; developmental milestones (girls achieve these earlier than boys).
   A. School-aged children: School performance, drug and alcohol history, especially if there has been a change in behavior (questions preferably asked when parent is out of the room).
   B. Adolescents: Drug history, contraceptive history and sexual history are best elicited when the parent is out of the room.
II. General exam: Measure head circumference and check age-specific norms (see Figures 8–11 and Tables 15 and 16). Examine the skin, morphology of the face and extremities, and cardiovascular system. In neonates, look for external trauma such as cephalhematoma or subgaleal hematoma. Retinal hemorrhages resulting from the birth process or trauma may be seen. Measure the size of the anterior and posterior

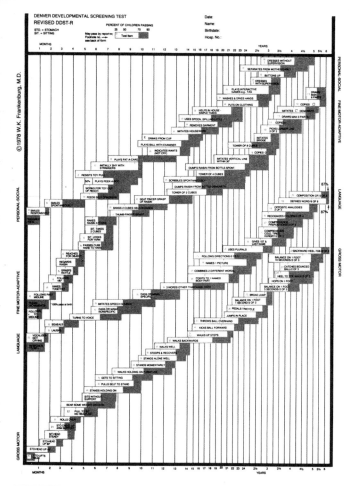

FIGURE 8

Denver Development Screening Test. (Courtesy of W.K. Frankenburg, MD.)
See foldout.

fontanels, and note whether they are bulging. Auscultate head for bruits. Transilluminate head.

III. Neurologic exam.

   A. Infants: Much of the information regarding the neonate is obtained through observation of level of alertness, posture, and spontaneous movements. Assess posture and muscle tone. Arching of the neck

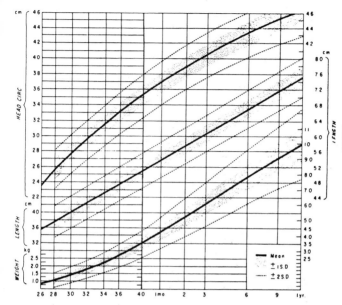

FIGURE 9

Fetal and infant norms: weight, length, and head circumference.

and back, scissoring of legs on vertical suspension, and contractures indicate increased tone. Hypotonic infants "slip through your fingers" at the shoulders, legs will flop apart in a frog-leg posture on vertical suspension, and head will "lag" as infant is pulled from supine to sitting by gentle arm traction.

1. *Premature infants* normally are hypotonic and have head lag. Prematures will not be able to turn the head from side to side when placed face down. Arms and legs are held in extension until 35 weeks' gestation.

2. *Full-term infants* should be able to lift their heads for short periods and turn them from a central face-down position to one side. When held at the axillae, facing the examiner, the normal full-term infant should flex arms and legs and hold head erect.

B. Older children: Do as much of the exam as necessary with the child on the parent's lap. Examining the hands and feet for tone and reflexes is often a nonthreatening way to begin. For a toddler, much motor information can be obtained while the child is playing with toys on the floor. Older children are typically quite cooperative and the exam is similar to an adult.

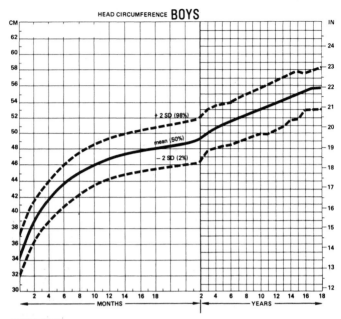

IV. Normal myelination begins during the fifth fetal month. It proceeds in a highly predictable and orderly manner: Caudal to cephalad, dorsal to ventral, and central to peripheral. Sensory tracts myelinate first.
   A. Birth (full term): Medulla, dorsal midbrain, inferior and superior cerebellar peduncles, posterior limb of internal capsule, ventrolateral thalamus.
   B. One month: Deep cerebellar white matter, corticospinal tracts, pre/postcentral gyrus, optic nerves, tracts.
   C. Three months: Brachium pontis, cerebellar folia, ventral brainstem, optic radiations, anterior limb of internal capsule, occipital subcortical U fibers, corpus callosum splenium.
   D. Six months: Corpus callosum genu, paracentral subcortical U fibers, centrum semiovale (partial).
   E. Eight months: Centrum semiovale (complete except some frontotemporal areas), subcortical U fibers (complete except for most rostral frontal areas).
   F. Eighteen months: Essentially like adults.
   G. Twenty years: Peritrigonal region.

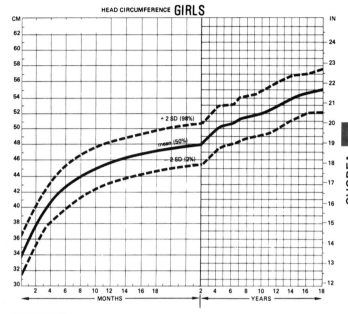

FIGURE 11

Head circumference, girls. (From Nellhaus G: *Pediatrics* 41:106, 1968. Used by permission.)

TABLE 15

PRIMITIVE REFLEXES IN NEONATES AND INFANTS

Reflex	Response	Appears (Age)	Disappears (Age in mo)
Palmar grasp		28 wk	4–5
Moro reflex (drop baby's head suddenly in relation to trunk)	Opens hands, extends and abducts upper extremities and draw them together	28–32 wk	4–5
Gag		32 wk	Persists
Suck		34 wk	4
Tonic neck (rotate infant's head to the side while chest is maintained flat)	Arm and leg extend on side toward which face is rotated, flexion of limbs on opposite side; Abnormal: asymmetric or obligatory and sustained pattern	34 wk	4

Table continued on following page

TABLE 15 —cont'd

PRIMITIVE REFLEXES IN NEONATES AND INFANTS

Reflex	Response	Appears (Age)	Disappears (Age in mo)
Reflex stepping (baby supported in upright position)		35 wk	5
Crossed adductor		35 wk	7
Plantar grasp		Birth	9–12
Extensor plantar response (Babinski)		Birth	10
Placing (dorsum of foot placed against edge of table)		1 day	Covered by voluntary action
Landau reflex (lift baby with one hand under its trunk, face downward)	Reflex extension of vertebral column → baby lifts head above horizontal	3 mo	24
Parachute response (suspend child horizontally about the waist, face down)	Arms extend and fingers spread	4–9 mo	Covered by voluntary action

TABLE 16

LANDMARK DEVELOPMENTAL MILESTONES (SEE DENVER DEVELOPMENT SCALE)

Age (Mo)	Gross Motor	Fine Motor	Language	Social
4	Rolls over	Moves arm in unison to grasp	Orients to voice	Enjoys looking around
6	Sits unsupported	Grasps with either hand, transfers	Babbles	Recognizes strangers
9	Crawls, pulls to stand	Pincer grasp, holds bottle	Understands no	Explores, plays pat-a-cake
12	Walks alone	Throws objects	Uses 2 words besides dada/mama	Imitates, comes when called
24	Walks up and down stairs alone	Turns single pages, removes clothes	Uses 2 word sentences; follows 2-step commands	Parallel play
36	Pedals tricycle	Dresses partially, draws a circle	Uses 3-word sentences, plurals	Group play, shares toys
48	Hops, skips	Buttons, catches ball	Knows colors, asks questions	Tells "tall tales"

REFERENCES

Menkes JH: *Textbook of child neurology*, Philadelphia, Lea and Febiger, 1990,
Osborn AG: *Diagnostic neuroradiology*, St. Louis, Mosby, 1994.

CHOREA

Chorea is involuntary, rapid, jerky, arrhythmic movements of muscle
groups. It can involve the upper or lower extremities, trunk, neck, or face
and may be generalized, symmetric, asymmetric, or unilateral. Chorea is
distinguished from other movement disorders by the random timing and
distribution. The movements are often incorporated into deliberate movements by the patient that may camouflage the disorder. Grimacing and
respiratory grunts may be manifestations.

Following are the most common causes of chorea:

1. Huntington's disease.
2. Drug-induced (see below).
3. Systemic lupus erythematosus.
4. Polycythemia vera.
5. Hyperthyroidism.
6. Pregnancy (chorea gravidarum) or oral contraceptive use.
7. Neuroacanthocytosis, a multisystem neurologic disease characterized
   by dementia, psychiatric disturbances, seizures, chorea, dystonia, tics,
   akinetic-rigid features, diminished deep tendon reflexes, muscle
   atrophy and weakness, and acanthocytes in peripheral blood.

Other causes by group include the following.

I. Age-related
   A. Physiologic chorea of infancy.
   B. Kernicterus.
   C. Cerebral palsy.
   D. Buccal-oral-lingual chorea of aging.
   E. "Senile" chorea.
II. Hereditary
   A. "Benign" familial (need to consider Huntington's disease).
   B. Amino acid, carbohydrate, and lipid disorders.
   C. Lesch-Nyhan syndrome.
   D. Wilson's disease.
   E. Hallervorden-Spatz syndrome.
   F. Ataxia-telangiectasia.
   G. Tuberous sclerosis.
   H. Sturge-Weber syndrome.
   I. Myoclonic epilepsy.
   J. Pelizaeus-Merzbacher disease.
   K. Sickle-cell disease.
   L. Leigh's disease.

M. Porphyria.

N. Paroxysmal kinesiogenic and dystonic choreas.

O. Familial basal ganglia calcification.

P. Olivopontocerebellar atrophy.

III. Drug-induced and toxic

A. Neuroleptics.

B. Antiparkinsonian agents: Dopaminergic, amantadine, anticholinergics.

C. Anticonvulsants: Carbamazepine, phenytoin, phenobarbital.

D. Noradrenergic stimulants: Amphetamine, methylphenidate, pemoline, aminophylline, theophylline, caffeine.

E. Anabolic steroids and oral contraceptives.

F. Opiates: Methadone, heroin.

G. Others: Antihistamines, lithium, tricyclics, isoniazid, reserpine, metoclopramide, digoxin, methyldopa, diazoxide, triazolam.

H. Toxins: Ethanol intoxication and withdrawal, carbon monoxide, mercury, manganese, thallium, toluene.

IV. Metabolic

A. Hyponatremia and hypernatremia.

B. Hypocalcemia.

C. Hypomagnesemia.

D. Hypoglycemia and hyperglycemia.

E. Hypoparathyroidism.

F. Addison's disease.

G. Pregnancy.

H. Hepatic encephalopathy.

I. Renal failure.

J. Vitamin deficiencies: thiamine (beriberi), niacin (pellagra), B_{12}.

V. Infectious or immunologic

A. Sydenham's chorea (St. Vitus' dance) post-rheumatic fever.

B. Diphtheria, pertussis, typhoid fever, including postvaccinal.

C. Viral encephalitis.

D. Neurosyphilis.

E. Lyme disease.

F. Legionnaires' disease.

G. Sarcoidosis.

H. Systemic lupus erythematosus, Henoch-Schönlein purpura, Behçet's syndrome, periarteritis nodosa; antiphospholipid antibody syndrome.

I. Multiple sclerosis.

VI. Cerebrovascular

A. Basal ganglionic infarction or hemorrhage.

B. Arteriovenous malformation.

C. Migraine.

VII. Miscellaneous

A. Posttraumatic.

B. Brain tumors: Primary, metastatic, lymphoma.

C. Epidural and subdural hematomas.

D. Electrical injury.

REFEFERENCE

Joseph AB, Young RR, eds: *Movement disorders in neurology and neuropsychiatry*, Boston, Blackwell Scientific Publications, 1992.

CHROMOSOMAL DISORDERS

Mental retardation (MR), often with microcephaly, is a characteristic of most chromosomal disorders. Partial deletions and partial trisomies have been described for almost every chromosome, but only trisomies 21, 18, and 13, and several sex chromosome anomalies have a recognizable clinical syndrome likely to be diagnosed prior to karyotyping. Karyotype analysis is indicated in the evaluation of most children with mental retardation, especially if they are associated with dysmorphic features.

A. *Trisomy 21 (Down's syndrome):* (1 in 660 births) MR, hypotonia, infantile spasms, oblique palpebral fissures, median epicanthal fold, Brushfield spots (accumulation of fibrous tissue appearing as light colored spots encircling the periphery of the iris), low-set ears, thick protruding tongue, bilateral simian creases, short extremities and digits, heart anomalies, GI anomalies (duodenal atresia), and upper cervical spine malformation. In later life, these patients develop Alzheimer's disease with progressive cognitive decline and pathological findings of neuritic plaques and neurofibrillary tangles. They are also at risk for stroke in childhood due to congenital heart disease. Seizures are also common in later adult life.

B. *Trisomy 13:* (1 in 5000 births) Severe MR, microcephaly, microphthalmos, arhinencephaly spectrum, median facial anomilies, low-set dysplastic ears, heart anomalies, polycystic kidneys.

C. *Trisomy 18 (Edward's syndrome):* (1 in 4500 births) Severe MR, brain grossly and microscopically normal in 50%, long narrow skull, low-set dysplastic ears, second finger overlies third, thumb distally implanted and retroflexible, heart anomalies, polycystic kidneys.

D. *XXY (Klinefelter's syndrome):* (1 in 500 males) Mild MR, learning disabilities, language disorder, behavior disorders, intention tremor, tall with long limbs, hypogonadism, hypogenitalism, increased follicle-stimulating hormone levels, gynecomastia.

E. *XYY:* Borderline MR, learning disabilities, behavior disorders, tall stature.

F. *Fragile X:* (1 in 2000 males) MR, long face, large floppy ears, *macroorchidism*. May have macrocephaly. Usually X-linked recessive pattern of inheritance, but some heterozygous females may have MR along with developmental Gerstmann's syndrome. Karyotype analysis shows an expanded number of CAG repeats on the relevant portion of X-chromosome.

G. *XXX:* MR without other specific findings.

H. *XO (Turner's syndrome):* Usually normal intelligence (but frequently have problems with visuospatial skills), short stature, broad chest with widely spaced nipples, low posterior hairline, webbed neck, congenital lymphedema, cubitus valgus, ovarian dysgenesis.

REFERENCE

Aicardi J: *Semin Pediatr Neurol* 5:15–20, 1998.

COMA *(see also Brain Death, Cardiopulmonary Arrest)*

Consciousness is the state of awareness of self and surroundings. Loss of awareness with concomitant defects in arousal constitutes coma, and when less pronounced, lethargy, stupor, and obtundation. Coma is neither a unitary state nor an etiologic diagnosis. Its presence suggests specific dysfunction of both hemispheres or dysfunction of the brainstem reticular activating system, or both. The mechanism of dysfunction may be a structural lesion (supratentorial or subtentorial), a metabolic disturbance, or psychogenic.

Coma evaluation requires a detailed medical history and a general physical examination to establish potential causes. In addition to complete chemistry tests, blood cell count, and coagulation panels, blood gas levels (observe color and request CO level), toxicology screens (on blood, urine, and gastric contents), thyroid function tests, cortisol level, and cultures should be obtained at the time of initial evaluation of coma of unknown cause. Emergency management is outlined in Table 17.

The neurologic examination is focused toward determining the pathophysiologic features by distinguishing the location and degree of CNS dysfunction, including the following.

I. Level of consciousness: Response to voice, shaking, or pain. Consider status epilepticus, akinetic mutism, vegetative state, locked-in (deefferented) syndrome, and psychogenic states (see below).

II. Brainstem function

A. Pupils: Light reflex tests for cranial nerves II and III (midbrain).

1. Anisocoria: With Horner's syndrome, suggests hypothalamic or lateral medullary dysfunction; without Horner's, and if there are associated ocular motility deficits, consider transtentorial herniation.

2. Miosis: Common in toxic or metabolic encephalopathy (preserved light reflex is a hallmark of metabolic coma) and central herniation with supratentorial mass lesion. Pinpoint, barely reactive pupils suggest acute pontine lesion or presence of opioids.

3. Mydriasis: In association with absent light reflex and (sometimes) irregular pupils, suggests dorsal midbrain dysfunction. Beware of atropine or sympathomimetics commonly given during resuscitation.

4. Fixed, midposition pupils suggest midbrain nuclear (third nerve) dysfunction.

TABLE 17

EMERGENCY MANAGEMENT OF COMA OF UNKNOWN CAUSE

1. Ensure oxygenation. Clear airway, suction, perform bag-valve-mask ventilation, and use intubation as needed. Immobilize cervical spine prior to neck extension until C-spine injury is excluded radiographically. Atropine, 1 mg IV, may prevent vagally mediated bradyarrhythmias during intubation.
2. Maintain circulation with fluids and pressors to keep mean arterial pressure above 100 mmHg. Continuous ECG monitoring is necessary.
3. Thiamine, 100 mg IV, followed by glucose 25 g (50 ml D50) IV, immediately after blood is drawn (large volume) for diagnostics.
4. Treat intracranial hypertension if suspected (see Intracranial Pressure).
5. Stop seizures when present (see Epilepsy).
6. Restore acid-base balance.
7. Treat drug overdose. For suspected narcotics give naloxone (Narcan) 0.4 mg IV, repeat as necessary if effective (short half-life) or in 5 min. For suspected anticholinergics (e.g., tricyclics), give physostigmine, 1 mg IV. For suspected benzodiazepine overdose, give Flumazenil starting at 0.2 mg IV over 30 seconds. Failure to respond to a total dose of 5 mg makes it unlikely that coma is due to benzodiazepines.
8. Exclude intracranial masses by CT (uncontrasted).
9. Normalize body temperature.
10. Treat infection if suspected (see Meningitis).
11. Specific therapy should be instituted as soon as a diagnosis is established.

B. Eye movements: Assess conjugacy, gaze deviation or preference, nystagmus, and spontaneous movements. Oculocephalic responses and vestibulo-ocular testing with ice water evaluate brainstem connections of cranial nerves III, IV, VI, and VIII. Presence of nystagmus without ocular deviation to the irrigated ear on caloric testing suggests psychogenic coma, since it indicates integrity of brainstem and hemispheric pathways. Roving eye movements suggest an intact brainstem. Ocular bobbing and its variants suggest pontine lesions.

C. Corneal or sternutatory reflexes test cranial nerves V and VII (pons).

D. Gag (pharynx) or cough (larynx-trachea) reflexes test cranial nerves IX and X (medulla).

III. Breathing patterns

    A. *Cheyne-Stokes respirations* consist of cyclically increasing, then decreasing respiratory depth and rate, separated by apneic phases. It results from the interaction of an increased ventilatory drive to pCO_2 and a decreased forebrain stimulus for respiration, when pCO_2 is decreased. It suggests bilateral cerebral hemispheric or diencephalic dysfunction but may be produced by any encephalopathic state. It is also common in severe congestive heart failure.

    B. *Central neurogenic hyperventilation* is attributed to brainstem injury. *Tachypnea* is more common and is usually associated with hypocapnia and hypoxemia. It often resolves with correction of the metabolic abnormalities, whereas central neurogenic hyperventilation does not. Tachypnea with brainstem disease may be associated with neurogenic pulmonary edema.

C. *Apneustic breathing* consists of prolonged "jamming" of respiration in inspiratory and expiratory phases. Although rare, it is seen with dorsolateral pontine lesions at the level of the sensory trigeminal nucleus.

D. *Ataxic breathing* consists of generally slow, irregular respirations with variable amplitude and can progress rapidly to complete apnea. It is due to bilateral lesions of the reticular formation in the caudal dorsomedial medulla, where the respiratory rhythm is generated. Medullary compression, usually caused by acute lesions, may result in respiratory arrest, leading to cardiovascular collapse.

E. These breathing patterns may be a false localizing sign in cases of coexisting metabolic derangement. For example, metabolic acidosis and hypoxia cause reactive hyperventilation, simulating neurogenic hyperventilation.

IV. Sensorimotor

A. Spontaneous activity. Assess for volitional movement, choreoathetosis, posturing (arms decorticate or flexor vs. decerebrate or extensor), asterixis, myoclonus, and seizures.

B. Response to noxious stimuli (listed in order of increasing severity of coma). Lateralizing features of response should be noted.
1. Purposeful.
2. Flexion withdrawal.
3. Abnormal flexion (decorticate posturing): Usually slow, stereotyped flexion of arm, wrist, and fingers with shoulder adduction and variable leg extension.
4. Abnormal extension (decerebrate posturing): Extension of wrist and arm with adduction and internal rotation of shoulder; extension and internal rotation of leg with plantar flexion of foot.
5. No response.

C. Tone: Assess for flaccidity, rigidity, spasticity, clonus, and paratonia.

V. Tendon reflexes: Assess for asymmetry, increase, or decrease in response.

The Glasgow coma scale quantitates level of consciousness. It is easy to use and reliable, with low interobserver variability (see Table 18). Since the scale does not assess brainstem reflexes, it does not communicate a complete neurologic assessment but is useful for rapid identification, reliable communication, serial quantitation, and aid in assessing prognosis, particularly when used in evaluation of posttraumatic coma.

CAUSES OF COMA

I. Accurate localization can identify likely causes of altered consciousness.

A. Supratentorial lesion.
1. Subcortical destructive lesions.
2. Hemorrhage: Epidural, subdural, subarachnoid, intracerebral; hypertensive, vascular malformation.

TABLE 18

GLASGOW COMA SCALE

		Score
Eye opening	Open spontaneously	4
	To verbal command	3
	To pain	2
	Do not open	1
Best motor response	Obeys to verbal command	6
	Localizes pain	5
	Flexion withdrawal	4
	Flexion-abnormal (decorticate)	3
	Extension-abnormal (decerebrate)	2
	No response	1
Best verbal response	Oriented and converses	5
	Disoriented and converses	4
	Verbalizes	3
	Vocalizes	2
	No response	1
	Total: (Range, 3 to 15)	—

C

COMA

3. Infarction: Thrombotic or embolic arterial occlusion, venous thrombosis.
4. Tumor: Primary, metastatic.
5. Abscess: Intracerebral, subdural.
6. Closed head injury.

B. Infratentorial lesion.
   1. Compressive: Cerebellar hemorrhage, infarct, tumor, or abscess; posterior fossa subdural, extradural hemorrhages, basilar aneurysm.
   2. Destructive: Brainstem hemorrhage, infarction, tumor, demyelination, or abscess.

C. Diffuse brain dysfunction.
   1. Intrinsic: Encephalitis, progressive multifocal leukencephalopathy, meningitis, concussion, ictal or postictal state, herniation.
   2. Hypoxic or metabolic: Anoxia, ischemia, nutritional (e.g., Wernicke's syndrome), hepatic encephalopathy, uremia, pulmonary disease.
   3. Endocrine: Nonketotic hyperglycemic hyperosmolar coma, ketoacidosis, DIC, hypoglycemia, Addison's disease, myxedema, thyrotoxicosis, panhypopituitarism.
   4. Toxic, drug-induced: Amphetamines, cocaine, psychedelics, tricyclics, phenothiazines, lithium, benzodiazepines, methaqualone, glutethimide, barbiturates, alcohol, opiates, ibuprofen, aspirin.

     5. Ionic and acid-base disorders: Hypo-osmolarity or hyperosmolarity; hyponatremia or hypernatremia, hypocalcemia or hypercalcemia, hypophosphatemia, lactic acidosis, cerebral edema.

     6. Hypothermia, hyperthermia.

     7. Remote effects of cancer (paraneoplastic): Limbic encephalitis, thalamic degeneration.

  D. Psychogenic coma.

     1. Conversion reaction, catatonic stupor, malingering.

II. The clinical course may also suggest localization and cause.

  A. Supratentorial mass with diencephalic or brainstem compression.

     1. Early focal cerebral dysfunction.

     2. Rostral to caudal progression with signs referrable to one area at a time.

     3. Asymmetric motor signs.

     4. Third-nerve palsy preceding coma (early herniation).

  B. Infratentorial mass or destruction.

     1. Early brainstem dysfunction or sudden onset of coma with accompanying brainstem signs.

     2. Vestibulo-ocular abnormalities present.

     3. Cranial nerve palsies usually present.

     4. Abnormal respirations common, appear early.

  C. Metabolic causes.

     1. Confusion and stupor precede motor signs.

     2. Motor signs usually symmetric.

     3. Pupillary reactions usually preserved (except with certain drugs and toxins; see Pupil).

     4. Asterixis, myoclonus, tremor, and seizures are common.

     5. Acid-base disturbance with hypoventilation or hyperventilation is common.

  D. Psychogenic unresponsiveness.

     1. Lids tightly closed.

     2. Pupils reactive or dilated (factitious mydriatics).

     3. Oculocephalic responses highly variable; nystagmus and arousal occur with caloric stimuli.

     4. Motor tone normal or inconsistent.

     5. Breathing normal or rapid.

     6. Reflexes nonpathologic.

     7. Normal EEG.

III. Other states that may resemble coma.

  A. Vegetative state: Subacute or chronic condition after severe brain injury characterized by wakefulness, sleep-wake cycles, and eye opening to auditory stimuli, without evidence of consistent cognitive function or response to stimuli. Blood pressure and respirations are maintained. Vegetative state may follow coma and persist for years (a duration longer than 1 month is called persistent vegetative state). About one-third of patients eventually become more responsive (more common in traumatic than in hypoxic cases). May occur with forebrain, occipital, hippocampal, or diffuse cerebral or cerebellar destruction.

B. Akinetic mutism: Subacute or chronic condition characterized by seeming alertness, yet minimal vocalization or movement even with noxious stimuli. May occur with cingulate, limbic, corpus striatum, globus pallidus, thalamic, or reticular formation damage.

C. Locked-in syndrome: Intact consciousness plus quadraplegia and lower cranial nerve dysfunction. Voluntary vertical, and sometimes horizontal, eye movements are preserved. Usually occurs with ventral pontine infarcts, tumors, hemorrhages, or myelinolysis; ventral midbrain infarction; head injury; or severe neuromuscular disease. May be transient or chronic.

IV. Prognosis in coma, excluding traumatic and drug-related causes, is usually poor. Prediction is less reliable in cases of intoxications and trauma but more precise after cardiopulmonary arrest (see Cardiopulmonary Arrest). In general, the longer coma lasts, the lower the chance for regaining independent function (i.e., "good recovery").

A. Prediction: Data obtained from 500 patients, excluding known trauma or drug intoxication (Levy et al, 1985).

1. At 6 hours after onset of coma, absence of any of the following was associated with less than 5% chance of good recovery.
   a. Pupillary light reflex.
   b. Corneal reflexes.
   c. Oculocephalic reflexes.
   d. Vestibulo-ocular reflexes (calorics).

2. At 1 day after onset, none of the patients with absent corneal reflexes had satisfactory recovery.

3. At 3 days after onset, no patient with absence of any of the following had satisfactory recovery.
   a. Pupillary reflexes.
   b. Corneal reflexes.
   c. Motor function.

4. Predictors of good outcome are less reliable than negative predictors.
   a. At 6 hours after onset, with moaning or better verbal response *plus* pupillary, corneal *or* oculovestibular responses: 41% of patients had good recovery.
   b. At 1 day after onset, with inappropriate or better words *plus* any three of pupillary, corneal, oculovestibular, or motor responses: 67% had good recovery.
   c. At 3 days after onset, with inappropriate or better words *plus* corneal *and* motor responses: 74% had good recovery.
   d. At 7 days after onset, with eye opening to pain *plus* localizing motor response: 75% had good recovery.

B. Overall outcome (at one year).

1. 16% of patients were back to independent life.

2. 11% were severely disabled.
3. 12% were in a vegetative state.
4. 61% died without recovery.

REFERENCES

American Neurological Association committee on ethical affairs: *Ann Neurol* 33:386–390, 1993.
Levy D et al: *JAMA* 253:1420–1426, 1985.
Plum F, Posner JB: *The diagnosis of stupor and coma*, ed 3, Philadelphia, FA Davis, 1982.

COMPLEX REGIONAL PAIN SYNDROME (REFLEX SYMPATHETIC DYSTROPHY)

Reflex sympathetic dystrophy (RSD), or more recently complex regional pain syndrome (CRPS), has been defined as "a complex disorder or group of disorders that may develop as a consequence of trauma affecting the limbs, with or without an obvious nerve lesion…". It can be associated with visceral or central nervous system diseases or could have a *no-background event*. Currently, RSD is equivalent to CRPS type I, different from CRPS type II, which includes a definable nerve lesion.

Clinical manifestations may include the following:

1. Autonomic symptoms: Swelling (more on the dorsal side), sweating, skin changes (reddish, cyanotic, or marbled) and temperature changes (warmer or colder limb).
2. Sensory symptoms: Spontaneous pain (increases by lowering limb and improves by its elevation), worse at night, may be constant or intermittent. Skin hyper- or hypoalgesia may be present. Mechanical allodynia is rarely observed.
3. Trophic disturbances: Occurs later in the course including osteoporosis, glossy skin, nail and hair growth abnormalities, and stiff joints.
4. Motor symptoms: Active limb movement is impaired, muscular strength is reduced. Postural or action tremor is frequent in hands more than in feet.

Three stages of the RSD can be identified: Stage I (acute phase) includes pain, temperature changes, and hyperalgesia. Stage II (dystrophic phase) has worsening of stage I symptoms. Stage III (atrophic phase) usually includes irreversible tissue damage with thin skin, thickened fascia, muscle contracture, joint stiffness, diffuse osteoporosis, limb movement reduction, and allodynia.

Diagnosis is confirmed by comparative x-ray examination, MRI, three-phase bone scan (scintigraphy), measurement of cutaneous temperature (thermography and/or infrared thermometer; difference of 1°C between affected and unaffected limb is present in 75% to 98% of patients with

RSD), autonomic testing (resting sweating output test and Quantitative Sudomotor Reflex Test; QSART), phentolamine test, local clonidine application, and sympathetic blocks.

Treatment: Analgesics and NSAIDS are not very effective but may be tried as adjuvants. Sodium channels blockers may be effective, such as carbamazepine, phenytoin, and mexiletine. Gabapentin and some antidepressant medications (Venlafaxine, Amitryptyline, Buproprion) may also help.

Blockage of sympathetic activity is usually needed to treat CRPS. Different techniques are in use:

1. Postganglionic blocks with intravenous regional block using guanethidine: This is contraindicated in cases of arthritis, phlebitis, and cardiac or coronary insufficiency. Other agents that have been used are reserpine, lidocaine+steroids, bretylate, ketanserin, yohimbine, prazosin, phenoxybenzamine (efficacy more than 6 months) and buflomedil.
2. Ganglion blocks: Lumber sympathetic and stellate ganglion blocks are frequently used with lidocaine 0.5%. Duration is short and repeated blocks are necessary. Continuous infusion via a catheter has been used.
3. Preganglionic blocks: Epidural blocks (cervical or lumber) can be used after failure of postganglionic or ganglion blocks, using either local anesthetics or opioids or both.
4. Sympathectomy: A surgical ablation of the paravertebral sympathetic ganglion can be considered if the effect of the various blocks are transient.

Team approach and other supportive care is vital in managing this difficult syndrome including physical and occupational therapy as well as psychotherapy and biofeedback.

REFERENCE
Harden RN: *Clin J Pain* 16:S26–S32, 2000.

COMPUTED TOMOGRAPHY (CT)

Computed tomography (CT) combines conventional x-ray with a digitized, computerized reconstruction technique that yields multiple two-dimensional images of the body. Tissues are assigned absorption coefficients by the computer (CT or Hounsfield numbers) and are displayed as shades of gray (see Table 19). The range of CT numbers displayed can be manipulated to focus on certain structures (e.g., bony structures or intracranial contents) by "windowing." The *window width* (WW) determines the range of CT numbers displayed, and the *window level* (WL) determines the center of the window width. Large windows, for example, one with a WW of less than 400, are used for evaluating bone, whereas smaller windows, such as when WW 200, are used for evaluating brain tissue.

C

COMPUTED TOMOGRAPHY (CT)

TABLE 19

CT DENSITY

Moiety	Hounsfield Units
Bone	1000
Calcification	100
Acute blood	85
Tumor	30–60
Gray matter	35–40
White matter	25–30
CSF	0
Adipose	−100
Air	−1000

From Woodruff WW: *Fundamentals of neuroimaging*, Philadelphia, WB Saunders, 1993.

TABLE 20

CT FINDINGS IN STROKE

Duration	Infarct Without Contrast	With Contrast
Hyperacute (<1 day)	Normal or blurring of gray-white junction and/or effacement of gyri	No enhancement
Acute (1–7 days)	Vaguely defined hypodensity, best seen after 3–4 days; maximal edema and mass effect	No enhancement
Subacute enhancement (8–21 days)	Hypodensity less evident; decreased mass effect and edema	Gyral (peaks at week 3)
Chronic (>21 days)	Hypodensity sharply defined and isodense to CSF	Enhancement usually in 6–7 weeks

In evaluating stroke a negative initial CT should be repeated in 2 to 3 days, when edema (and hypodensity) is maximal, as appropriate.

Duration	Intraparenchymal Hemorrhage Appearance	Mass Effect
Acute	Homogeneous hyperdensity	Mass effect
Subacute		
Early (3 days to 3 weeks)	Enlarging hypodense periphery with hyperdense center	Mass effect
Late (3–5 weeks)	Hypodense periphery; isodense center	Mass effect
Chronic (>5 weeks)	Hypodense periphery; hypodense center	Mass effect resolves after several months

Ring enhancement is present from week 1 to week 7.

From Woodruff WW: *Fundamentals of neuroimaging*, Philadelphia, WB Saunders, 1993.

Iodinated IV contrast material enhances (brightens) many normal vascular structures (large vessels, choroid plexus, tentorium, and falx) as well as highly vascular pathologic structures (meningiomas, pituitary adenomas, chordomas, medulloblastomas, lymphomas, sarcomas, metastases, optic nerve gliomas, acoustic neuromas, and late infarcts) (see Table 20). "Ring" enhancement (white rim or dark core) is seen with abscess capsules, glioblastomas, metastases, dermoid cysts, and other lesions. Little or no enhancement is usually seen in normal brain tissue, oligodendrogliomas, astrocytomas, ependymomas, fresh infarcts, or edema. Variable degrees of enhancement may be seen in glioblastomas, craniopharyngiomas, basilar meningitis, encephalitis, and metastases.

CT is preferred to MRI for imaging *acute* hemorrhage. However, CT is generally less sensitive than MRI, especially in visualizing the posterior fossa and the temporal lobes, where bony artifact degrades CT images. CT combined with myelography is an alternative for spinal imaging, albeit with less resolution of neural structures than with MRI. CT also remains the imaging modality of choice for those unable to undergo MRI either due to metal devices (aneurysm clips, cochlear implants, pacemakers) or those too claustrophobic or agitated to obtain adequate MRI images.

REFEERENCE

Wooodruff WW: *Fundamentals of neuroimaging*, Philadelphia, WB Saunders, 1993.

CONFUSIONAL STATE

Acute confusional states are also known as delirium. It may affect between 20–70% of hospitalized patients depending on the definition. Clinical features are disturbance of attention with (1) disturbance of vigilance, (2) inability to maintain a stream of thought, and (3) inability to carry out goal-directed movements. Mild anomia, dysgraphia, dyscalculia, and constructional deficits may be seen. Perceptual distortions may lead to illusions and hallucinations. Tremor, myoclonus, or asterixis may accompany acute confusional states.

Metabolic disturbances, toxic exposure, drugs, infection (systemic and CNS), head trauma, and seizures are common causes of confusional states. Unilateral or bilateral damage to the fusiform and lingual gyri as well as lesions of the nondominant posterior parietal and inferior prefrontal regions may produce a confusional state.

CONGENITAL MALFORMATIONS OF THE BRAIN AND SPINE

I. Dorsal induction
   A. Primary neurulation: 3 to 4 weeks age of gestation (AOG); notochord, chordal mesoderm induce neural plate, neural plate closes forming neural tube, tube closes beginning at medulla, proceeds rostrally and caudally.

Defects at this stage may cause: craniorachischisis, myeloschisis (failure of closure of neural tube or vertebral arch); anencephaly (absent calvaria and brain; brainstem and cerebellum present); encephalocele (meninges and brain parenchyma protrude through skull defect); myelomeningocele (meninges and spinal cord protrude through defect in vertebral arch); Chiari malformation; hydromyelia (focal dilation of central spinal cord canal).

    B. Secondary neurulation: 4 to 5 weeks AOG; notochord, mesodermal interactions form dura, pia, vertebrae, skull.

Defects at this stage may cause: myelocystocele; diastomyelia (splitting of spinal cord by mesodermal band); meningocele/lipomeningocele; lipoma; dermal sinus with or without cyst; tethered cord/tight filum terminale; anterior dysraphic lesions (neurenteric cyst); caudal regression syndrome.

II. Ventral induction: 5 to 10 weeks AOG; prechordal mesoderm induces face, forebrain; cleavage of prosencephalon; formation of optic vesicles, olfactory bulbs/ tracts; telencephalon gives rise to cerebral hemispheres, ventricles, caudate, putamen; diencephalon gives rise to thalami, hypothalamus, and globus pallidus; rhombencephalon gives rise to cerebellar hemispheres, vermis; myelencephalon gives rise to medulla and pons.

Defects at this stage may cause: holoprosencephaly (failure of cleavage of embryonic forebrain into paired cerebral hemispheres→absent interhemispheric fissure, large single ventricle, and marked absence of cerebral parenchyma); septo-optic dysplasia (rudimentary septum pellucidum, hypoplasia of optic nerve, and chiasm); arhinencephaly; olfactory bulb, and tract aplasia; facial anomalies; cerebellar hypoplasias/dysplasias (Joubert syndrome, rhombencephalosynapsis; tectocerebellar dysplasia); Dandy-Walker malformation.

III. Neuronal proliferation, differentiation, histogenesis: 2 to 4 months AOG; germinal matrix forms at 7 weeks; cellular proliferation forms neuroblasts, fibroblasts, astrocytes, endothelial cells; choroid plexus is formed; CSF production begins.

Defects at this stage may cause: microcephaly, megalencephaly, aqueductal stenosis, arachnoid cysts, congenital vascular malformations.

IV. Cellular migration: 2 to 5 months AOG; neuroblast migrate from germinal matrix along radial glial fibers; cortical layers form from deep to superficial; gyri, sulci form; commissural plates form corpus callosum, hippocampal commissure.

Defects at this stage may cause: schizencephaly (lateral clefts through cerebral hemispheres extending from cortex to ventricles); lissencephaly (absence of gyri); pachygyria (abnormally wide and thick gyri); micro/polymicrogyria (small gyri with increased number and abnormal lamination); heterotropias (ectopic collections of gray matter); Lhermitte-Duclos sign; callosal agenesis.

V. Neuronal organization: 6 months postnatal; neuronal alignment, orientation, layering; dendrites proliferate; synapses form.

VI. Myelination, maturation: 6 months—adulthood; oligodendrocytes produce myelin; peak myelin formation from 30 weeks gestation to 8 months postnatal; corpus callosum develops further; attains adult configuration at birth.

Defects at this stage may be due to: metabolic and demyelinating disorders.

VII. Acquired degenerative, toxic, inflammatory lesions: any stage; secondarily acquired injury to otherwise normally formed structures

Defects at this stage may cause: hydranencephaly (remnant cerebral hemisphere is paper-thin membrane sac composed of glial tissue filled with CSF covered with leptomeninges); hemiatrophy; multicystic encephalomalacia; periventricular leukomalacia.

ARNOLD-CHIARI MALFORMATIONS

Type 1: Cerebellar tonsils herniated below foramen magnum; associated with syringomyelia and bony deformities; symptoms develop during adolescence or adulthood.

Type 2: Cerebellar vermis, fourth ventricle, and medulla are displaced inferiorly and deformed; associated with spina bifida and lumbar meningomyelocele, polymicrogyria, heterotropias, syringomyelia, hydromyelia, enlargement of the foramen magnum, elongation of the cervical arches, platybasia, basilar invagination, assimilation of the atlas, and Klippel-Feil anomaly; symptoms begin in infancy or early childhood, most commonly presenting as hydrocephalus.

Type 3: Includes cervical spina bifida, cerebellar herniation through the defect, and a dystrophic posterior fossa; rarely compatible with postnatal life.

Type 4: Cerebellar hypoplasia; may be related to or the equivalent of the Dandy-Walker malformation, incomplete vermian fusion, and enlarged fourth ventricle

REFERENCE

Bradley WG, Daroff RB, Fenichel GM, Marsden CD. *Neurology in clinical practice*, ed 3, Boston, Butterworth-Heinemann, 2000.
Osborn AG: *Diagnostic neuroradiology*, St. Louis, Mosby, 1994.

CRAMPS

Cramps are painful muscle spasms. When pathologic, they may represent abnormalities of muscle, nerve, or CNS. Although the following disorders do not have true cramps, patients with myotonia, neuromyotonia, tetany, tetanus, and stiff-person syndrome often complain of "cramps"; therefore they are included in the differential diagnosis.

I. Myopathic disorders
   A. The painful muscle spasms associated with glycogenoses (most commonly phosphorylase or phosphofructokinase deficiency), disorders of lipid metabolism, and carnitine palmityltransferase (CPT) deficiency are designated *contractures*, and there is severe, intermittent, sharp

muscle pain with palpable shortening and hardening of the affected muscles. Contractures may be precipitated by exercise (glycogenoses and CPT deficiency) or fasting (CPT deficiency); they are associated with increased weakness and are unaffected by curare or nerve block. The EMG is electrically silent during contractures. Treatment includes a high-carbohydrate diet for phosphorylase deficiency and a high-carbohydrate, low-fat diet for CPT deficiency.

B. The "cramps" associated with myotonic disorders are painless (see Myotonia).

II. Disorders of peripheral nerves

A. *Tetany* results from hypocalcemia and alkalosis. Hypomagnesemia and hyperkalemia may cause carpopedal spasm. Severe tonic spasms are painful only during prolonged attacks. They may be provoked by hyperventilation or limb ischemia causing a lowered depolarization threshold of motor nerve fibers. EMG reveals asynchronous, grouped motor unit potentials discharging at a rate of 5 to 15 per second and separated by periods of electrical silence. Treatment is the correction of the underlying cause.

B. *Neuromyotonia* (generalized myokymia, continuous muscle fiber activity, and Isaac's syndrome) manifests as muscle stiffness. In severe cases stiffness is present at rest and impedes movement. Neuromyotonia occurs at any age and is usually sporadic. The defect is in the distal portion of the nerve, and the motor activity is not altered by spinal or proximal nerve block. The EMG shows short bursts of motor unit activity at 10 to 100 Hz. Treatment is with phenytoin, carbamazepine, or dantrolene.

C. *Motor neuron disease* and *muscle denervation* of any cause may be associated with cramps.

III. Central disorders

A. *Stiff-person syndrome* is characterized by the adult onset of rigid, uncontrolled proximal and axial muscle contractions that are present only during wakefulness. Proximal muscle contractions are usually greater than distal contractions. The cramps are extremely painful and may be precipitated by movement, noise, or other sensory stimuli; they are blocked by curare, general anesthesia, and nerve block. The EMG shows continuous activity in agonist and antagonist muscles with normal motor unit morphology. Treatment is with diazepam, clonazepam or other muscle relaxants. Stiff-person syndrome is now felt to be an autoimmune disorder with antibodies to glutamate decarboxylase in serum and CSF.

B. *Tetanus* is characterized by acute, rapidly progressive, generalized, continuous tonic contractures with superimposed painful spasms caused by loss of inhibitory postsynaptic potentials in the spinal cord. Tonic spasms of the masticatory muscles (trismus or lockjaw) are common. The spasms may be stopped with curare and during sleep. EMG is similar to that in stiff-person syndrome. Treatment

includes ventilatory support, tetanus antitoxin, diazepam, chlorpromazine, phenobarbital, or curare.

IV. Physiologic cramps

Painful muscle cramps may occur in normal individuals, usually at rest or
after extreme exercise. EMG shows a high-voltage, high-frequency burst of
motor unit potentials. Passive stretching of the muscle usually stops the cramp.
Occasionally quinine, phenytoin, carbamazepine, or diazepam is helpful.

REFERENCES

Darnell RB et al: *Neurology* 43:114–121, 1993.
Layzer RB, Rowland LP: *N Engl J Med* 285:31–40, 1971.

CRANIAL NERVES

Nerve	CNS Nucleus	Function/Innervation
I	Olfactory bulb	Smell
II	Lateral geniculate nucleus	Vision
III	Oculomotor nucleus	Extraocular muscles except superior oblique and lateral rectus
	Edinger-Westphal nucleus	Sphincter pupillae and ciliary muscle
IV	Trochlear nucleus	Superior oblique muscle
V	Spinal and main sensory nucleus	Sensory from face, deep tissues of head and neck, dura mater, and tympanic membrane
	Mesencephalic nucleus	Muscle spindles; mechanoreceptors of face and mouth
	Trigeminal motor nucleus	Muscles of mastication and tensor tympani
VI	Abducens nucleus	Lateral rectus muscle
VII	Facial motor nucleus	Muscles of facial expression and stapedius
	Spinal trigeminal nucleus	Sensory from external ear and tympanic membrane
	Solitary nucleus	Taste from anterior two-thirds of tongue
	Superior salivatory nucleus	Salivary and lacrimal glands
VIII	Cochlear and vestibular nuclei	Balance and hearing
IX	Nucleus ambiguous	Muscles of pharynx
	Spinal trigeminal nucleus	Sensory from external ear, tympanic membrane, and posterior one-third tongue
	Solitary nucleus	Taste from posterior one-third of tongue
	Solitary and spinal trigeminal	Carotid body and sinus; sensation from nasal nuclei and oral pharynx
	Inferior salivatory nucleus	Parotid gland
X	Nucleus ambiguous	Muscles of larynx and pharynx
	Spinal trigeminal nucleus	Sensory from external ear
	Solitary nucleus	Taste buds of epiglottis
	Solitary and spinal trigeminal	Parasympathetics from thoracic and abdominal viscera; sensory from larynx and pharynx

Table continued on following page

C

CRANIAL NERVES

Nerve	CNS Nucleus	Function/Innervation
	Dorsal motor nucleus	Parasympathetics to thoracic and abdominal viscera
XI	Nucleus ambiguous	Muscles of larynx and pharynx
	Accessory nucleus	Sternocleidomastoid and trapezius
XII	Hypoglossal nucleus	Intrinsic tongue muscles

REFERENCE

Kandel ER et al: *Principles of neural science*, New York, The McGraw-Hill Companies, 2000.

CRANIOCERVICAL JUNCTION

Dysfunction resulting from lesions at the foramen magnum or craniocervical junction is usually produced by compression or shearing. Signs and symptoms are usually chronic, since acute lesions usually become evident with respiratory arrest, and may include various combinations of the following: spastic quadriparesis; cranial nerve palsies such as dysphagia, dysarthria, absent gag, hearing loss, vocal cord paralysis, nystagmus (downbeat and periodic alternating), vertigo, facial weakness or diplopia; hydrocephalus; head and neck pain; extremity weakness or paresthesias; facial pain; drop attacks; syringomyelia; ataxia; papilledema; dorsal column signs; and recurrent apnea or stridor. Some individuals with abnormalities of the craniocervical junction may be asymptomatic.

CRANIOSYNOSTOSIS

Premature closure of suture(s) while the brain is still growing, resulting in abnormal skull shape:

1. Sagittal: scaphocephaly; 60%; may be familial, boys more than girls; neurologically normal.
2. Coronal: brachycephaly; 20%; girls more than boys; if untreated, may have neurologic abnormalities; affected in Apert's and Crouzon's disease.
3. Single coronal or lambdoidal: plagiocephaly.
4. Metopic: trigonocephaly; +/- mental retardation.
5. Multiple: oxycephaly (pointed head); correction should be undertaken at age 1 to 2 months to prevent neurologic damage from increased ICP; seen in Carpenter syndrome.

Most cases are sporadic and of uncertain etiology. It may be one feature of a larger syndrome of genetic or chromosomal abnormality. Craniosynostosis may be seen in association with metabolic disorders (rickets, mucopolysaccharidoses, hyperthyroidism, hypercalcemia, hypophosphatemia) or hematologic disorders (sickle cell, thalassemia, polycythemia vera). Presentation depends on the underlying cause, but most cases are associated with hydrocephalus. Evaluation includes palpation of the calvarial bones (palpable ridging) and skull x-rays (band of increased density at site of prematurely closed suture) and CT or MRI. Management depends on the underlying etiology; some cases may require surgery or ventriculoperitoneal shunting.

REFERENCE

Fenichel GM: *Clinical pediatric neurology: a signs and symptoms approach*, Philadelphia, WB Saunders, 1997.

DEGENERATIVE DISEASES OF CHILDHOOD

I. Diseases that predominantly affect white matter (present with long tract signs [spasticity and hyperreflexia], optic atrophy, cortical blindness and/or deafness)
   A. Metachromatic leukodystrophy: Autosomal recessive (AR); arylsulfatase deficiency; metachromatic granules; onset 2 to 5 years; with peripheral neuropathy; MRI—arcuate fibers spared.
   B. Krabbe's disease: AR; beta-galactosidase deficiency; globoid cells; onset 4 to 6 months; optic atrophy, hyperacusis; with peripheral neuropathy; MRI—arcuate fibers spared and parieto-occipital lobes involved early, high-density basal ganglia.
   C. Adrenoleukodystrophy: X-linked recessive; acyl-Co-A synthetase deficiency and long-chain fatty acids accumulate; single peroxisomal enzyme deficiency; childhood ALD—neurologic symptoms before adrenal insufficiency; adrenoleukomyeloneuropathy—spinal cord and nerves involved, onset in 20 to 30s, paraparesis and adrenal dysfunction almost at the same time; MRI—occipital lobes and corpus callosum splenium affected, marked contrast enhancement. Pathologically three zones are identified: innermost zone with necrosis, intermediate zone of active demyelination and inflammatory changes, and peripheral zone of demyelination without inflammation.
   D. Pelizaeus-Merzbacher disease: X-linked recessive; deficient proteolipid protein expression; newborn—hypotonia, tongue fasciculations; childhood onset—dementia and choreoathetosis; MRI—perivascular white matter spared producing a "tigroid pattern,"; involves arcuate fibers.
   E. Alexander disease: Sporadic; Rosenthal fibers; macrocephaly; MRI—frontal lobe hyperintensities, (+) contrast enhancement.
   F. Canavan disease: AR; N-acetyl-aspartylase deficiency; widespread vacuolation macrocephaly; MRI—near or total lack of myelin, involves arcuate fibers.

DEGENERATIVE DISEASES OF CHILDHOOD

G. Cockayne's syndrome: AR; defective DNA repair; large ears, sunken eyes; onset 2 years; retinitis pigmentosa progeria; MRI—demyelination, perivascular calcification in basal ganglia and cerebellum.

H. Chediak-Higashi syndrome: Neutrophil dysfunction leading to defective bacterial killing; intracytoplasmic inclusions in neutrophils and neurons, most prominent in pons and cerebellum; albinism, nystagmus, hepato-splenomegaly; mental retardation, cerebellar, and long-tract signs, cranial and peripheral neuropathy.

I. Neuroaxonal dystrophy: Neuroaxonal spheroids along axons, especially neuromuscular junction; onset 2 years, upper and lower motor neuron signs

J. Phenylketonuria: AR, phenylalanine hydroxylase deficiency. MRI—arcuate fibers spared, optic radiations affected the most. Treatment with low phenylalanine diet, mental retardation results if not treated early.

II. Diseases that predominantly affect gray matter (present with myoclonus, seizures, and cognitive impairment)

A. Lipidoses

1. Tay-Sachs disease (GM2 gangliosidosis): AR; hexosaminidase A deficiency; onset 3 to 6 months, excessive startle, macrocephaly, retinal cherry-red spot; MRI—hyperintense signal in caudate, thalamus, and putamen on T2-weighted images.

2. Gaucher's disease: AR; glucocerebrosidase deficiency; type III—early to mid-childhood, seizures, dementia, subacute neuronopathy; hepatosplenomegaly.

3. Niemann-Pick's disease: AR; sphingomyelinase deficiency; type A—infantile, hypotonia, pulmonary interstitial disease, organomegaly, retinal cherry-red spot. Type B—neurologically normal. Type C—more than 1 to 2 years of age, presents with spasticity, seizure, vertical gaze paresis, and ataxia.

B. Neuronal lipofuscinosis: "Fingerprint" inclusions of lipofuscin within cytosomes on electron microscopy of leukocytes. Presents with dementia, vision loss, ataxia, myoclonus, seizures; infantile, late infantile (photoconvulsive response at 3 Hz on EEG), juvenile (Batten disease), adult (Kufs disease).

C. Mucopolysaccharidoses

1. Hurler syndrome: AR; Alpha-L-Iduronidase deficiency; mucopolysaccharides accumulate in neurons (meganeurites) and in histiocytes (gargoyle cells) in perivascular spaces; Gargoyle-like facies, dwarfism, kyphosis, hepatosplenomegaly, severe psychomotor deterioration, death between 5 and 10 years; MRI—macrocrania, thick dura, perivascular "pits"; concave or "hooked" thoracolumbar vertebrae.

2. Hunter: X-linked recessive; iduronate-2-sulfatase deficiency; thick dura, perivascular "pits."

3. Sanfilippo: AR; heparan-N-sulfatase deficiency; normal until age 2 to 8 years then progressive dementia, hyperactive, aggressive, spastic and movement disorder. Death in second to third decade of life.

III. Diseases that primarily affect gray and white matter

A. Leigh's disease (subacute necrotizing encephalopathy): Mitochondrial; spongiosis, demyelination, astrogliosis and capillary proliferation in basal ganglia, brainstem and spinal cord; Infantile—onset at 2 years of hypotonia, vomiting and seizures; childhood; adult—fifth to sixth decade; MRI—hyperintense foci in globus pallidus, putamen, and caudate.

B. Myoclonic epilepsy with ragged-red fibers (MERRF): Mitochondrial; muscle biopsy—ragged red fibers; myoclonic epilepsy, myopathy, progressive external ophthalmoplegia, multiple infarcts in cortex and white matter.

C. Mitochondrial encephalomyopathy with lactic acidosis and stroke (MELAS): Mitochondrial; myopathy, encephalopathy, lactic acidosis, strokelike episodes, large and multifocal infarcts mainly in occipital lobes.

D. Kearns-Sayre syndrome: Mitochondrial; elevated pyruvate; progressive external ophthalmoplegia, cerebellar ataxia, heart block, and pigmentary retinopathy. Treatment is supportive with pacemaker and coenzyme q10; prognosis is poor and patients rarely survive past the second decade.

E. Alper's disease: Etiology is uncertain, hypoxic injury versus AR inheritance. Onset before 6 years; myoclonic seizures appear early, then mental retardation and spasticity or opisthotonus.

F. Menke's disease: XLR; defective transmembrane copper transport; seizures, hypotonia develops into spastic quadriparesis; light-colored and brittle hair, hyperextensible joints, skeletal anomalies; susceptible to sepsis, heat-intolerant.

G. Zellweger syndrome: AR; multiple peroxisomal enzymes; MRI—heterotropia, patchy/polymicrogyria.

IV. Diseases that predominantly affect basal ganglia (present with movement disorders)

A. Huntington's disease: AD; CAG repeat; chorea and personality changes; atrophy of caudate and enlarged frontal horns of lateral ventricle.

B. Hallervorden-Spatz: Iron deposits in globus pallidus (GP) and substantia nigra (SN); mental retardation, stiff gait, equinovarus; low signals in GP and SN on T2-weighted images MRI, low signal surrounds region of high signal "eye of tiger" sign.

C. Fahr disease: AR; first 2 years mental retardation and movement disorder; MRI—prominent calcification in dentate nuclei, centrum semiovale, and subcortical white matter.

D. Wilson disease: Chromosome 13, AR; P-type ATPase deficiency, with decrease in ceruloplasmin and serum copper. Copper deposits in liver and basal ganglia; onset 8 to 16 years. Parkinsonism, seizures, ataxia, dementia, hemolytic anemia, liver dysfunction. Treatment is Penicillamine and zinc.

E. Dystonia musculorum deformans (See Dystonia).

F. Aminoacidurias.

   1. Glutaric aciduria I: AR; glutaryl-CoA dehydrogenase (lysine to tryptophan); dystonia and dyskinesia; MRI—high-signal changes in basal ganglia and caudate; affects mitochondrial activity and preferentially involves basal ganglia leading to "bat wing" dilatation of sylvian fissures.

   2. Methylmalonic academia: AR; secondary to blockage of conversion of methyl malonic acid (MMA) to succinyl-CoA leading to MMA accumulation. Hyperammonemia and ketoacidosis. MRI—hyperdensities in globus pallidus.

REFERENCES

Bradley WG, Daroff RG, Fenichel GM, Marsden CD: *Neurology in clinical practice*, ed 3, Boston, Butterworth-Heinemann, 2000.

Menkes JH: *Textbook of child neurology*, Philadelphia, Lea and Febiger, 1990.

Osborn AG: *Diagnostic neuroradiology*, St. Louis, Mosby, 1994.

DEMENTIA

Dementia is a clinical syndrome characterized by loss of function in multiple cognitive and emotional abilities in an individual with previously normal intellectual level and occurring in clear consciousness (i.e., in the absence of delirium). *DSM IV-R diagnostic criteria* require memory impairment and abnormalities in at least one of these areas: language, judgment, abstract thinking, praxis, constructional abilities, or visual recognition. This deficit must be sufficient to interfere with activities of daily living, work duties, or other social activities. The term "dementia" does not imply a specific underlying cause, a progressive course, or irreversibility. The definition also excludes patients with isolated deficits such as aphasia or apraxia, or if symptoms occur during delirium.

Prevalence is about 1% percent at age 60 years and doubles every 5 years, to reach 30% to 50% by the age of 85.

Examination for suspected dementia should include assessment of multiple areas of cognitive performance, including memory, language, perception, praxis, attention, judgment, calculation, and visuospatial functions. The presence of psychiatric features (affective disorder, hallucinations, delusions, and anxiety) must also be sought. Questions about the patient's activities and self-care capabilities should be obtained from collateral sources of information (caregiver). Acquiring family history is essential. Short, standardized mental status tests such as Mini-Mental Status Examination and the Short Blessed Dementia Scale are widely used. Mild cognitive deficits may require more extensive neuropsychologic testing.

Laboratory evaluation should include electrolyte and screening metabolic panel, complete blood cell count, thyroid function tests, syphilis serology, and vitamin B_{12}. CT or MRI scan of the brain are used to rule out structural lesions. Other tests (EEG, lumbar puncture, HIV titer, serologic testing for vasculitis, heavy metal screening, angiography, brain biopsy, and formal psychiatric assessment) are indicated only if suggested by the history or examination. In younger adults dementia may be caused by late onset childhood metabolic diseases, and special studies may be required.

Conditions causing dementia can be divided into the following groups: degenerative disorders (Alzheimer's disease [AD], Pick's disease, Huntington's disease, Parkinson's disease, and diffuse Lewy body disease); degenerative disease with specific tau mutation (familial frontotemporal dementia and parkinsonism, progressive supranuclear palsy, familial progressive subcortical gliosis, corticobasal ganglionic degeneration, familial multiple system tauopathy with presenile dementia); metabolic and deficiency disorders (hypothyroidism, hepatic encephalopathy, Cushing syndrome, porphyria, Wilson's disease, and vitamin B_{12} deficiency); cerebrovascular disease, and infections (syphilis, viral and postviral encephalitic syndromes, chronic meningitis, progressive multifocal encephalopathy, HIV infection, and Creutzfeldt-Jakob disease); systemic disorders (lupus erythematosus, sarcoidosis, and Sjögren's syndrome); toxins and drugs (heavy metals, carbon monoxide, and anticholinergic, psychoactive, and other medications); head trauma; brain tumors; psychiatric disorders (depression); multiple sclerosis; and normal-pressure hydrocephalus.

The most common cause of dementia in adults is AD (50% to 60%), followed by vascular dementias (20%); in another 15% to 20% of patients, vascular dementias coexist with AD. Potentially treatable causes account for about 10% of cases.

ALZHEIMER'S DISEASE

Alzheimer's disease (AD) is the most common cause of dementia. Incidence is 1% per year for individuals over 65 years of age, and prevalence in people 85 years of age and older is about 50%.

Risk factors: Increased age and family history are the most important risk factors for AD. Less well-defined risks include smoking, stroke, female gender, head trauma, endocrine dysfunction, and low educational level. Lower risk have been suggested in those taking nonsteroidal anti-inflammatory drugs (NSAIDs) and postmenopausal women on estrogen replacement therapy.

Genetic risk: These chromosomes have been linked to AD—early-onset: 21q21, 14q24.3, and 1q; early and late-onset: 1q and 19q13.2. Apolipoprotein E4 (see Table 21) is associated with both early and late-onset familial AD. Some families have autosomal dominant inheritance. All individuals with Down's syndrome develop pathological evidence of AD if they live past 35 years of age.

TABLE 21

GENETIC FACTORS LINKED TO ALZHEIMER'S DISEASE RISK

Genetic Factor	Chromosome Involved	Age at Onset (yr)
Down's syndrome	21	>35
Amyloid precursor protein mutation	21	45–66
Presenilin 1 mutation	14	28–62
Presenilin 2 mutation	1	40–85
Apolipoprotein E ε4 allele	19	>60

From Martin JB: *N Engl J Med* 340(25):1970–1980, 1999.

Pathological hallmarks of AD are neurofibrillary tangles, neuritic plaques with amyloid deposition, amyloid angiopathy, and neuronal loss. Secondary association cortex is most heavily involved. The most widespread neurochemical change is a 50% to 90% decline in choline acetyltransferase activity.

Clinical features of AD are variable but include *cognitive decline* due to recent memory loss. The ability to focus attention and recall remote events may initially be subtle and worsens with time and is usually associated with progressive disorientation to time and place. *Language decline* (particularly finding words in spontaneous speech), anomia (especially for parts of objects), and other types of language difficulties appear. *The ability to perform activities of daily living (ADLs)* may be impaired by visuospatial dysfunction, apraxia, or other motor dysfunction such as rigidity or gait disorder. *Behavioral symptoms* are common and include depression and anxiety, personality changes, delusions, and hallucinations but can occur in later stages of otherwise typical AD. *Other features* such as extrapyramidal signs (rigidity and tremor) may indicate atypical dementia, such as "Lewy body variant," and myoclonus and seizures may indicate Creutzfeldt-Jakob disease.

Diagnosis of Alzheimer's disease is by the typical clinical features and exclusion of other causes of dementia. Definite AD can be diagnosed by autopsy. When strict diagnostic criteria (see Table 22) are followed, accuracy of antemortem diagnosis of AD reaches 80% to 90%.

Differential diagnosis: Pick's disease, which is characterized by early disinhibited behavior and frontal lobe dysfunction. CT or MRI may show asymmetric frontal or temporal lobe atrophy. Rapidly progressive dementia with myoclonus must be differentiated from Creutzfeldt-Jakob disease. Vascular dementia, the second most common cause of dementia, can be distinguished based on evidence of strokes on neuroimaging. Key clinical differentiating factors include abrupt onset, stepwise deterioration, focal neurologic signs and symptoms, and risk factors for stroke.

Treatment: Donepezil (Aricept) is a reversible selective anticholinesterase inhibitor with minimal peripheral side effects. It is indicated in mild-moderate dementia. Dosage is 5 mg daily, which may be increased to 10 mg after 4 to 6 weeks. The most frequent adverse effects are nausea, diarrhea, vomiting, and insomnia. Rivastigmine (Exelon) is a pseudo-irreversible cholinesterase

TABLE 22

CRITERIA FOR CLINICAL DIAGNOSIS OF ALZHEIMER'S DISEASE (NINCDS–ADRDA)

I. Criteria for *probable* Alzheimer's disease include:
   A. Dementia established by clinical examination and documented by Mini-Mental Test, Blessed Dementia Scale, or some similar examination and confirmed by neuropsychological test.
   B. Deficit in two or more areas of cognition.
   C. Progressive worsening of memory and other cognitive functions.
   D. No disturbance of consciousness.
   E. Onset between ages 40 and 90, most often after age 65.
   F. Absence of systemic disorders or other brain diseases that in and of themselves could account for the progressive deficits in memory and cognition.

II. The diagnosis of *probable* Alzheimer's is supported by:
   A. Progressive deterioration of specific cognitive functions such as language (aphasia), motor skill (apraxia), and perception (agnosia).
   B. Impaired activities of daily living and altered patterns of behavior.
   C. Family history of similar disorders, particularly if confirmed neuropathologically.
   D. Laboratory results of:
      1. Normal lumbar puncture as evaluated by standard techniques.
      2. Normal pattern or nonspecific changes in EEG, such as increased slow wave activity.
      3. Evidence of cerebral atrophy on CT with progression documented by serial observation.

III. Other clinical features consistent with the diagnosis of *probable* Alzheimer's disease, after exclusion of causes of dementia other than Alzheimer's disease, include:
   A. Plateaus in the course of progression of the illness.
   B. Associated symptoms of depression, insomnia, incontinence, delusions, illusions, hallucinations, catastrophic verbal, emotional, or physical outbursts, sexual disorders, and weight loss.
   C. Other neurologic abnormalities in some patients, especially with more advanced disease and including motor signs such as increased muscle tone, myoclonus, or gait disorder.
   D. Seizures in advanced disease.
   E. CT normal for age.

IV. Features that make the diagnosis of *probable* Alzheimer's disease uncertain or unlikely include:
   A. Sudden, apoplectic onset.
   B. Focal neurologic findings such as hemiparesis, sensory loss, visual field deficits, and incoordination early in the course of the illness.
   C. Seizures or gait disturbances at the onset or very early in the course of the illness.

V. Clinical diagnosis of *possible* Alzheimer's disease:
   A. May be made on the basis of the dementia syndrome in the absence of other neurologic, psychiatric, or systemic disorders sufficient to cause dementia, and in the presence of variations in the onset, in the presentation, or in the clinical course.
   B. May be made in the presence of a second systemic or brain disorder sufficient to produce dementia, which is not considered to be the cause of the dementia.
   C. Should be used in research studies when a single, gradually progressive severe cognitive deficit is identified in the absence of other identifiable cause.

Table continued on following page

TABLE 22 —cont'd

CRITERIA FOR CLINICAL DIAGNOSIS OF ALZHEIMER'S DISEASE (NINCDS–ADRDA)

VI. Criteria for diagnosis of *Definite* Alzheimer's disease are:
    A. The clinical criteria for *probable* Alzheimer's disease and histopathologic
       evidence obtained from a biopsy or an autopsy.
VII. Classification of Alzheimer's disease for research purposes should specify features
    that may differentiate subtypes of the disorder, such as:
    A. Familial occurrence.
    B. Onset before age 65.
    C. Presence of trisomy-21.
    D. Coexistence of other relevant conditions such as Parkinson's disease.

From McKhann G et al: *Neurology* 34:939, 1984.

---

inhibitor. Dosage is 1.5 to 6 mg BID and side effects are similar to donepezil if titrated slowly. Galanthamine (Reminyl) is started at 4 mg BID and can be increased slowly to 12 mg BID. Efficacy and side effects are similar to these other medications. Tetrahydroaminoacridine (Tacrine) is a reversible nonacetyl-cholinesterase inhibitor. It is rarely used due to the need for frequent dosing and hepatotoxicity.

    Behavioral symptoms are disruptive and require careful investigation. Treatment for any underlying medical condition (e.g., urinary tract infection) and thorough review of the medication list should be sought before starting any psychoactive drugs. Depression can be treated with tricyclic antidepressant agents (e.g., imipramine, amitriptyline) or selective serotonin-reuptake inhibitors (e.g., fluoxetine, sertraline). Neuroleptics can be used to treat psychosis and delusions. Oxazepam is useful for episodic anxiety, but benzodiazepines are sometimes associated with paradoxical effect. Chloral hydrate is useful for insomnia. Counseling and social planning in the face of increasing disability is an important facet of long-term management.

VASCULAR DEMENTIA

Diagnostic criteria for vascular dementias include dementia with evidence of cerebrovascular disease demonstrated by history, clinical examination, or brain imaging; the two conditions must be temporally related, with onset of dementia within 3 months after a recognized vascular event. Vascular dementias can be divided into several types. Multi-infarct dementia (MID) is caused by multiple infarcts, which may affect both cortical and subcortical areas. The modified *Hachinski scale* (see Table 23) may help to differentiate multi-infarct dementia from Alzheimer's disease. Small vessel disease with dementia includes bilateral lacunae in the white matter; *Binswanger's disease* (subacute arteriolar encephalopathy) is one subtype of small vessel disease. Dementia can also be caused by a strategically localized infarction involving an area concerned with cognition (e.g., angular and fusiform gyrus syndrome). Hypoperfusion resulting from cardiac arrest can cause global cognitive decline. CADASIL (cerebral autosomal dominant arteriopathy with subcortical infarcts and leukoencephalopathy) is an autosomal dominant

TABLE 23

CLINICAL FEATURES OF THE ISCHEMIC SCORE (MODIFIED HACHINSKI SCALE)*

Feature	Point Value
Abrupt onset	2
Stepwise deterioration	1
Fluctuating course	2
Nocturnal confusion	1
Relative preservation of personality	1
Depression	1
Somatic complaints	1
Emotional incontinence	1
History of presence of hypertension	1
History of strokes	2
Evidence of associated atherosclerosis	1
Focal neurologic symptoms	2
Focal neurologic signs	2

Adapted from Rosen WG et al: *Ann Neurol* 7:486–488, 1980
*Score ≤ 4 suggests primary degenerative dementia; score >7 suggests vascular dementia.

form of vascular dementia localized to chromosome 19 with onset between the third and fourth decade. Treatment of vascular dementia is directed at prevention of further vascular events.

DIFFUSE LEWY BODY DEMENTIA (DLBD)

DLBD is the second most commonly encountered type of degenerative dementia after AD. Age of onset is 50 to 70 years. Clinical diagnosis is often suspected in patients with *parkinsonism and dementia, particularly those with visual hallucinations or excess sensitivity to the extrapyramidal effects of neuroleptics*. The disease course typically shows considerable fluctuation, prominent depression, visual hallucinations, and delusions during the initial stages. Definitive diagnosis is by autopsy. Cortical Lewy bodies contain α-synuclein, a presynaptic protein of unknown function. Mutations of this gene are associated with familial forms of Parkinson's disease.

FRONTOTEMPORAL DEMENTIA (FTD)

FTD is dementia characterized by selective loss and atrophy of neurons in the frontal and temporal lobes. It includes:

1. Classic Pick's disease, the third most common degenerative dementia after AD and DLBD. Both sexes are affected; onset is 40 to 80 years. There is marked personality deterioration with antisocial behaviors. Visuospatial skills are remarkably preserved until late in the disease. Ballooned neurons and Pick's bodies are classic pathological findings.
2. Pick's disease with extrapyramidal signs, which includes corticobasal degeneration (CBD) and frontotemporal dementia with parkinsonism. The latter is mostly sporadic, but a subgroup of this is familial caused

by mutation of the chromosome 17 "tau gene" and is also known as a "*tauopathy*." Initially, behavioral abnormalities appear without memory loss, followed by progressive dementia and later on, parkinsonism.
3. Progressive nonfluent aphasia is characterized by effortful speech production and phonologic and grammatical errors in the absence of decline of other aspects of cognition. Difficulties in reading and writing may also occur, but comprehension is relatively preserved.
4. Semantic dementia is characterized by loss of semantic memory with severe naming and word comprehension impairment in the context of fluent, effortless speech output.

PRION DISEASES

Prions are protease-resistant proteinaceous infectious agents causing several transmissible and fatal neurodegenerative diseases in mammals. These proteins are conformational variants of the prion protein, a physiologic sialoglycoprotein, a copper-binding protein of the cell surface. It is unknown how these agents undergo the conformational changes to a self-replicable infectious isoform of the prion protein and subsequently cause neuronal cell death. None of these agents evoke immune response. Human diseases caused by prions include the following:

1. *Creutzfeldt-Jakob disease (CJD)*. Sporadic CJD occurs worldwide with an incidence of 0.5 to 1.5 per million population per year. Men and women are equally affected and onset of disease is between 50 and 70 years of age. There is no evidence of geographical or seasonal clustering. Familial forms (15% to 20% of CJD cases) affect younger patients and have autosomal dominant transmission (short arm of chromosome 20). Infectious transmission was reported after intracranial transplantation and depth EEG electrode, inoculation, corneal grafting, and cadaver-derived human growth hormone. Initially, CJD presents with fatigue, disordered sleep, cognitive decline, confusion, ataxia, aphasia, visual loss, hemiparesis, or amyotrophy. Signs of cerebellar, pyramidal, and extrapyramidal involvement develop in most patients.

    Diagnosis is suggested by rapid course of progression and development of myoclonic jerks, particularly startle myoclonus in response to acoustic or tactile stimulus. EEG findings may be normal in the early stages. Later in the course, periodic biphasic or triphasic (classically 1 Hz activity) synchronous complexes over a slow background rhythm may develop. Periodic complexes carry sensitivity of 67% and specificity of 86%, and they are less likely to be present in the familial cases. Cerebrospinal fluid examination is usually normal or may show mildly elevated protein. Immunoassay for 14-3-3 protein in the CSF has a sensitivity of 96% and specificity of 99% (false-positive in stroke and meningoencephalitis). Diagnosis is based on pathological findings of spongiform changes, neuronal loss, and gliosis. There is no therapy and the mean survival time is 5 months, with 80% dying within 1 year.

2. *Atypical CJD* with prominent amyotrophic or ataxic features and longer duration or absence of typical EEG changes can cause diagnostic uncertainty. Differential diagnosis includes amyotrophic lateral sclerosis, multiple sclerosis, or paraneoplastic cerebellar degeneration. Rapid progressive dementia with myoclonus should be differentiated from other degenerative disease such as Alzheimer's disease with myoclonus, infectious diseases such as HIV in young age, tertiary syphilis or subacute sclerosing panencephalitis, and encephalopathies due to heavy metal or other toxins.

3. *Variant Creutzfeldt-Jakob disease [bovine spongiform encephalopathy (BSE)]*, also called "mad-cow disease," caused an epidemic in the United Kingdom and France. Patients acquire the disease by eating meat or meat products contaminated with BSE. It affects younger adults and presents with prominent behavioral manifestations, persistent paresthesias and dysesthesias, and similar periodic EEG pattern.

4. *Kuru* is an endemic form of prion disease formerly associated with cannibalism in the Fore tribe of New Guinea.

5. *Gerstmann-Straussler-Scheinker disease*. Most cases are familial with autosomal dominant inheritance (point mutation of PrP gene on chromosome 20) and present with ataxia, dementia, aphasia, and extrapyramidal symptoms. The course is similar but slower than CJD, and death occurs in 4 to 10 years.

6. *Fatal familial insomnia* is characterized by disordered sleep, ataxia, and dementia. The disease affects mainly the thalamic nuclei and is associated with mutation of codon 178 of the PrP gene.

REFERENCES

Collinge J: *Lancet* 354(9175):317–323, 1999.
Cummings JL, Benson DF: *Dementia: a clinical approach*, ed 2, Boston, 1992, Butterworth-Heinemann.
Dickson DW: *Brain Patrol* 8(2):339–354, 1998.
Geldmacher DS, Whitehouse PJ: *N Engl J Med* 335(5):330–336, 1996.
Johnson RT, Gibbs CJ Jr: *N Engl J Med* 339(27):1994–2004, 1998.
Luis CA et al: *Neuropsychology* 9(3):137–150, 1999.
Mayeux R, Sano M: *N Engl J Med* 341(22), 1999.
Neary D et al: *Neurology* 51(6):1546–1554, 1998.
Prusiner SB: *Curr Opin Neurobiol* 2:638–647, 1992.
Roman G et al: *Neurology* 43:250–260, 1993.

DEMYELINATING DISEASE

These CNS disorders—demyelinating disease, neuropathy, and multiple sclerosis (MS)—involve destruction of normally formed myelin and oligodendroglia, in contrast to the dysmyelinating diseases (e.g., leukodystrophies) in which myelin is abnormally formed. Multiple sclerosis is the most common. MS and the related acute disseminated encephalomyelitis (ADEM) appear to be immune mediated, although etiopathogenesis remains an enigma.

CLASSIFICATION

I. Autoimmune
   A. Primary diseases of myelin.
      1. Multiple sclerosis (MS).
      2. Devic's disease, possibly a variant of MS, consists of optic neuritis and transverse myelitis.
      3. Schilder's disease, a rapidly progressive sporadic disease, results in bilateral, massive hemispheric demyelination and is seen mainly in children and adolescents.
      4. Balo's sclerosis, also a possible variant of MS, results in acute demyelination in a concentric pattern.
   B. Parainfectious or postvaccination.
      1. ADEM, a uniphasic, inflammatory demyelinating disorder, occurs shortly after measles, varicella, rubella, or other viral illnesses, after vaccination, or after immunizations.
      2. Acute hemorrhagic leukoencephalitis, a hyperacute necrotizing form of ADEM, occurs usually after upper respiratory tract infections, and pathologic features are more tissue-destructive.
      3. Site-restricted, uniphasic, acute inflammatory demyelinating disorders include transverse myelitis, optic neuritis, cerbellitis, and Bickerstaff's brainstem encephalitis.
      4. Chronic or recurrent parainfectious or postvaccination encephalomyelitis (possibly related to MS).
II. Infectious
   A. Progressive multifocal leukoencephalopathy.
   B. Subacute sclerosing panencephalitis.
III. Nutritional
   A. Alcohol or tobacco amblyopia.
   B. Central pontine myelinolysis.
   C. Marchiafava-Bignami syndrome.
   D. Vitamin B_{12} deficiency.
IV. Toxic or metabolic
   A. Anoxia or hypoxia.
   B. Carbon monoxide poisoning.
   C. Mercury intoxication (Minamata disease).
   D. Radiation therapy.
   E. Methotrexate, especially with radiation therapy.
V. Hereditary
   A. Familial spastic paraplegia.
   B. Hereditary ataxias.
   C. Leber's disease.

REFERENCES

Baker D, Davison AN: *Neurochem Res* 16:1067–1072, 1991.
Francis GS, Antel JP, Duquette P: In Bradley WG et al: *Neurology in clinical practice,* Boston, Butterworth-Heinemann, 1991.

DERMATOMES (See Inside Front Cover and Figures 12 and 13)

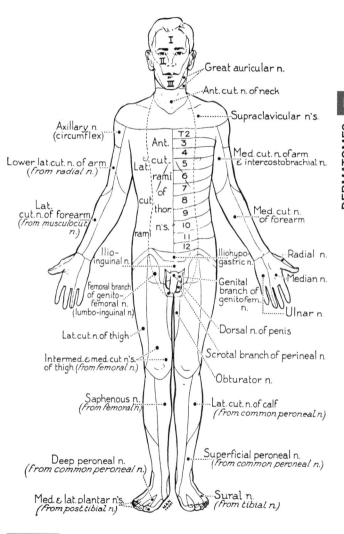

Great auricular n.

Ant. cut. n. of neck

Supraclavicular n's.

Axillary n.
(circumflex)

Ant.
cut.
rami
of
cut.
thor.
n's.
rami

Lat.

Med. cut. n. of arm
& intercostobrachial n.

Lower lat. cut. n. of arm
(from radial n.)

Lat.
cut. n. of forearm
(from musculocut.
n.)

Med. cut. n.
of forearm

Ilio-
inguinal n.

Iliohypo-
gastric n.

Radial n.

Femoral branch
of genito-
femoral n.
(lumbo-inguinal n.)

Genital
branch of
genitofem.
n.

Median n.

Ulnar n.

Lat. cut. n. of thigh

Dorsal n. of penis

Intermed. & med. cut. n's.
of thigh (from femoral n.)

Scrotal branch of perineal n.

Obturator n.

Saphenous n.
(from femoral n.)

Lat. cut. n. of calf
(from common peroneal n.)

Deep peroneal n.
(from common peroneal n.)

Superficial peroneal n.
(from common peroneal n.)

Med. & lat. plantar n's.
(from post. tibial n.)

Sural n.
(from tibial n.)

FIGURE 12

Cutaneous sensory distribution of peripheral nerves (anterior). (From Haymaker W, Woodhall B: *Peripheral nerve injuries: principles of diagnosis,* Philadelphia, WB Saunders, 1953.)

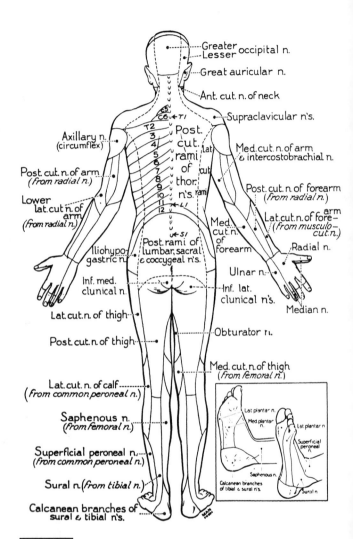

FIGURE 13

Cutaneous sensory distribution of peripheral nerves (posterior). (From Haymaker W, Woodhall B: *Peripheral nerve injuries; principles of diagnosis,* Philadelphia, WB Saunders, 1953.)

DIALYSIS

Two neurologic syndromes are related to dialysis:

1. *Dialysis disequilibrium syndrome* is the acute onset of neurologic manifestations during or after hemo- or peritoneal dialysis. *Clinical features:* Seizures (generalized more often than focal), headache, anorexia, nausea, disorientation, cramps, and even coma. *Etiology:* It is probably an accumulation of urea and idiogenic osmoles in the brain during renal failure. With dialysis, plasma osmolality decreases and the subsequent osmotic gradient results in obligatory retention of water by the brain and subsequent brain edema. Slower dialysis offers the brain more time to clear the idiogenic osmoles. EEG changes reflect the degree of uremia before dialysis and consist of bursts of rhythmic delta waves and occasionally spike-and-wave complexes. *Management:* It is usually self-limited and recovery usually occurs in a few days.
2. *Dialysis dementia syndrome* is now rare and occurs almost exclusively in chronic hemodialysis patients. *Clinical features:* Subacute development of personality changes, memory difficulties, dysarthria, myoclonus, and seizures. *Dialysis dementia* in part is defined by EEG. There may be 2- to 4-second bursts of high-voltage, irregular, frontally dominated generalized delta waves, accompanied by frontal sharp waves, spikes, and triphasic waves on normal or minimally slow background. *Etiology* may be related to elevated aluminum levels in the dialysate fluid. Removal of aluminum from dialysis baths by deionization has markedly reduced the frequency of this syndrome. *Treatment* is with desferrioxamine.
3. *Dialysis encephalopathy* may be part of a multisystem disease that includes vitamin D-resistant osteomalacia, myopathy, and anemia.
4. *Others:* Subdural hematomas, confusional states from hyperosmolarity, hypercalcemia, hypophosphatemia, drug intoxication, and Wernicke's encephalopathy. Patients with chronic renal failure often have multiple risk factors for cerebrovascular disease.

REFERENCES

Daly DD, Pedley TA: *Current practice of clinical electroencephalography*, ed 2, New York, Raven, 1990, 376.
Dhondt JL: *N Engl J Med* 318:582–583, 1988.

DISSEMINATED INTRAVASCULAR COAGULATION (DIC)

A clotting disorder complicating many diseases, most commonly associated with obstetric catastrophes, malignancies, massive trauma, and bacterial sepsis. It is less commonly associated with immunologic disturbances, diabetic ketoacidosis, tissue damage (*stroke, brain hemorrhage, meningitis* etc.), or shock. In each case, potent thrombogenic stimuli, such as tissue factor or endotoxin, trigger the coagulation cascade and activate platelets.

Fibrin then deposits in the microcirculation, causing ischemia, red blood cell (RBC) damage, hemolysis, and secondary fibrinolysis.

DIC can be either an explosive and life-threatening bleeding disorder or relatively mild and subclinical. Most often, patients have hemorrhagic or thrombotic complications in venipuncture sites or distal extremities. *Neurologic complications* can affect any portion of the brain or spinal cord with hemorrhage or thrombosis, producing a fluctuating encephalopathy, commonly with focal findings. Confusion, delirium, stupor, and coma may occur with hemiparesis, hemianopsia, ataxia, aphasia, seizures, and focal brainstem disease.

Laboratory manifestations include an elevated prothrombin and partial thromboplastin times, low platelets, falling fibrinogen (consumptive), and elevated fibrin split products and D-dimer (due to fibrinolysis). Anemia, fragmented RBCs, and schistocytes may be found.

Treatment consists of correcting the underlying cause. Active bleeding requires fresh-frozen plasma and cryoprecipitate to replenish clotting factors and platelet transfusions to correct thrombocytopenia. Thrombotic complications may be treated with heparin. Heparin is sometimes used to treat hemorrhage, when platelets and plasma fail. *Prognosis* is variable, and patients with severe deficits may completely recover.

REFERENCES

Aminoff MJ: *Neurology and general medicine*, Edinburgh, Churchill Livingstone, 1989, 204–205.
Bick RL, Arun B et al: *Hemostasis* 29:111–134, 1999.

DIZZINESS

Dizziness is a nonspecific term commonly used to describe a variety of subjective experiences. An accurate description of what the patient means, a detailed medical history, and reproduction of the patient's symptoms by means of provocative maneuvers such as hyperventilation, Barany's maneuver, and stooping over, as well as measuring orthostatic blood pressures, help suggest the following more specific etiologic categories:

I. *Vertigo:* The illusion of self-motion or environmental motion (see Vertigo).

II. *Syncope or presyncope:* The sensation of impeding faint or loss of consciousness. Causes include cardiac arrhythmia, carotid sinus hypersensitivity, postural hypotension (diabetic autonomic neuropathy or side effect of antihypertensive, diuretic, dopaminergic, or other drugs), anemia, and Addison's disease (see Syncope).

III. *Disequilibrium:* Loss of balance without various subjective movement sensations of head. May occur with cerebellar or proprioceptive disturbances or with muscle weakness.

IV. Dizziness that is due to causes other than those previously mentioned may be described as lightheadedness, floating, wooziness, faintness, or some other sense of altered consciousness. Causes include the following.

A   Hyperventilation syndrome. One of the most common causes of dizziness or lightheadedness. Circumoral and digital paresthesias are frequently associated. Symptoms may be reproduced during hyperventilation. Occasionally a patient has positional vertigo with hyperventilation (see Hyperventilation, Vertigo).

B. Multiple sensory deficits. Two or more of the following are usually present: visual impairment (often caused by cataracts), neuropathy, vestibular dysfunction (see Vertigo), cervical spondylosis, and ortho-pedic disorders that interfere with ambulation. Patients may complain of lighheadedness when walking and turning. Holding the examiner's finger lightly may provide enough additional sensory input to relieve the symptoms. Patients are often elderly or diabetic, or both.

C. Psychogenic dizziness (not associated with hyperventilation). Patients complain of vague lightheadedness, mental fuzziness, or difficulty thinking. They may be depressed or anxious. Dizziness is usually con-tinuous rather than episodic. Patients may state that all or none of the maneuvers performed during physical examination produce dizziness.

D. Severe anemia or polycythemia may cause symptoms of lighthead-edness or dizziness.

E. Drugs may produce symptoms of dizziness that are not necessarily related to orthostatic changes in blood pressure or presyncope. These include antiarrhythmics, anticonvulsants, antidepressants, antihista-mines, antihypertensives, antiparkinsonian agents, hypnotics, hypo-glycemics, phenothiazines, alcohol, and tobacco.

F. Endocrinologic disorders (hypoglycemia, Addison's disease, hypopi-tuitarism, and insulinoma).

Treatment of dizziness depends on the underlying cause. For evaluation and management of vertigo, see Vertigo.

DYSARTHRIA

A disorder of speech produced by disturbances of the muscles of articula-tion. Six patterns of dysfunction have been distinguished: flaccid, spastic, ataxic, hypokinetic, hyperkinetic, and mixed. Although each has differing sound characteristics to the trained ear, most clinicians rely on associated neurologic signs such as limb ataxia, involvement of cranial nerve VII, IX, X, or XII, or brisk jaw jerk or gag reflex to distinguish the speech patterns (ataxic, flaccid, and spastic respectively).

DYSKINESIA

A nonspecific term that refers collectively to the abnormal involuntary movements ascribed to movement disorders. Most commonly the term is utilized to describe the involuntary *nontremorous hyperkinetic* movements associated with L-dopa and dopamine agonist and postneuroleptics (tardive dyskinesia).

DYSPHAGIA

Swallowing can be divided into three phases: oral, pharyngeal and esophageal. Dysfunction at any of these levels is called dysphagia. Dysphagia can lead to aspiration of liquids or solids which can lead to pneumonia or death.

Problems swallowing primarily liquids, are typical of neurologic disorders whereas dysphagia mainly for solids is typical of mechanical obstruction but can be seen with pharyngeal muscle weakness. Coughing or choking on swallowing suggests laryngeal weakness; nasal regurgitation of liquids suggests palatal weakness.

Local structural lesions of the upper GI tract may cause dysphagia by mechanical obstruction. Neurologic causes of dysphagia involve lesions anywhere along the pathways subserving swallowing, coordination of which depends on sensation from the tongue, mouth, pharynx, and larynx, and voluntary and reflex motor activity of cranial nerves V, VII, IX, X, and XII. The "swallowing center" is in the medulla, near the respiratory center. Lesions of the inferior precentral gyrus or posterior inferior frontal gyrus both cause severe dysphagia without buccolingual apraxia, speech impairment, or weakness. Bilateral upper motor neuron disease manifesting as pseudobulbar palsy is usually associated with dysphagia. Lesions of cerebellar and extrapyramidal pathways may also cause dysphagia. Dysphagia is seen in peripheral nervous system diseases such as Guillain-Barré syndrome, myasthenia, polymyositis, and oculopharyngeal dystrophy. Thus, dysphagia is nonlocalizing and associated with lesions from muscle to cerebral cortex.

Swallowing evaluation by a speech therapist should be obtained in cases of suspected aspiration. Silent aspiration is frequently underdiagnosed, because of the lack of overt swallowing difficulties. The presence/absence of a gag reflex cannot solely differentiate patients at risk. For patients in whom oral feeding is unsafe, a nasogastric tube or a percutaneous gastrostomy tube can be used. Regulation of food and liquid consistency is an essential component of ongoing management in conjuction with speech pathologists and dieticians.

REFERENCE

Hughes TA, Wiles CM: *J Neurol Neurosurg Psychiatry* 64:569–572, 1998.

DYSTONIA

Dystonia is an involuntary contraction of muscle groups that manifests as a jerking or twisting movement, or *sustained* abnormal postures. Dystonia is categorized into primary and secondary forms. Primary dystonias refers to those dystonic disorders that are not associated with a presumed or known metabolic, structural, or degenerative abnormality. Primary dystonias in general are worsened with stress or anxiety and are often alleviated with rest, relaxation, or "sensory tricks" i.e., light touching. Acute onset of dystonia in an adult is often attributable to the initiation of neuroleptics or, less commonly, antidepressants. Hyperglycemia, hypothyroidism, hypoparathyroidism, systemic lupus erythematosus (SLE) and polycythemia rubra vera are a few of the metabolic abnormalities that can be associated with acute onset of dystonia as well as other dyskinesias. Cytologic and chemical evaluation may give a clue to other less common etiologies for acute onset dystonia and should be obtained in the initial investigations. One should also consider evaluation for Huntington's and Wilson's disease because of the options and implications regarding a positive diagnosis.

I. Primary generalized dystonia: idiopathic torsion dystonia (ITD)/dystonia musculorum deformans (DMD).

Hereditary/sporadic: DYT1 gene, chromosome 9q32-34, AD/AR, familial forms often found in Ashkenazi Jews. Deep tendon reflexes are preserved and no long tract signs found. There is also an X-linked form Xq13.1 (DYT 3 gene), which has been described in Filipino males. Patients typically develop symptoms in late childhood involving one limb and progress to include the other limbs, torso, and neck.

II. Periodic dystonia: AR/AD, hereditary/sporadic, dystonic symptoms precipitated by movement or startle (kinesigenic) or nonkinesigenic.

III. Focal/segmental.
   A. Meiges syndrome (cranial dystonia), oro-facial/mandibular manifestations of dystonia. Occurs more frequently in women.
      1. Blepharospasm: Involuntary spasmodic closure of the eyelids preceded and associated with increased force and frequency of blinking.
      2. Oromandibular dystonia (lingual dystonia): Jaw clenching, forced jaw opening, or tongue protrusion, painful grimacing, chewing, lip smacking.
      3. Spasmodic dysphonia (laryngeal dystonia): Spasms of the laryngeal muscles that produce strained, harsh, and breathy voice.
   B. Spasmodic torticollis: Dystonia limited to the neck muscles, primarily trapezius and sternocleidomastoid. Symptoms manifest as posturing of head in flexion (anterocollis), extension (retrocollis), or to the side (laterocollis) or painful phasic spasmodic alternations. DYT7 is responsible for autosomal dominant familial torticollis.
   C. Writer' cramp: focal dystonia of the hand precipitated by writing. Symptoms may progress up the arm or include a violent tremor. Symptoms disappear with cessation of attempt to write. This is one example of task-specific dystonia.

IV. Dystonia-plus syndromes: Rapid-onset dystonia-parkinsonism, dopa-responsive dystonia, and myoclonus-dystonia.

V. Secondary dystonias: Cerebral palsy, pachygyria, encephalitis, AIDS, Creutzfeldt-Jakob disease, head trauma, anoxia, stroke, multiple sclerosis, hypoparathyroidism, drug induced (dopamine D_2 antagonists, levodopa, ergotamine, anticonvulsants), toxins (Mn, CO, cyanide, methanol, disulfiram).

A

DYSTONIA

VI. Psychogenic: Occur in less than 5% of all dystonias.

Preliminary laboratory evaluation for dystonia may include:

CBC with differential—wet mount to rule out acanthocytes
Chemistry panel, including, glucose, BUN/Cr, electrolytes including
    Ca^{++}, Mg^{++}
ESR, LFTs, PTH, thyroid tests, VDRL, ANA profile, LAC, ACL
Lactate, pyruvate
Serum Cu/ceruloplasmin
Cholesterol/trig
Acute streptolysin, Slit lamp eye exam, EKG, CT/MRI of head

Further investigation may be indicated in the childhood or adolescent onset of dystonic symptoms. Other electrophysiologic tests may be indicated if preliminary tests are inconclusive. EEG may be indicated to exclude epileptic mechanism.

Treatment for dystonia remains symptomatic. In addition to correcting underlying metabolic abnormalities and deficits, certain pharmacologic therapies have proven effective. Anticholinergic agents, dopaminergic agents (*dopa-responsive dystonia*), benzodiazepines, and muscle relaxants (baclofen) have been moderately efficacious in the symptomatic relief of sustained and painful dystonias. Botulinum toxin injections have been found to be very effective in the treatment of focal dystonias. Botulinum injection needs to be repeated every 3 months, and antibodies may develop in 5% against the toxins. Tests are available commercially to detect these antibodies. Generalized dystonia responds well to stereotactic surgery, i.e., pallidotomy and thalamotomy.

REFERENCE

Thyagarajan D: *J Clin Neurosci* 6:1–8, 1999.

ELECTROCARDIOGRAM (ECG)

Changes in electrocardiographic rhythm and morphology may occur with acute CNS disease in the absence of other etiologies. Although most frequently reported in subarachnoid hemorrhage (SAH), ECG changes can be seen in migraine, brain tumor, head injury, and stroke. In epileptic patients, cortical stimulation of the left insula leads to bradycardia and depressor effects, with the opposite effect with right-sided stimulation.

CNS disease is associated with both ventricular and supraventricular dysrhythmias, the former occurring more frequently in the presence of elevated cardiac enzymes. Morphologic changes include Q-waves, ST elevation or depression, and U waves. *In SAH, large upright or deeply inverted T waves and prolonged QT intervals are characteristic.* These changes may be mediated by increased sympathetic tone associated with hypothalamic involvement and can cause myocardial ischemia and infarction with CK elevations and regional wall motion abnormalities. Both ischemic and hemorrhagic myocardial damage have been noted in association with SAH.

Abnormal cardiac rhythms are associated with embolic strokes, leading to significant mortality and morbidity. The prevalence of atrial fibrillation below age 55 years in the United States is less than 0.5%, rising to 6% for individuals older than 65 years. Stroke may also lead to atrial fibrillation, brady-tachyarrhythmias, and myocardial damage.

REFERENCES

Devinsky O et al: *Neurology* 48:1712–1714, 1997.
Fine DG et al: *JACC* 15:215A, 1990.
Oppenheimer MB et al: *Neurology* 42:1727, 1992.
Vingerhoets F et al: *Stroke* 24:26, 1993.
Wilterdink JL et al: *Neurology* 51:S23–S26, 1998.

ELECTROENCEPHALOGRAPHY

The electroencephalogram (EEG) is a recording of electrical activity originating from extracellular current flow in the superficial layers of cerebral cortex. This activity reflects the major influence of subcortical structures, especially the brainstem reticular formation and intralaminar and reticular nuclei of the thalamus, generating the three normal states of consciousness: waking, non-rapid eye movement sleep (NREM), and rapid eye movement sleep (REM). EEG is useful clinically in large part because it provides real-time information regarding brain physiology, rather than structure.

I. The normal adult waking EEG may contain the following.
   A. Alpha rhythm (8 to 13 Hz): This is present occipitally in nearly all adults. It appears during relaxed wakefulness with eyes closed, and attenuates with eye opening or mental effort; these characteristics distinguish it from *alpha activity*, which merely satisfies the frequency criterion (see alpha coma, below). The alpha rhythm reaches 8 Hz by about age 3 and stays at or above that frequency in the vast majority of normal elderly individuals.
   B. Beta activity (>13 Hz): A normal finding unless its amplitude consistently exceeds 25 millivolts, which may suggest the presence of benzodiazepines, barbiturates, or chloral hydrate. Beta is enhanced over skull defects (breach rhythm, sometimes quite "spiky" appearing) and depressed in areas of focal brain injury and over subdural, epidural, or subgaleal fluid collections.
   C. Theta activity (4 to 7 Hz): Admixed and of low voltage in normal records, theta becomes more sustained and prominent during

drowsiness. Normal elderly individuals may have a limited amount of shifting temporal theta. *Activity slower than 4 Hz (delta) should not be present in the waking adult record*.

D. Mu rhythm: This is a rhythm of alpha frequency that is located centrally, appears with eyes open, and blocks with contralateral extremity movement. It originates from sensorimotor cortex.

E. Lambda waves: These sharp, surface-negative transients appear over occipital regions, only with eyes open, especially upon looking at a strong visual pattern.

F. Other benign patterns appearing during waking or drowsiness include: rhythmic temporal theta bursts of drowsiness (psychomotor variant), subclinical rhythmic electrographic discharge of adults (SREDA), benign epileptiform transients of sleep (BETS), positive occipital sharp transients of sleep (POSTS), 14- and 6-Hz positive bursts, 6-Hz phantom spike and wave, and wicket spikes.

G. Hyperventilation (HV) response: A physiologic increase in generalized slowing occurs with prolonged HV, particularly in children, and is accentuated with hypoglycemia. Abnormalities during HV include focal slowing or epileptiform discharges.

H. Photic stimulation response: Normal photomyoclonic responses consist of muscular contractions, typically orbicularis oculi, elicited by each flash. Abnormal photoparoxysmal responses, bursts of generalized epileptiform discharges that may outlast the flash stimuli, are indicative of generalized epilepsy or an inherited EEG trait.

II. The normal adult sleep EEG may contain the following.

A. Stage I sleep (drowsiness) is defined by dropout of the waking alpha rhythm, accentuation of frontocentral theta activity, and slow rolling eye movements. *Vertex waves*, large-amplitude, sharp, surface-negative transients maximal at the central vertex, may occur.

B. Stage II sleep is marked by the appearance of sleep spindles, rhythmic 12- to 15-Hz waves with a waxing and waning morphology, and K complexes, large biphasic sharp transients maximal over the vertex, often precipitated by external stimuli.

C. Stages III and IV sleep are defined by the presence of delta waves 2 Hz or slower, greater than 75 μv, occurring between 20% and 50% of a 30-second epoch (stage III) or over 50% (stage IV).

D. REM sleep is defined by relatively low-voltage desynchronized EEG, muscular atonia, and bursts of rapid eye movements.

III. EEG abnormalities.

A. Epilepsy: Interictal epileptiform activity, consisting of spikes, sharp waves, or spike-wave complexes, are strongly but not absolutely correlated with epilepsy. Thus, their presence does not unequivocally indicate a diagnosis of epilepsy nor does their absence exclude it. Nevertheless, their presence, in combination with clinical information, frequently allow one to make a diagnosis in terms of recognized electroclinical syndromes (see Epilepsy). Ictal discharges, or electrographic seizures, provide irrefutable evidence of an epileptic seizure disorder. In generalized epilepsies, electrographic seizures may consist of a pronged run of otherwise typical interictal discharges, but in partial epilepsies this is rarely the case and the ictal patterns have their own morphology. The absence of an ictal EEG pattern during a typical generalized convulsion provides strong evidence of a nonepileptic seizure (see Epilepsy), but this is less true for auras, focal motor or sensory seizures, or complex partial seizures.

B. Focal brain lesions: The presence of continuous, focal, polymorphic delta activity, especially in combination with depression of ipsilateral background rhythms, strongly suggests a focal lesion. However, an area of focal dysfunction, as may be seen following complicated migraine or a focal seizure, should also be considered. Periodic lateralized epileptiform discharges (PLEDS) are frequently associated with irritative lesions such as acute cerebral infarcts or encephalitis.

C. Diffuse encephalopathies: The EEG has a high sensitivity for detecting global cerebral dysfunction, but is nonspecific as to etiology. Exceptions include Alzheimer's disease and HIV encephalopathy, in which the EEG may remain normal until late in the course of the disease. Early changes include slowing of the alpha rhythm and the appearance of generalized theta activity; more severe cases show generalized polymorphic delta, frontal intermittent rhythmic delta activity (FIRDA), and lack of normal reactivity. Triphasic waves are seen in hepatic or other metabolic encephalopathies and may be periodic. Other conditions associated with periodic discharges include Creutzfeldt-Jakob disease (most patients have periodic sharp discharges, occurring with a period of about 1 second, within 12 weeks of diagnosis) and subacute sclerosing panencephalitis (periodic, generalized slow waves, or sharp and slow complexes, with a period of about 5 to 10 seconds).

D. Coma: Findings include lack of normal background, reactivity, or state changes, in combination with continuous generalized polymorphic delta activity, FIRDA, low-voltage patterns, periodic discharges including PLEDS or triphasic waves, or burst-suppression pattern (bursts of electrical activity separated by periods of diffuse voltage suppression, indicative of severe diffuse cerebral dysfunction). In patients with coma following seizures, electrographic status epilepticus should be ruled out. Alpha coma, with generalized invariant unreactive alpha frequency activity, is associated with toxic or metabolic insults and cerebral anoxia, and must be distinguished from normal alpha rhythms present in those with a "locked in state."

E. Brain death: Confirmatory evidence includes the demonstration of electrocerebral silence (ECS), under proper technical conditions, in the appropriate clinical context. Conditions associated with reversible

E

ELECTROENCEPHALOGRAPHY

ECS include overdose of CNS depressants, hypothermia, cardiovascular shock, metabolic and endocrine disorders, and very young age.

ELECTROLYTE DISORDERS

Symptoms are usually more severe with acute changes in electrolyte levels. Occasionally, chronic disturbances may produce signs and symptoms opposite from the acute state. In general, central nervous system dysfunction occurs with abnormalities of sodium, peripheral nervous system dysfunction with abnormal potassium levels, and combinations of both with abnormalities of calcium, magnesium, and phosphate. Management is directed at treatment of the primary disorder and correction of the electrolyte abnormality. Neurologic findings usually disappear with appropriate therapy (see Table 24 for signs and symptoms).

SODIUM

Sodium is the main determinant of serum osmolality (Osm) and extracellular fluid volume. Therefore, neurologic symptoms are dependent on the time lag necessary for the brain to compensate for rapid changes in serum Na^+ concentration, and thus, Osm.

Hyponatremia: Acute decreases of Na^+ levels to 130 mEq/L may produce symptoms. Chronic changes to 115 mEq/L may be asympto-

TABLE 24

NEUROLOGIC SIGNS AND SYMPTOMS OF ELECTROLYTE DISTURBANCES

	$\downarrow Na^+$	$\uparrow Na^+$	$\downarrow K^+$	$\uparrow K^+$	$\downarrow Ca^{++}$	$\uparrow Ca^{++}$	$\downarrow Mg^{++}$	$\uparrow Mg^{++}$	Acute $\downarrow PO_4^=$	Chronic $\downarrow PO_4^=$
Muscle weakness	−	−	+(1)	+/−	−	+/−	+/−	+(2)	+	+(1)
Reflexes	0	0	0	0	0→↑	↑	↑	↓	↓	0→↑
Cognitive changes	+(3)	+(3)	−	−	+(4)	+(3)	+(4)	+(3)	+(4)	−
Seizures	+	+	−	−	+	+/−	+	−	+/−	−
Tetany	−	−	+(5)	−	+	−	+	−	−	−
Focal signs	+/−	−	−	−	−	+/−	−	−	+(6)	−
Abnormal movements	−	+(7,8,9)	−	−	−	−	+(8,9)	−	−	−
Other	A,B	B(10)		C	D	E				

(1) Proximal > distal.
(2) May be severe.
(3) Lethargy to coma.
(4) Variable or unpredictable.
(5) When associated with alkalosis.
(6) Cranial nerve palsies.
(7) Rigidity.
(8) Tremor.
(9) Myoclonus.
(10) May occur with rehydration.

(A) Cramps.
(B) Cerebral edema.
(C) Cardiac toxicity.
(D) Pseudotumor cerebri.
(E) Headache.
　+　Usually present.
　−　Usually absent.
　+/−　Occasionally present.
　↑　Usually increased.
　↓　Usually decreased.
　0　Usually normal.

matic. EEG abnormalities are common but nonspecific, with slowing that correlates with decreased Na^+ levels. Acute hyponatremia (<115 mEq/L) with seizures carries a high mortality rate and necessitates rapid (over a 6-hour period) correction to 120 to 125 mEq/L (with hypertonic saline or normal saline and furosemide). *Rapid correction to levels greater than 120 to 125 mEq/L may result in central pontine myelinolysis (CPM),* a disorder described in alcoholics but also occurring in children and adults with liver disease, severe electrolyte imbalances, malnutrition, anorexia, burns, cancer, Addison's disease, and sepsis. There is symmetric focal myelin destruction predominantly involving the basal central pons.

Asymptomatic chronic hyponatremia usually requires no immediate intervention and is managed by correction of the underlying condition.

Hypernatremia: Neurologic symptoms develop when the serum Na^+ level rises above 160 mEq/L or the serum Osm is greater than 350 mOsm/kg. Level of consciousness correlates well with the degree of hyperosmolality. Sudden increases in serum Osm may produce decreased brain cell volume, with mechanical traction on cerebral vessels causing subcortical, subdural, or subarachnoid hemorrhage. CSF protein levels may be high without pleocytosis, and the EEG is normal or mildly slowed.

Hypernatremia resulting from diabetes insipidus may occur with tumors involving the hypothalamus or pineal region, as well as with basilar meningitis, encephalitis, ruptured aneurysms, sarcoidosis, trauma, or surgery.

Treatment with *isotonic solutions* should be given to reduce the serum Na^+ level by no more than 1 mEq/L every 2 hours during the first 2 days of treatment. Rapid infusion of hypotonic solutions may cause cerebral edema and seizures.

POTASSIUM

Almost 60% of total body K^+ is located within muscle, therefore predominantly muscular symptoms occur with altered K^+ levels.

Hypokalemia most commonly occurs with diuretic use but also occurs with GI losses, mineralocorticoid excess, and rarely, thyrotoxicosis. Muscle weakness usually develops with serum levels of 2.5 to 3.0 mEq/L, with structural muscle damage occurring at levels below 2.0 mEq/L. Hypokalemia and hypocalcemia frequently coexist, with cancellation of neuromuscular manifestations. Treatment of one condition in isolation may produce symptoms of the other. ECG and cardiac abnormalities are common and may require ICU monitoring and treatment.

Treatment involves increasing dietary K^+, supplements of KCl, and the use of K^+-sparing diuretics.

Hyperkalemia is relatively uncommon, but may occur in familial hyperkalemic periodic paralysis (see Periodic Paralysis). Quadriparesis may develop with levels greater than 6.8 mEq/L, and levels greater than 7.0 mEq/L are life-threatening and require ICU monitoring with immediate therapy, which may include administration of glucose and insulin, cation exchange resins, or calcium gluconate.

E

ELECTROLYTE DISORDERS

CALCIUM

Plasma Ca^{++} is a stabilizer of excitable membranes in the central and peripheral nervous systems and in muscle. Ca^{++} concentrations are closely controlled through the combined effects of parathyroid hormone, calciferol, and calcitonin on intestine, kidney, and bone.

Hypocalcemia is relatively rare, except in neonates, in patients with renal failure, and after thyroid or parathyroid surgery. The "tetany syndrome" originates in the peripheral nerve axon and initially becomes evident with distal and perioral tingling. Distal tonic spasms (carpopedal spasms) may progress to laryngeal stridor and opisthotonus if severe.

The EEG is diffusely slow with an exaggerated response to photic stimulation. ECG abnormalities are also common.

Treatment of mild cases is accomplished with oral calcium supplements. Tetany or seizures may require 10% IV solutions of calcium gluconate or CaCl. Underlying disorders should be corrected, if possible. Hypocalcemia often coexists with hypomagnesemia. In such cases, total serum calcium levels may be normal, but ionized calcium levels may be low.

Hypercalcemia: Malignant neoplasms are the most common cause of increased serum Ca^{++} levels. Mental status alterations occur with total serum levels greater than 14 mg/dl. Myopathy or carpal tunnel syndrome may occur in association with hyperparathyroidism.

Treatment of symptomatic patients consists of saline hydration and furosemide. Occasionally, mithramycin (suppresses bone resorption) or calcitonin (suppresses bone resorption and increases urinary Ca^{++} excretion) is required.

MAGNESIUM

Ninety-eight percent of Mg^{++} is intracellular. It is necessary for the activation of various enzymes. Extracellular Mg^{++} affects central and peripheral synaptic transmission. Changes in serum levels may not reflect total body stores.

Hypomagnesemia occurs most commonly as a result of excess renal loss (chronic alcoholism, diuretics), but may also be the result of decreased intake or absorption. Neurologic symptoms usually develop at levels below 0.8 mEq/L.

The presence of seizures requires treatment with parenteral $MgSo_4$. Oral Mg^{++} supplements may suffice in less severe cases. Calcium gluconate should be available when giving IV $MgSo_4$, as transient hypermagnesemia may cause respiratory muscle paralysis (see also hypocalcemia, above).

Hypermagnesemia, an uncommon disorder, usually occurs with increased intake and renal failure. Deep tendon reflexes may be lost at levels of 5 to 6 mEq/L, and CNS depression occurs at levels above 8 to 10 mEq/L. Muscular paralysis is due to neuromuscular blockade. Treatment of paralysis may be accomplished by small amounts of parenteral calcium gluconate and hydration. Otherwise, discontinuation of Mg^{++}-containing preparations is indicated. If renal function is severely impaired, dialysis may be necessary.

Magnesium infusions are often given as treatment for seizures associated with eclampsia. Serum magnesium levels need to be closely monitored in this situation.

PHOSPHATE

Hypophosphatemia is often complicated by multiple abnormalities of electrolytes, nutrition, and acid-base balance. The syndrome commonly occurs in malnutrition and chronic alcoholism, especially after the infusion of glucose or hyperalimentation solutions.

Acute hypophosphatemia may not reflect decreased total body stores and may produce neurologic symptoms if severe (<1.5 mEq/L). Chronic hypophosphatemia is usually moderate (1.5 to 2.5 mEq/L) and may not be symptomatic unless acute stresses (alcohol withdrawal, burns, binding of $PO_4^=$ in the gut) cause sudden decreases below the moderate level.

REFERENCE

Riggs JE: In Aminoff MJ, ed: *Neurology and general medicine,* New York, Churchill Livingstone, 1989.

RESPIRATORY ALKALOSIS

This condition is frequently observed in patients with bronchial asthma, hepatic cirrhosis, salicylate intoxication, hypoxia, sepsis, pneumonia, and acute anxiety (hyperventilation syndrome). Acute respiratory alkalosis constricts the cerebral arterioles and decreases the cerebral blood flow. Confusion accompanied by a slow EEG may develop.

More severe alkalosis (pH 7.52 to 7.65) in patients with respiratory insufficiency and hypoxia may result in a symptom complex of hypotension, seizures, asterixis, myoclonus, and coma. Other neurologic manifestations of milder respiratory alkalosis include paresthesias, dizziness, cramps as a result of coexistent tetany, hyperreflexia, and muscle weakness.

RESPIRATORY ACIDOSIS

Acute respiratory acidosis is a condition of low pH and high pCO_2, occurring as a result of impairment of the rate of alveolar ventilation. Lethargy and confusion occur as the pCO_2 rises above 55 mmHg. Seizures, stupor, or coma may occur with levels greater than 70 mmHg. The serum bicarbonate level is either normal or high, depending on how rapidly the respiratory failure developed.

Neurologic manifestations resulting from cerebral vasodilation include headache, increased intracranial pressure, and papilledema. Hyperreflexia or hyporeflexia and myoclonus may also occur. Causes of acute respiratory acidosis include sedative drugs, brainstem injury, neuromuscular disorders, chest injury, airway obstruction, and acute pulmonary disease.

Chronic respiratory acidosis generally occurs in patients with chronic bronchitis, emphysema, extreme kyphoscoliosis, or extreme obesity (pickwickian syndrome). It is most often symptomatic with acute exacerbations of disease. Compensatory polycythemia often results from chronic hyper-capneic states. Hypoventilation or Pickwickian syndrome may manifest as excessive daytime somnolence.

Therapy involves ventilatory support and treating the underlying dis-order. The possibility of sedative or narcotic drug ingestion must be sus-pected in otherwise healthy patients who suddenly develop acute respiratory depression.

METABOLIC ALKALOSIS

Metabolic alkalosis may result from either excessive ingestion of base or excessive loss of acid. Delirium and stupor owing to this condition are rarely severe. Severe metabolic alkalosis produces a blunted confusional state rather than stupor or coma and may result in cardiac arrhythmias and severe compensatory hypoventilation.

Neurologic manifestations include paresthesias, cramps (due to tetany), muscle weakness (due to associated hypokalemia), and hyporeflexia. Causes of hypokalemic metabolic alkalosis include Cushing's syndrome, vomiting or gastric drainage, diuretic therapy, and primary aldosteronism. Treatment depends on the underlying cause.

METABOLIC ACIDOSIS

Metabolic acidosis occurs when a decrease in plasma bicarbonate level lowers pH. Cardinal features are hyperventilation and, when severe, "Kussmaul's respiration." In chronic metabolic acidosis, hyperventilation may be difficult to detect on clinical examination. The presence of neuro-logic symptoms depends on various factors, including the type of systemic metabolic defect, whether the fall in systemic pH affects the pH of the brain and CSF, the rate at which acidosis develops, and the specific anion causing the metabolic disorder. All metabolic acidosis produce hyperpnea as the first neurologic symptom. Other manifestations include lethargy, drowsiness, confusion, and mild, diffuse skeletal muscle hypertonus. Extensor plantar responses occur at a later stage. Stupor, coma, or seizures generally develop only preterminally.

The most common causes of metabolic acidosis sufficient to produce coma and hyperpnea include uremia, diabetes, lactic acidosis, and ingestion of acidic poisons. Ketoacidosis occasionally develops in severe alcoholics after prolonged drinking episodes. In diabetics treated with oral hypoglycemic agents, lactic acidosis and diabetic ketoacidosis must be considered.

Since metabolic acidosis is a manifestation of a variety of different diseases, the treatment varies depending on the underlying process and on the acuteness and severity of the acidosis.

REFERENCES

Layzer RB: *Neuromuscular manifestations of systemic disease,* Philadelphia, FA Davis, 1985.

Plum F, Posner JB: *The diagnosis of stupor and coma,* ed 3, Philadelphia, FA Davis, 1982.

ELECTROMYOGRAPHY AND NERVE CONDUCTION STUDIES (EMG/NCS)

Nerve conduction studies and EMG examination are used to localize lesions in the peripheral nervous system, to provide further information regarding the underlying pathophysiology of peripheral nervous system disorders, and to access the severity and temporal course of the disorder.

Nerve conduction studies are performed by recording the action potentials with a surface electrode over the skin. Motor nerve conduction studies involve stimulating a peripheral nerve and recording the action potential from a muscle innervated by that nerve (see Table 25). Sensory nerve conduction studies are done by stimulating a mixed sensory/motor nerve proximally and recording a nerve action potential from a cutaneous sensory nerve distally, or vice versa. The amplitude, duration, shape, and latency of compound muscle action potentials (CMAP) and sensory nerve action potentials (SNAP) are noted. Conduction velocities are calculated from distance and latency differences between proximal and distal stimuli. Normal values of nerve conduction studies vary with different physiologic factors, most importantly with temperature and age. Normal nerve conduction velocities are approximately 50 m/sec in the upper extremities and 40 m/sec in the lower extremities. In addition to the routine nerve conduction studies, the effect of repetitive stimulation, exercise, and rest may also be studied in special circumstances.

The *F wave* is a late motor response that occurs after the CMAP. The pathway of the F response occurs with supramaximal stimulation to a motor nerve, causing an antidromic action potential up toward the spinal

TABLE 25

ROUTINE NERVE CONDUCTION STUDIES IN NEUROMUSCULAR DISORDERS

Disorder	Amplitude	Distal Latency	Conduction Velocity	F and H Wave Latencies
Polyneuropathy				
Axonal	↓	NL	>70%	Mild ↑
Demyelinating	NL or ↓	NL or ↑	<50%	↑
Myopathy	NL or ↓ motor	NL	NL	NL
Radiculopathy	NL or ↓ motor NL sensory	NL	>80%	NL or ↑
Neuromuscular transmission defect				
Presynaptic type	NL or ↓ motor NL sensory	NL	NL	NL
Postsynaptic type	NL	NL	NL	NL
Motor neuron disease	↓ motor N1 sensory	NL	>70%	NL or ↑
Upper motor neuron disease	NL	NL	NL	NL

cord to reach the alpha motor neuron. This then causes backfiring of a small population of motor neurons, generating an orthodromic action potential, which travels back down the nerve and reaches the muscles. It is recorded as a low-amplitude motor response occurring after the initial CMAP (*M wave*) and is a means of evaluating the entire length of motor nerves. The F response usually occurs at a latency of 25 to 32 msec in the upper extremities and 45 to 56 msec in the lower extremities. In theory, abnormal F wave latencies are very nonspecific and occur with any disease that affects motor nerves, such as polyradiculopathies, entrapment neuropathies, and hereditary motor and sensory polyneuropathy. However, prolonged F wave latencies have their greatest usefulness in detecting early polyradiculopathies such as seen in Guillain-Barré syndrome, in which prolonged or impersistent F waves may be the only abnormalities on nerve conduction studies early on.

The *H wave* is a late response occurring from a monosynaptic reflex arc, with the Ia fiber from muscle spindle as a sensory afferent and the alpha motor neuron and motor axons as a motor efferent. Because of practical and anatomic considerations, the tibial H reflex (S1 dorsal and ventral roots) is the only one routinely recorded. The typical H reflex latency is approximately 30 msec. Since the H reflex is the electrical equivalent of the ankle reflex, the responses are prolonged or absent in peripheral neuropathies, proximal tibial or sciatic neuropathy, lumbosacral plexopathy, or S_1 radiculopathy. It can be absent in normal people for more than age 60 years.

Repetitive stimulation focuses on the decremental or incremental response of the CMAP after repetitive nerve stimulation. Repetitive stimulation is useful in diagnosis and differential diagnosis of disorders of neuromuscular transmission. With slow repetitive stimulation (2 to 5 Hz), which creates progressive decrement of the number of acetylcholine (ACh) vesicles released from the presynaptic nerve terminal, a >10% CMAP amplitude decrement is seen in myasthenia and Lambert-Eaton myasthenic syndrome. The decrement is worse 2 to 4 minutes after prolonged (1 minute) exercise, but this decrement can be corrected after brief (10 sec) exercise (post-tetanic or post-exercise facilitation). With fast repetitive stimulation (30 to 50 Hz), which causes accumulation of calcium in the presynaptic nerve terminal and results in increased numbers of ACh vesicles being released, a >100% CMAP amplitude increment can be seen in presynaptic disorders such as Lambert-Eaton myasthenic syndrome and to a lesser extent in botulism. A brief period of exercise (10 sec) also can be used to elicit the incremental response with the same mechanism as in rapid repetitive stimulation.

The electromyographic needle examination records electrical activity in muscle, yielding more information on the localization and pathophysiology of the peripheral nervous system disorders. For each of the muscles being studied, the first part of the examination is to access insertional and spontaneous activity at rest. Once the insertional and spontaneous activity has been accessed, the examiner will ask the patient to slowly contract the muscle, and the motor unit action potentials (MUAP) are evaluated. MUAP are accessed for duration, amplitudes, and numbers of phases. Then, the number of MUAP and their relationship to the firing frequency (recruitment and activation pattern) are evaluated.

The remainder of this chapter outlines disorders associated with specific abnormalities found on the needle examination.

INSERTIONAL ACTIVITY

Insertional activity occurs when a needle is quickly moved through the muscle and creates depolarization of muscle fiber in a brief burst for several hundred milliseconds; activities lasting longer than 300 msec indicate increased insertional activity. Increased insertional activity may be seen in neuropathic disorders that result in denervation and several myopathic conditions that result in necrosis of the muscle fibers, such as inflammatory myopathies. It is decreased in periodic paralysis during paralytic phases and when normal muscle tissue is replaced by fibrous tissue.

SPONTANEOUS ACTIVITY

Recognition of abnormal spontaneous activity can lead to several helpful information for the diagnosis:

1. The distribution of abnormal spontaneous activity may suggest the neuroanatomical localization of the lesion, e.g., mononeuropathy, radiculopathy.
2. Certain types of spontaneous activity are associated with specific disorders, e.g., myotonic discharges in myotonic dystrophy and hyperkalemic periodic paralysis (see below).
3. The amount of spontaneous activity or the presence of spontaneous activity may provide information regarding the time course and severity of the lesion, e.g., presence of fibrillation potentials are seen beginning 2 to 3 weeks after the acute nerve injury.

Abnormal Spontaneous Activity Originating from Muscle Fibers

Fibrillation potentials (brief, regular-firing, muscle fiber action potentials) and *positive sharp waves* (longer duration with initial positive deflection, regular-firing, muscle fiber action potentials) are due to spontaneous depolarization of the muscle fibers and are electrophysiologic markers of denervation. These typically occurs 2 to 3 weeks after denervation in neurogenic disorders (neuropathies, radiculopathies, motor neuron disease, etc.). They may also be seen in muscle disorders, especially in inflammatory myopathy and muscular dystrophies, and can rarely be seen in severe disorders of the neuromuscular junction, as in botulism.

Complex repetitive discharges (high-frequency, regular-firing, multi-serrated repetitive discharges with abrupt onset and termination, creating a characteristic "machine-like" sound) result from the depolarization of a single muscle fiber followed by ephaptic spread to adjacent denervated fibers. This occurs in a wide variety of chronic neurogenic disorders (poliomyelitis, motor neuron disease, radiculopathies, neuropathies) and myopathic disorders (Duchenne and limb-girdle dystrophy, polymyositis, hypothyroidism).

Myotonic discharges are also spontaneous discharges of a muscle fiber characterized by a waveform with waxing and waning amplitude and frequency, creating a "dive bomber" sound on the recording. They are typically seen in myotonic dystrophy, myotonia congenita, paramyotonia congenita, hyperkalemic periodic paralysis, acid maltase deficiency, diazocholesterol toxicity, clofibrate toxicity, and rarely in polymyositis and colchicine toxicity.

Abnormal Spontaneous Activity Originating from the Motor Unit

Fasciculation potentials are random single spontaneous discharges from the individual motor unit. On EMG, fasciculations have the morphology of simple MUAP or they can be complex and large if they represent a pathologic motor unit. They are most common in chronic neurogenic disorders (motor neuron disease, peripheral neuropathies, radiculopathies, entrapment neuropathies). Fasciculations may also be seen in normal individuals.

Myokymic discharges are rhythmic, grouped, spontaneous repetitive discharges of the same motor unit. They may be recorded in facial muscles (facial myokymia) associated with brainstem lesions from multiple sclerosis, brainstem glioma, or vascular disease. Appendicular myokymia is associated with radiation plexopathy. Rarely, it may be seen in Guillain-Barré syndrome, radiculopathy, chronic entrapment neuropathy, and gold toxicity.

Neuromyotonia is high-frequency (150 to 250 Hz) decrementing, repetitive discharges of a single motor unit that create a characteristic "pinging" sound on EMG recording. These are rare and are seen only with chronic neuropathic diseases (e.g., polio and adult-onset spinal muscular atrophy) and syndromes of continuous motor unit activity, such as in Isaac's syndrome.

Cramp potential is a painful involuntary muscle contraction that trends to occur with a muscle in shortened position or contracting. Electrically, cramps are high-frequency discharges of motor units. Cramps occur commonly in normal individuals and in many neurogenic and metabolic disorders, including electrolyte imbalances, hypothyroidism, pregnancy, and uremia (see Cramps).

Voluntary Motor Unit Potentials

The pattern of MUAP abnormalities will allow determination whether the disorder is a neuropathic or a myopathic process and often helps to determine the time course and severity of the lesion. Assessment of MUAP can be divided into two parts.

1. Morphology
Short-duration, small-amplitude motor unit action potentials occur in disorders with atrophy or loss of muscle fibers in the motor unit. Thus, they

are present in all myopathic disorders. In severe cases of neuromuscular transmission disorders (e.g., botulism), the MUAP can also be small amplitude and short duration due to the majority of the neuromuscular junctions being blocked. In early reinnervation, after severe denervation in which the newly sprouting axons only begin to reinnervate a few muscle fibers, the MUAP will also be small, short duration, and polyphasic but with reduced recruitment ("nascent" MUAP).

Long-duration, large-amplitude motor unit action potentials occur with increased number or density of muscle fibers, or a loss of synchrony of fiber firing within a motor unit such as in chronic neuropathic processes, e.g., motor neuron disease, chronic radiculopathies, chronic axonal neuropathies, and chronic entrapment neuropathy.

Polyphasic motor unit action potentials (five or more phases). Polyphasia is a measure of synchrony of the firing of muscle fibers within the same motor unit. This is a nonspecific measure and may be abnormal in both myopathic and neurogenic disorders. Increased polyphasia may be seen in up to 5% to 10% of the MUAPs in any muscle and still be normal.

Unstable motor unit action potentials are fluctuations of amplitude, duration, or shape of a given motor unit potential from moment to moment, which are usually due to blocking of individual muscle fiber action potentials in the motor unit. This may be seen in disorders of neuromuscular transmission, myositis, muscle trauma, reinnervation, and rapidly progressive neurogenic atrophy.

2. Recruitment and Activation
Recruitment refers to the relation of firing rate of individual potentials to the total number of motor units firing. *Decreased recruitment* (small number of units firing with a high frequency) occurs when there is a decreased number of available motor units; the remaining motor units will fire at a faster frequency to increase the muscle force as in any neurogenic disorder or severe myopathy. *Early recruitment* (an excess of motor units for a given force) occurs in myopathies; when the force generated by each individual motor unit is decreased, more motor units are recruited to generate the same amount of force.

Activation refers to the ability to increase the firing rate, which is a central process. Poor activation of motor unit action potentials (small number of units firing slowly) is generally due to upper motor neuron lesions or lack of effort.

REFERENCES

Katirji B: In *Electromyography in clinical practice: A case study approach*, St. Louis, Mosby, 1998.

Preston DC, Shapiro BE: *Electromyography and neuromuscular disorders: Clinical-electrophysiologic correlations*, Boston, Butterworth-Heinemann, 1998.

E

ELECTROMYOGRAPHY AND NERVE CONDUCTION STUDIES (EMG/NCS)

ENCEPHALITIS

An inflammation of brain related to infectious, postinfectious, or demyelinating states. It can occur as an acute febrile illness associated with headache, seizures, lethargy, confusion, coma, ocular motor palsies, ataxia, abnormal movements, and myoclonus. Alternatively it may present as a slowly progressive afebrile disease. With viral infections, the meninges (meningoencephalitis) or the spinal cord (encephalomyelitis) are often involved. Compared to the high frequency of systemic viral infection, encephalitis is an uncommon complication. Prognosis of viral encephalitis depends upon the causative agent and the use of antiviral agents. Variable degrees of residua include impaired cognition and memory, behavioral changes, hemiparesis, or seizures.

Transmission of viruses can be from humans (e.g., HIV), animals (e.g., rabies), mosquitoes (e.g., St. Louis and Japanese encephalitis), ticks (e.g., Central European encephalitis), or other arthropods. Endemic causes in the United States are herpes simplex, West Nile virus (WNV), and rabies. Japanese B encephalitis is the most common epidemic infection outside North America. Arthropod-born viruses (Arboviruses) can be sporadic or epidemic. Viruses enter the central nervous system (CNS) by one of two routes—hematogenous (most common) or neuronal.

Diagnosis is difficult to confirm and sometimes is made by history alone. The season may help determine the pathogen. CSF usually shows a pleocytosis (mostly mononuclear cells) and mildly elevated protein. Glucose tends to be normal. Red blood cells (RBCs) can be found in certain encephalitis (e.g., herpes simplex). Acute and convalescent antibody levels from serum and CSF typically are only useful retrospectively. Polymerase chain reaction (PCR) testing facilitates the identification of causative agents.

I. Viral encephalitis.
    A. Herpes simplex encephalitis (HSV type 1).
        The most common cause of fatal viral encephalitis in the western world. Most cases represent reactivation of latent trigeminal ganglion infection. Onset is subacute with fever, headache, behavioral changes, seizures, and focal signs. Stupor and coma may result. EEG usually shows periodic lateralizing epileptiform discharges (PLEDS) between the second and 15th day of the illness. Spike and slow waves are common and often localized to the temporal lobe. CT scan, although less sensitive than EEG, may show temporal or insular low densities and focal hemorrhages or enhancement. MRI is the neuroimaging procedure of choice and may show increased signal intensity on T2WI in the medial and inferior temporal lobe extending to the insula. CSF usually shows 5 to 500 cells, elevated protein, normal or mildly decreased glucose, and elevated opening pressure. RBCs may be seen. Antibodies to HSV are detected in the CSF 8 to 12 days after onset of the disease and increase during the first 2 to 4 weeks. Viral cultures are not useful. PCR is >95% sensitive and 100% specific. False-negative results

may occur if there are RBC in the CSF to inhibit PCR reaction or if CSF is collected in the first 24 to 48 hours of symptoms or after 10 days of onset. Untreated, mortality is about 70%, with severe neurologic sequelae in most of the survivors. *Treatment* with acyclovir, 10 milligrams per kg q 8 hr for 2 to 3 weeks significantly reduces morbidity and mortality, especially if started early. Acyclovir-resistant HSV infection has been identified in immunodeficient patients. Brain biopsy should be considered in those who do not respond to therapy or in whom other diagnoses are possible. HSV-2 causes most cases of encephalitis in newborns. The risk of intrapartum transmission is 30% to 50% in primary maternal infection and <3 % with recurrent infection.

B. Rabies.

Carriers include skunks, foxes, dogs, bats, and raccoons. The virus is present in saliva and is transmitted by bite. Incubation is from days to months. Not everyone bitten by rabid animals contracts the disease. However, once the infection is established, death almost invariably occurs (usually within 18 days). The prodrome usually consists of headache, malaise, agitation, mental changes, seizures, dysphagia (causing hydrophobia), dysarthria, facial numbness, and spasm. The medulla and pons are most frequently and extensively involved, and paralysis may be secondary to spinal cord involvement. *Treatment* consists of mechanically scrubbing wound sites with soap and benzalkonium solution and administrating human rabies immunoglobulin or human diploid cell line rabies vaccine. Death is invariable once CNS manifestations occur.

C. Epidemic encephalitis.

Mostly arthropod transmitted. Peak incidence in late summer and fall. In the United States, St. Louis encephalitis and La Crosse virus (California encephalitis) are the most common. St. Louis encephalitis is found in the Ohio-Mississippi River basin, with a fatality of 10% to 20%. The La Crosse virus is the most common cause of pediatric arboviral encephalitis. Venezuelan equine encephalitis is found in the southeastern United States, with very low mortality; most infections result in flu-like illnesses. Eastern equine encephalitis occurs along the Gulf of Mexico and Atlantic seaboard, usually affects horses and birds, and is rare among humans. It has a 25% to 70% mortality, attacking the young and very old with a fulminant course. Western equine encephalitis occurs in west, southwest, and central North America. Treatment is aimed at brain edema and seizures.

WNV is a flavivirus that has birds as a reservoir and is transmitted by mosquitoes. It is endemic in the Middle East, Africa, and southwest Asia. Clinically it is characterized by abrupt onset of flulike illness. A maculopapular rash occurs in half of the patients. Meningitis or encephalitis is most common in older individuals and happens in less than 15% of patients. *Diagnosis* is by PCR or CSF culture, or identification of antibody in the serum and CSF. WNV was first identified in the United States in New York in 1999 and an increase in death of birds, particularly crows, can be observed during an outbreak. There is no specific treatment, and death may occur in older individuals.

D. Nonepidemic viral encephalitis

Enterovirus, ECHO, Coxsackievirus, polio, measles, mumps, Epstein-Barr virus (EBV), rubella, varicella zoster virus (VZV), and lymphocytic choriomeningitis virus can all cause sporadic encephalitis.

1. Slow latent viral infections cause slowly progressive disease with insidious onset and lack of fever. These include subacute sclerosing panencephalitis (SSPE), a form of chronic measles virus infection, progressive multifocal leukoencephalopathy (see PML below), and progressive rubella panencephalitis.

   SSPE has had dramatically decreased prevalence in countries with widespread use of the measles vaccine, but prevalence has increased with the occurrence of AIDS. Usually occurring in children or young adults, onset is insidious, with changes in cognition, vision, and behavior. Malaise and lethargy are common. Myoclonus can occur. Deterioration progresses over weeks to months, with patients becoming markedly demented. CSF shows a mild pleocytosis, increased protein, and occasionally decreased glucose. Neuroimaging shows generalized cortical atrophy. The EEG pattern of periodic discharges is characteristic. Pathological studies show changes suggestive of viral invasion of gray and white matter, with the hypothalamus and brainstem usually not involved.

2. AIDS and immune deficiency-related encephalitis.

   PML caused by a papovavirus designated JC virus (not associated with Creutzfeldt-Jakob disease), usually occurs in patients with lymphoproliferative (leukemia, lymphoma) or granulomatous disease, or during immunosuppression. It is characterized by multifocal white matter signs, such as impaired speech, vision, and cognition, progressing to death in 1 to 18 months. PCR for JC virus in CSF has a sensitivity of 72% to 92% and specificity of 92% to 96%. MRI shows multifocal white matter lesions.

   Encephalitis in immunosuppressed patients may also be caused by VZV, HSV-1, EBV, HHV-6, cytomegalovirus (CMV), measles virus, or enterovirus. In VZV encephalitis, patients may have a history of shingles for days or months previously. Encephalitis CMV is rare in immunocompetent individuals, and a combination of ganciclovir and foscarnet has been used in treatment.

II. Nonviral causes of encephalitis or encephalomyelitis.

A. Prion infections.

Prion (Proteinaceous infectious particle) diseases are sometimes confused with encephalitides, but they are slowly progressive with insidious onset and absence of fever. They include Creutzfeldt-Jakob disease, Gerstmann-Straussler-Scheinker syndrome, and Kuru (see Creutzfeldt-Jakob disease).

B. Rickettsia
Epidemic, murine and scrub typhus, Rocky Mountain spotted fever, Q fever.

C. Bacteria.
Listeria, brucellosis, pertussis, Legionnaire's disease, tuberculosis, tularemia, typhoid fever, bubonic plague, dysentery, cholera, melioidosis, psittacosis, leprosy, scarlet fever, rheumatic fever.

D. Spirochetes.
Relapsing fever, syphilis (meningovascular), rat bite fever, leptospirosis, Lyme disease.

E. Protozoa/metazoa.
Entamoeba, Naegleria, trypanosomiases, leishmaniasis, malaria, toxoplasmosis.

F. Helminthic.
Ancylostomiasis, angiostrongyliasis, ascariasis, cysticercosis, echinococcosis, filariasis, schistosomiasis, toxocariasis, trichinosis.

G. Miscellaneous.
Behçet's disease, CNS Whipple's disease, vasculitis, Rasmussen's syndrome (chronic focal encephalitis).

III. Postinfectious encephalomyelitis.

This may follow a CNS or systemic viral infection, nonviral infection, or immunization. In the United States, varicella and upper respiratory infections (especially influenza) are most commonly associated, whereas worldwide it most commonly follows measles. A disturbance of the immune system is the presumed cause, with an irreversible monophasic, demyelinating syndrome. Limited CNS forms may include acute transverse myelitis, acute cerebellitis, and postinfectious optic neuritis. Acute hemorrhagic encephalitis (Hurst's disease) is a severe and usually fatal form. The clinical symptoms and CSF profile are similar to that seen during direct viral infections. *Treatment* is with high doses of intravenous methylprednisolone. Acyclovir and ganciclovir are used if encephalitis by VZV and Human Herpes Virus 6 (HHV-6) are in the differential.

REFERENCES

Marra CM: *Semin Neurol* 20:323–327, 2000.
Roos KL: *Neurol Clin* 17:813–833, 1999.

ENCEPHALOPATHY

A nonspecific term for diffuse brain dysfunction, usually the result of a systemic condition. Initially, there is impaired attention, confusion, and disorientation. Later, there may be progression to stupor and coma, or it may present as coma of unknown cause. Associated features may include agitation, hallucination, myoclonus, asterixis, generalized seizures, or EEG slowing or triphasic waves. Additional evaluation should include review of recent medications, metabolic screening, consideration of systemic or CNS infection and neuroimaging.

ENCEPHALOPATHY, PERINATAL HYPOXIC-ISCHEMIC

Hypoxic-ischemic encephalopathy (HIE) is caused by either diminished oxygen delivery or diminished brain perfusion. Timing of insult may be antepartum (20%; maternal cardiac arrest or hemorrhage), intrapartum (35%; abruptio placenta, uterine rupture, or traumatic delivery), both (35%; maternal DM or infection, intrauterine growth retardation [IUGR]), or postnatal (10%; cardiovascular compromise, persistent fetal circulation, recurrent apnea; more common in premature infants).

Clinical features: The signs of HIE correlate with the severity of the insults. Mild encephalopathy lasts less then 24 hours. It is characterized by hyperalertness or by mild depression of the level of consciousness, which may be accompanied by uninhibited Moro and deep tendon reflexes, signs of sympathetic overdrive, or only slightly abnormal EEG. Infants with moderate to severe encephalopathy show variation in level of alertness in the first 12 to 24 hours. Seizures occur in 70% of these infants during this period. Coma may supervene and progress to brain death by 72 hours. If the infant survives, marked hypotonia and bulbar and autonomic dysfunction persist. Term infants may demonstrate quadri-paresis with predominant proximal and arm weakness. This pattern represents involvement of border zones of circulation between ACA-MCA and MCA-PCA. Premature infants manifest spastic diplegia primarily due to injury of motor fibers to the leg that lie dorsal and lateral to the external angles of the lateral ventricles.

Neuropathology: Patterns of injury are influenced by the nature of the insult and the gestational age of the infant at the time of injury. Patterns that occur in term infants include selective neuronal necrosis (CA1 region of hippocampus, deep layers of cerebral cortex, and cerebellar Purkinje fibers), status marmoratus of basal ganglia and thalamus, parasagittal cerebral injury, and focal and multifocal ischemic brain injury. Periventricular leukomalacia (PVL) represents the primary ischemic lesion of the premature infant.

Diagnostic tests: In preterm infants, head ultrasound (HUS) demon-strates periventicular echoes in the first day or two. After 1 to 3 weeks, lateral ventricles enlarge as these areas become cystic and gliosis super-venes. HUS in the term infant is especially accurate when used consecu-tively in the first weeks of life. Compared to HUS, MRI visualizes HIE injuries of basal ganglia better. Diffusion-weighted sequence on MRI detects focal cerebral ischemic injury very early in its course.

Management: Supportive care includes ensuring adequate oxygentation and perfusion, and seizure control.

Prognosis: Predictors of poor neurologic outcome include (1) acidosis at birth, (2) persistent moderate or severe HIE, (3) neonatal seizures, (4) interictal background abnormalities such as burst-suppression, persistently low-voltage, or electrocerebral inactivity, (5) HUS findings of periventricular intraparenchymal echodensities, and (6) extensive brain edema with effacement of cerebral cortex on MRI.

REFERENCE

Rivkin MJ: *Clin Perinatol* 24:607–625, 1997.

E

EPILEPSY

EPILEPSY

DEFINITIONS AND CLASSIFICATIONS

The epilepsies are a group of conditions marked by recurrent seizures, which are the clinical manifestations of abnormal brain electrical discharges. Epileptic seizures are classified as focal (partial, local), beginning in a part of one hemisphere, *generalized*, beginning bilaterally, or *unclassified* as to focal or generalized. Focal seizures that subsequently evolve to generalized seizures are said to exhibit secondary generalization.

INTERNATIONAL CLASSIFICATION OF EPILEPTIC SEIZURES

I. Partial.
   A. Simple partial seizures.
      1. With motor signs.
      2. With somatosensory or special sensory symptoms.
      3. With autonomic symptoms or signs.
      4. With psychic symptoms.
   B. Complex partial seizures.
      1. Simple partial onset.
      2. With impairment of consciousness at onset.
   C. Partial seizures evolving to secondarily generalized seizures.
      1. Simple partial seizures evolving to generalized seizures.
      2. Complex partial seizures evolving to generalized seizures.
      3. Simple partial seizures evolving to complex partial seizures evolving to generalized seizures.
II. Generalized seizures (convulsive or nonconvulsive).
   A. Absence seizures.
      1. Typical absence.
      2. Atypical absence.
   B. Myoclonic seizures.
   C. Clonic seizures.
   D. Tonic seizures.
   E. Tonic-clonic seizures.
   F. Atonic seizures (astatic seizures).
III. Unclassified seizures.

REVISED INTERNATIONAL CLASSIFICATION OF EPILEPSIES, EPILEPTIC SYNDROMES, AND RELATED SEIZURE DISORDERS

I. Localization-related (focal, local, partial).
  A. Idiopathic (primary).
    1. Benign childhood epilepsy with centrotemporal spikes ("benign rolandic epilepsy").
    2. Childhood epilepsy with occipital paroxysms.
    3. Primary reading epilepsy.
  B. Symptomatic (secondary).
    1. Temporal lobe epilepsies.
    2. Frontal lobe epilepsies.
    3. Parietal lobe epilepsies.
    4. Occipital lobe epilepsies.
    5. Chronic progressive epilepsia partialis continua of childhood (Kojewnikoff's syndrome).
    6. Syndromes characterized by seizures with specific modes of precipitation (e.g., reflex epilepsy or startle epilepsies).
  C. Cryptogenic, defined by:
    1. Seizure type.
    2. Clinical features.
    3. Etiology.
    4. Anatomic localization.
II. Generalized.
  A. Primary (idiopathic), in order of age of onset.
    1. Benign neonatal familial convulsions.
    2. Benign neonatal convulsions.
    3. Benign myoclonic epilepsy in infancy.
    4. Childhood absence epilepsy (pyknolepsy).
    5. Juvenile absence epilepsy.
    6. Juvenile myoclonic epilepsy (of Janz).
    7. Epilepsy with generalized tonic-clonic convulsions on awakening.
    8. Other generalized idiopathic epilepsies.
    9. Epilepsies with seizures precipitated by specific modes of activation.
  B. Cryptogenic or symptomatic, in order of age of onset.
    1. West's syndrome.
    2. Lennox-Gastaut syndrome.
    3. Epilepsy with myoclonic-astatic seizures.
    4. Epilepsy with myoclonic absences.
  C. Symptomatic (secondary).
    1. Nonspecific etiology.
      a. Early myoclonic encephalopathy.
      b. Early infantile epileptic encephalopathy with suppression bursts.
      c. Other symptomatic generalized epilepsies.
    2. Specific syndromes.
      a. Neurologic diseases with seizures as a prominent feature.

III. Epilepsies undetermined whether focal or generalized.
  A. With both focal and generalized seizures.
    1. Neonatal seizures.
    2. Severe myoclonic epilepsy of infancy.
    3. Epilepsy with continuous spike waves during slow-wave sleep.
    4. Acquired epileptic aphasia (Landau-Kleffner syndrome).
    5. Other undetermined epilepsies.
IV. Special syndromes.
  A. Situation-related seizures.
    1. Febrile convulsions.
    2. Isolated seizures or isolated status epilepticus.
    3. Seizures occurring only with acute metabolic or toxic events due to factors such as alcohol, drugs, eclampsia, and nonketotic hyperglycemia.

DIFFERENTIAL DIAGNOSIS OF EPILEPSY

Conditions producing symptoms or signs that may be mistaken for epileptic seizures include the following: (1) syncope, (2) transient ischemic attacks, (3) migraine, (4) metabolic derangements (e.g., hypoglycemia), (5) parasomnias, (6) transient global amnesia, (7) paroxysmal movement disorders (e.g., paroxysmal kinesigenic choreoathetosis), and (8) nonepileptic seizures (pseudo-seizures).

Nonepileptic seizures are common and may coexist in patients with epileptic seizures. They are associated with a variety of psychiatric syndromes, including somatoform disorders, panic disorders, dissociative disorders, psychotic disorders, factitious disorders, and malingering. They may be difficult to distinguish from epileptic seizures, especially of mesial temporal, basal frontal, and supplementary motor area origin. Seizures originating from these areas may not be associated with scalp ictal EEG changes (see EEG).

SELECTED EPILEPSY SYNDROMES
Idiopathic Syndromes

Benign childhood epilepsy with centrotemporal spikes (Benign Rolandic epilepsy) is a common autosomal dominant syndrome producing nocturnal generalized convulsions in otherwise normal children. Focal motor or sensory seizures, often involving the face, may occur. The EEG shows characteristic interictal centrotemporal spikes. Seizures are easily controlled with phenytoin or carbamazepine, and spontaneously disappear before adulthood.

Childhood absence epilepsy (pyknolepsy) occurs in genetically predisposed but otherwise normal children and is marked by typical absence seizures with a corresponding 3-Hz generalized spike-and-wave EEG discharge. Typical absences are not preceded by an aura nor followed by postictal confusion. Generalized tonic clonic seizures may also occur. Treatment consists of ethosuximide, effective for absence seizures only, and valproic acid, effective for both isolated absence seizures or absences complicated by or with generalized tonic clonic seizures. Absence seizures rarely persist into adulthood.

Juvenile myoclonic epilepsy (of Janz) is a genetic epilepsy syndrome whose gene has been mapped to chromosome 6. It presents in normal teenagers with early morning myoclonic jerks and generalized tonic clonic seizures. Sleep deprivation and photic stimulation are often activating influences. The interictal EEG typically shows 4- to 6-Hz generalized irregular spike-wave or polyspike-wave discharges with normal background. Valproate is highly effective, but relapses are the rule following drug discontinuation.

Symptomatic or Cryptogenic Syndromes

West's syndrome consists of the triad of infantile spasms, developmental arrest, and the interictal EEG pattern hypsarrhythmia, consisting of very high voltage multifocal spikes, sharp waves, and slow waves in a chaotic distribution. The syndrome may be cryptogenic or symptomatic of a variety of brain insults and is generally treated with ACTH (typically 40 units IM daily, increasing by 10 units per week as needed to a maximum of 80 units daily) or other corticosteroids. Prognosis is unfavorable and is worse in the cryptogenic than in the symptomatic group. *Lennox Gastaut syndrome* is characterized by multiple, difficult to control seizure types, especially atonic seizures and atypical absences in addition to generalized convulsions, mental retardation, and an abnormal interictal EEG with generalized 2- to 2.5-Hz slow spike and wave discharges. The syndrome often follows West's syndrome in an affected child and is associated with a poor prognosis. Valproate is the drug of choice because of its efficacy against the multiple seizure types, and felbamate is also beneficial. Polytherapy may be necessary. Surgical section of the corpus callosum is sometimes effective in controlling drop attacks.

Symptomatic Syndromes

Temporal lobe epilepsy (TLE), the most common symptomatic, localization-related epilepsy, causes simple partial, complex partial, and secondarily generalized seizures as a result of ictal discharges typically arising from mesial temporal structures such as the hippocampus or amygdala. The interictal EEG often shows unilateral or bilateral, usually anterior, temporal spikes. The most common associated lesion is hippocampal (mesial temporal) sclerosis; others include hamartomas, neoplasms (especially low-grade gliomas), cortical dysplasia, and vascular malformations. MRI scanning, using thin coronal sections through temporal structures, is the imaging modality of choice and may show unilateral hippocampal atrophy with enlargement of the ipsilateral temporal horn and increased hippocampal signal on T2-weighted images, suggestive of hippocampal sclerosis. Phenytoin and carbamazepine are equally effective in treating symptomatic partial epilepsies such as TLE. Valproate is as effective in treating secondarily generalized seizures but not as effective for partial seizures. Newer anticonvulsants are also indicated for treating partial complex seizures. Surgical resection, typically anterior temporal lobectomy, eliminates seizures in about 70% of medically refractory patients in whom the epileptogenic lesion can be accurately localized. Vagal nerve stimulation is also effective in treating this syndrome.

Posttraumatic epilepsy typically begins 6 months to 2 years following head trauma. Risk factors include intracranial hemorrhage, depressed skull fracture, early seizures, or duration of posttraumatic amnesia greater than 24 hours. Phenytoin reduces the incidence of seizures within the first week following head trauma but is not effective as prophylaxis against the development of posttraumatic epilepsy.

Other Syndromes

Febrile seizures are typically generalized convulsions, occurring in children between 3 months and 5 years of age, associated with fever but without evidence of intracranial infection or defined cause. They are common, occurring in 2% to 5% of children in this country, and tend to run in families. They usually occur during the early, rising temperature phase of an infectious illness. Most febrile seizures are *simple*, lasting less than 15 minutes and without focality; if the seizure is prolonged or focal, it is *complex* and associated with a higher risk of subsequent afebrile epilepsy. Other risk factors for seizure recurrence include more than one seizure in 24 hours, abnormal neurologic exam, and afebrile seizures in a parent or sibling. Overall, 6% to 13% of patients with two or more risk factors will develop afebrile epilepsy, compared to 0.9% without risk factors. There is no evidence that prophylactic treatment with anticonvulsants prevents future epilepsy. Phenobarbital, diazepam, and valproate (but not phenytoin or carbamazepine) reduce the rate of recurrent febrile seizures, but in most cases they are not recommended, since two-thirds of children will never have another febrile seizure and there is no evidence of mental or neurologic impairment due to febrile seizures. Rectal benzodiazepines may be useful for prevention of recurrent complicated febrile seizures.

Neonatal seizures are nearly always symptomatic, occurring as a result of a large number of brain insults; idiopathic syndromes are rare. The most common causes include hypoxic-ischemic encephalopathy, hypoglycemia, hypocalcemia, hyponatremia and hypernatremia, intraventricular or periventricular hemorrhage, central nervous system infections, cerebral malformations, inborn errors of metabolism, and drug withdrawal or intoxication. Neonatal seizures are classified clinically as subtle, tonic, clonic, and myoclonic (Volpe, 1989); generalized tonic-clonic convulsions are rare in the neonatal period. Neonatal seizures commonly occur electrographically without clear clinical change and may occur clinically without a clear EEG ictal pattern. Jitteriness is a benign nonepileptic phenomenon consisting of rapid, stimulus-sensitive movements of all four extremities, abolished by passive restraint of the limbs. Treatment of neonatal seizures most commonly involves phenobarbital (loading dose 20 mg/kg followed by maintenance dose of 3 to

4 mg/kg/day to achieve blood level of 16 to 40 mg/ml) or phenytoin (loading dose 15 to 20 mg/kg followed by maintenance dose 3 to 5 mg/kg/day to achieve blood level of 6 to 14 mg/ml). Hypocalcemia is treated with 5% calcium gluconate, 4 ml/kg IV, and hypomagnesemia with 50% magnesium sulfate, 0.2 ml/kg IV. Pyridoxine 50 to 100 mg IV should be given if seizures continue and the cause is uncertain. Duration of treatment once seizures are controlled is controversial.

STATUS EPILEPTICUS

A. Generalized tonic-clonic status epilepticus (GTCSE) is a medical emergency diagnosed either when two or more discrete seizures occur without complete recovery of consciousness or when a continuous seizure lasts at least 5 minutes. The likelihood of brain damage or death is directly related to the duration of GTCSE. GTCSE is more easily controlled when no new structural brain insult has occurred, as in withdrawal from anticonvulsants, drugs, or alcohol. More refractory cases may be seen in anoxic encephalopathy, stroke, hemorrhage, neoplasm, trauma, infection, or metabolic derangement. In general, the longer the duration of GTCSE, the more difficult it is to treat. A characteristic progression of EEG patterns in GTCSE has been described: (1) discrete seizures, (2) waxing and waning ictal discharges, (3) continuous ictal discharges, (4) continuous ictal discharges punctuated by flat periods, and (5) bilateral periodic epileptiform discharges on a flat background. In the latter stages, the patient may exhibit only subtle or no motor activity. Management of GTCSE must be carried out quickly. Treatment protocols are based on the following pharmacological properties of commonly used drugs (see Tables 26–31).

B. *Absence status epilepticus (spike-wave stupor)* constitutes continuous generalized spike-wave discharges with alteration of consciousness. It occurs more commonly in children with secondarily generalized epilepsy such as Lennox-Gastaut syndrome rather than with pyknolepsy. It may also occur sporadically in adults with no prior history of epilepsy. Treatment of the childhood condition consists of IV diazepam (0.3 to 0.5 mg/kg, no faster than 1 to 2 mg/min) followed by valproic acid. The adult form responds to the protocol listed for GTCSE. Because this condition is not life-threatening and residual brain damage is unproven, use of general anesthesia is not generally recommended.

Text continued on page 142

TABLE 26

COMPARISON OF MEDICATIONS COMMONLY USED TO TREAT STATUS EPILEPTICUS

Time	Diazepam	Lorazepam	Phenytoin	Phenobarbital
To reach brain	10 sec	2–3 min	1 min	20 min
To peak brain concentration	<5 min	30 min	15–30 min	30 min
To stop status	1 min	<5 min	15–30 min	20 min
Effective half-life	15 min	6 hr	>22 hr	50–120 hr

TABLE 27

AN APPROACH TO THE TREATMENT OF GTCSE

Action	Cumulative Time Frame
1. *Stabilization and diagnosis:* Secure an airway, administer oxygen, and be prepared to intubate quickly; assess vital signs, including rectal temperature, and treat hyperpyrexia appropriately; Insert 2 large bore IVs; obtain EKG, blood glucose, anticonvulsant levels, CBC, BUN, electrolytes, calcium, magnesium, phosphorus, serum and urine toxicology screens, and arterial blood gases; administer 100 mg thiamine IV and 50 ml of 50% glucose IV if necessary; obtain history and perform neurologic examination; consider possibility of nonconvulsive seizures.	0–15 min
2. *Stop seizures:* Through one IV, administer phenytoin 20 mg/kg no faster than 50 mg/min. Contraindications to phenytoin include documented allergy, significant heart block, or severe bradycardia. (If phenytoin is contraindicated, administer phenobarbital as described below or valproic acid at 20–25 mg/kg IV). EKG should be monitored continuously, and blood pressure taken frequently. If significant rhythm disturbances or hypotension occur during phenytoin infusion, reduce the rate to 25 mg/min. Fosphenytoin, a prodrug, can be used IM or IV, infusing at 20 mg/kg phenytoin equivalents, with a maximum rate of 150 mg/min. If additional seizures occur while phenytoin is being infused, administer either diazepam (no faster than 2 mg/min, to maximum 20 mg) or lorazepam (the preferred agent due to its longer half-life) no faster than 2 mg/min, to maximum 0.1 mg/kg, no more than 8 mg through the second IV, to avoid interrupting the phenytoin infusion. Benzodiazepines may cause respiratory depression.	15–60 min
3. *If seizures persist:* Following infusion of phenytoin, administer an additional 10 mg/kg phenytoin/fosphenytoin IV, no faster than 50 mg/min or try valproic acid at 20–25 mg/kg IV, at a maximum rate of 50–100 mg/min.	60–120 min
4. *If seizures persist:* Intubate the patient, if not already done. Obtain emergency EEG monitoring; administer phenobarbital IV 20 mg/kg at a rate of 50–75 mg/min, until seizures stop. Carefully monitor blood pressure and EKG.	120 min
5. *If seizures persist:* Induce general anesthesia with short (thiopental) or intermediate (pentobarbital) half-life barbiturates. Pentobarbital is given IV as a 5- to 10-mg/kg loading dose (no faster than 25 mg/min), followed by initial maintenance dose of 1–3 mg/kg/hr. Midazolam (loading dose 0.2–0.3 mg/kg, with maintenance of 0.1–0.2 mg/kg/hr or propofol (loading dose 1–2 mg/kg with a maintenance of 2–10 mg/kg/hr) anesthesia can also be employed in refractory cases. Adjust doses to achieve burst-suppression pattern on EEG with minimal blood pressure reduction. Pressor support may be required. Infusions should be utilized for at least 12 hours and used in conjunction with other antiepileptic agents.	
6. *Other maneuvers:* Concurrently with above, treat metabolic or toxic conditions; ensure adequate hydration, keep blood glucose between 100 and 150 mg/dl and core body temperature <37.5°C. If there is clinical suspicion for new brain insult, obtain neuroimaging once GTCSE is aborted. Perform LP following neuroimaging and treat appropriately in cases suggestive of CNS infection.	

E

EPILEPSY

TABLE 28

COMMON ANTIEPILEPTIC DRUGS: PRESCRIBING INFORMATION

Drug	Preparations	Average Target Plasma Concentrations (mg/L)*	Monotherapy Dose	Approximate Half-Life	Protein Binding
Phenytoin (Dilantin)	30 mg, 100 mg caps, 50 mg tabs, 30 or 125 mg/5 mg elixirs	10–20 (6–14 in neonates to 12 weeks)	Neonates: 15–20 mg/kg, then 3–5 mg/kg/day in divided doses Infants: 15 mg/kg, then 3–5 mg/kg/day in 3–4 doses Children: 15 mg/kg, then 5–15 mg/kg/day in 2 doses Adults: 15 mg/kg, then 5 mg/kg/day, once daily	Variable	90%
Phenobarbital (Luminal)	15, 30, 60, 130 mg tabs 20 mg/5 ml elixir	15–40	Infants, children: 6–16 mg/kg, then 3–8 mg/kg/day Adults: 4–8 mg/kg, then 2–4 mg/kg/day, single dose	40–70 hr 50–120 hr	50%
Primidone (Mysoline)	50, 250 mg tabs 250 mg/5 ml elixir	5–12 (metabolized also to phenobarbital)	Children: 50 mg/day, increasing 50 mg q 3 days to 15–25 mg/kg in 2–4 doses Adults: 250 mg/day in 2 doses; start with 100 mg at bedtime and increase by 100 mg q 3 days to 10–20 mg/kg/day in two to four doses	10–12 hr	<5%

Carbamazepine (Tegretol)	100, 200 mg tabs 100 mg/5 ml suspension	4–12	Children: 100 mg bid, increasing 100 mg qod to 15–20 mg/kg/day in three to four doses	5–27 hr	75%
			Adults: 200 mg bid, increasing 100 mg qod to 7–15 mg/kg/day in three to four doses		
Ethosuximide (Zarontin)	250 mg caps 250 mg/5 ml elixir	40–100	Children: 250 mg/day, increasing 250 mg q 4–7 days to 15–40 mg/kg/day in three to four doses	30 hr 50–60 hr	0%
			Adults: 250 mg bid, increasing 250 mg q 4–7 days to 15–30 mg/kg/day in three to four doses		
Valproic acid (Depakene)	250 mg tabs 250 mg/5 ml elixir	50–100	Children: 10–15 mg/kg/day, increasing 5–10 mg/kg/day q 1 week to 15–100 mg/kg/day in three to four doses	4–14 hr 6–16 hr	75–90% (inverse to concentration)
			Adults: 10–15 mg/kg/day, increasing 5–10 mg/kg/day q 1 week to 15–45 mg/kg/day in three to four doses		
Divalproex Sodium (Depakote)	125, 250, 500 mg tabs	50–100	Same as valproic acid except given in two to three doses	Same	75–90% (inverse to concentration)

Table continued on following page

E

EPILEPSY

TABLE 28 —cont'd
COMMON ANTIEPILEPTIC DRUGS: PRESCRIBING INFORMATION

Drug	Preparations	Average Target Plasma Concentrations (mg/L)*	Monotherapy Dose	Approximate Half-Life	Protein Binding
Clonazepam (Klonopin)	0.5, 1, 2 mg tabs	Not usually monitored	Children: 0.01–0.03 mg/kg/day, increasing 0.25–0.5 mg q 3 days to 0.1–0.2 mg/kg/day in three doses Adults: 0.5 mg/day, increasing 0.5–1.0 mg/day q 3 days	18–50 hr 18–50 hr	85%
Felbamate (Felbatol)	400, 600 mg tabs 600 mg/5 ml elixir	Not usually monitored	Children (adjunctive): 15 mg/kg/day three or four times daily Adult: 1200 mg/day, increasing 600 mg q 2 weeks up to 3600 mg/day	14–20	25%
Lamotrigine (Lamictal)	25, 50,100, 200 mg tabs	0.5–3.0 mg/ml	50 mg q HS increasing 50 mg q 2 weeks, as tolerated, divided into two doses	12–50 hr	55%
Levitoracetam (Keppra)	250, 500, 750 mg tabs	Not usually monitored	Children: 20–40 mg/kg Adults: 500 mg bid increasing up to 1500 mg bid	6–8 hr	<10%
Tiagabine (Gabitril)	2, 4, 12, 16, 20 mg tabs	Not usually monitored	4 mg q days, increasing at weekly intervals by 4–8 mg up to 56 mg/day	4–9 hr (shorter if on hepatic inducing AEDS)	95%
Topiramate (Topamax)	25, 100, 200 mg tabs 15, 25 mg sprinkle capsules	Not usually monitored	Initial 25–50 mg/day increasing by 25–50 mg increments to 20 mg bid as tolerated	20 hr	

Oxcarbazine (Trileptal)	150, 300, 600 mg tabs	4–12 (10-monohydroxy metabolite)	Children: 8–10 mg/kg/day increasing up to 20–40 mg/kg/day Adults: 150–300 mg bid up to 1200 mg bid	2 hr	40%
Zonisamide (Zonegran)	100 mg capsules	Not usually monitored	Children: 2–4 mg/kg/day Adults: 100–200 mg/day increasing up to 400–600 mg/day	60 hr	<10%
Gabapentin (Neurontin)	100, 300, 400 mg tabs 600, 800mg tabs	Not usually monitored	300 mg/day, increasing up to 900–1800 mg/day over 2–3 days divided into three to four doses	5–7 hr	0%

* Many patients will respond at different plasma concentrations, below or above the average plasma concentrations.

EPILEPSY

E

TABLE 29

DOSE-RELATED ADVERSE EFFECTS OF ANTIEPILEPTIC DRUGS

Drug	Side Effects
Phenytoin	*Acute*: Drowsiness, ataxia, diplopia, GI complaints, choreoathetosis, nausea, hypotension (after parenteral use), heart block *Chronic*: Gingival hyperplasia, hirsutism, folate deficiency, megaloblastic anemia, osteomalacia with vitamin D deficiency, peripheral neuropathy, encephalopathy, cerebellar dysfunction, pseudolymphoma, hemorrhage in the newborn
Phenobarbital	*Acute*: Sedation, behavior disturbance, ataxia *Chronic*: Attentional difficulty, hemorrhage in the newborn rheumatic syndrome
Primidone	*Acute*: Sedation, nausea, vertigo, ataxia *Chronic*: Behaviour disturbances (in children), loss of libido, attentional difficulties, hemorrhage in the newborn
Carbamazepine	*Acute*: Diplopia, vertigo, blurred vision, sedation, dry mouth stomatitis, hyponatremia (SIADH), headache, diarrhea, constipation, paresthesias *Chronic*: Liver enzyme induction, leukopenia, nervousness, hemorrhage in the newborn
Ethosuximide	*Acute*: Nausea, vertigo, vomiting, hiccups, headache *Chronic*: Insomnia, nervousness
Valproate	*Acute*: Sedation, GI disturbances *Chronic*: Weight gain, hepatic enzyme elevation, hyperammonemia, granulopenia, thrombocytopenia, alopecia, tremor
Clonazepam	*Acute*: Sedation, ataxia, irritability, hypersalivation *Chronic*: Behavior disturbances, tolerance, and withdrawal syndrome
Felbamate	*Acute*: GI disturbances, insomnia, headache, fatigue, nausea, vomiting *Chronic*: Weight loss
Lamotrigine	Rash, diplopia, sedation, dizziness, ataxia, headache, nausea, vomiting
Topiramate	Somnolence with confusion, psychomotor slowing, weight loss, speech disorders, ataxia, paresthesias, renal calculi
Oxcarbazine	Hyponatremia, headache, somnolence, nausea, vomiting, diplopia
Tiagabine	Somnolence, dizziness, attentional difficulties
Levetiracetam	Dizziness, somnolence, fatigue
Zonisamide	Renal calculi, kidney dysfunction, somnolence, fatigue, confusion, anorexia, ataxia, dizziness
Gabapentin	Sedation, fatigue, dizziness, nausea, weight gain, ataxia, headache and diplopia

TABLE 30
FACTORS AFFECTING SERUM CONCENTRATIONS OF ANTICONVULSANTS AND OTHER DRUG INTERACTIONS

Drug	Increased by AEDs	Increased by Other Drugs	Increased in Clinical State	Decreased by AEDs	Decreased by Other Drugs	Decreased by Clinical State	Interacts with Other Drugs
Phenytoin	Diazepam Ethosuximide Felbamate Oxcarbazine Phenobarbital Primidone Topiramate Valproic acid	Alcohol (acute) Amiodarone Amphetamines Aspirin Chloramphenicol Chlordiazepoxide Chlorpheniramine Cimetidine Diazepam Disulfiram Dicumarol Estrogens H2 antagonists Isoniazid Methylphenidate Omeprazole Phenylbutazone Phenothiazines Propoxyphene Sulfonamides Tolbutamide Trazodone	Hepatic disease	Phenobarbital Carbamazepine Clonazepam	Alcohol (chronic) Antineoplastics Loxepine Nicotine Nitrofurantoin Sucralfate Theophylline Tube feedings	Acute hepatitis Mononucleosis Pregnancy Renal disease	Corticosteroids Cyclosporine Ketoconazole Methadone Oral contraceptives Protease inhibitors Rifampin Tacrolimus Trazodone Warfarin
Phenobarbital	Valproid acid Phenytoin Felbamate	Alcohol MAO inhibitors	Acidic urine Hepatic disease Renal disease	Clonazepam	Chloramphenicol Dicumarol Phenylbutazone	Alkaline Urine	Chloramphenicol Cimetidine Folic acid Haloperidol Oral contraceptives Phenylbutazone

Table continued on following page

E

EPILEPSY

TABLE 30 —cont'd

FACTORS AFFECTING SERUM CONCENTRATIONS OF ANTICONVULSANTS AND OTHER INTERACTIONS

Drug	Increased by AEDs	Increased by Other Drugs	Increased in Clinical State	Decreased by AEDs	Decreased by Other Drugs	Decreased by Clinical State	Interacts with Other Drugs
Primidone	Valproic acid Clonazepam	—	—	Carbamazepine Phenytoin	—	—	Same list as Phenytoin
Carbamazepine	Felbamate (↑10, 11 Epoxide)	Cimetidine Diltiazem Erythromycin Fluoxetine Fluvoxamine Grapefruit juice Isoniazid Propoxyphene Sertraline Verapamil	Hepatic disease	Ethosuximide Felbamate Phenobarbital Phenytoin Primidone Valproic acid	—	Pregnancy	Corticosteroids Doxycycline Ketoconazole Lithium Oral contraceptives Protase inhibitors Quinidine Rifampin Tacrolimus Thyroid hormone Warfarin
Valproic acid	Felbamate	Salicylates	Hepatic disease	Carbamazepine Phenytoin Phenobarbital Primidone	Rifampin	—	Amitryptyline Nortriptyline Tolbutamide Warfarin Zidovudine
Ethosuximide	—	—	—	Carbamazepine Phenytoin Phenobarbital Primidone Valproic acid	—	—	—

Clonazepam	—	—	—	—	Antifungal agents (possibly)	—
Felbamate	—	—	Carbamazepine Phenytoin Phenobarbital	Phenytoin Carbamazepine All hepatic inducing AEDs	—	—
Lamotrigine	Valproic acid	Hepatic disease Renal failure	Phenytoin Carbamazepine	—	—	Methotrexate
Topiramate	—	Renal disease Hepatic disease (Possibly)	Phenytoin Carbamazepine	—	—	Carbonic Anhydrase inhibitors
Tiagabine	—	Hepatic disease	Phenytoin Phenobarbital Carbamazepine	—	—	—
Zonisamide	—	—	Phenytoin Carbamazepine Lamotrigine	—	—	—
Levetiracetam	—	Renal failure	—	—	—	—
Oxcarbazepine	—	Renal failure	Phenytoin Carbamazepine Lamotrigine Phenobarbital Valproic acid	—	—	Oral contraceptives See list for Carbamazepine
Gabapentin	—	Renal failure	—	Antacids	—	—

AED, Antiepileptic drugs.

TABLE 31

IDIOSYNCRATIC ADVERSE EFFECTS OF ANTIEPILEPTIC DRUGS*

Effect	Drug Type
Skin rash	All antiepileptic drugs
Erythema multiforme	All; more likely with ethosuximide
Stevens-Johnson syndrome	All
Exfoliative dermatitis	All
Systemic lupus erythematosus	Phenytoin, ethosuximide
Bone marrow depression	Most, including phenytoin, primidone, carbamazepine, ethosuximide, valproic acid, felbamate
Thrombocytopenia	Valproic acid; rare with phenytoin, phenobarbital, clonazepam
Lymphadenopathy	Phenytoin, ethosuximide
Hepatic toxicity	Valproic acid (usually in first 6 months of therapy), phenytoin, carbamazepine
Pancreatic toxicity	Valproic acid

Adapted from Dreifuss FE: In Ward AA, Penry JK, Purpura D, eds: *Epilepsy*, ed 1, New York, Raven, 1983.

C. *Simple partial status epilepticus (epilepsia partialis continua)* most commonly involves continuous clonic focal motor seizures, but other manifestations such as aphasia, head and eye deviation, somatosensory changes, visual disturbances, and autonomic symptoms may occur. Ictal EEG may be normal. Focal motor status is often seen in the setting of metabolic derangements, particularly nonketotic hyperglycemia. Treatment in this case consists of correcting metabolic abnormalities. Slow loading with IV diazepam or lorazepam to avoid respiratory depression, followed by phenytoin, may also be used.

D. *Complex partial status epilepticus* may consist of repeated discrete complex partial seizures without full clearing of consciousness or as a more continuous clouding of consciousness, mimicking a confusional state. EEG is diagnostic. Treatment initially is identical to the protocol listed for GTCSE, although the use of general anesthesia (e.g., thiopental, midazolam, propofol) if initial maneuvers may be indicated.

E. *Generalized convulsive status epilepticus* in children is treated as in adults with the following modifications: use diazepam 0.25 mg/kg IV, no faster than 1 to 2 mg/min. If there is a delay in obtaining an IV in a small child, this dose may be administered rectally via a feeding tube flushed with saline. Phenytoin 18 to 20 mg/kg is given IV over 20 minutes. If seizures persist, be prepared to intubate, and give phenobarbital 15 to 20 mg/kg IV no faster than 60 mg/min, with additional doses of 10 mg/kg as needed to control seizures. Recent studies have shown the benefit of valproic acid at 20 to 25 mg/kg IV in patients allergic to dilantin or phenobarbital, or as an adjunct to these agents in convulsive status epilepticus.

F. *Neonatal status epilepticus* must be diagnosed using EEG monitoring because of the frequent dissociation between electrographic and clinical seizure activity. Treatment is as outlined for neonatal seizures, above. Diazepam 0.3 to 0.5 mg/kg IV or lorazepam 0.1 mg/kg IV may be given in refractory cases but are contraindicated in jaundiced neonates.

ANTIEPILEPTIC DRUGS (AED)

Selection of an AED is based on clinical and electrographic identification of seizure type. The dose is increased until seizures are controlled or clinical toxicity develops. If the drug is ineffective when taken in toxic doses, it is generally recommended to switch to another monotherapy with another agent before using drug combinations. Drug levels may be useful to answer specific questions regarding compliance, toxicity, or individual pharmacokinetics. Free levels of highly protein—bound drugs such as phenytoin, carbamazepine, or valproic acid may be helpful during hypoalbuminemic states, renal or hepatic disease, pregnancy, malignancy, sepsis, burns, or in the presence of other drugs that displace protein binding. The use of serial laboratory monitoring to prevent serious idiosyncratic reaction is of little value. It may be implemented in high-risk patients (children under age 2, especially treated with polytherapy, patients with urea cycle defects, organic acidurias, mitochondrial disorders, GMI gangliosidosis, and neurodegenerative diseases) and in those with a history of adverse drug reactions. Abnormalities such as mild leukopenia or elevated hepatic enzymes are not predictive of severe complications. Current recommendations include the following: (1) obtain initial baseline blood work prior to initiation of therapy, including CBC with differential, liver and kidney function tests, lipid profile, PT, PTT; (2) refrain from subsequent routine monitoring in asymptomatic patients; (3) counsel patients and family to notify you immediately should any of the following develop: bruising, bleeding, rash, abdominal pain, vomiting, jaundice, lethargy, coma, or marked increase in seizure frequency; (4) for multiply handicapped, institutionalized patients who may not be able to communicate the above, annual routine blood monitoring may be of value.

REFERENCES

Browns TR: *Neurology* 40:S28–S32, 1990.
Dodson WE: *Neurology* 39:1009–1010, 1989.
Engel J Jr: *Seizures and epilepsy*, Philadelphia, FA Davis, 1989.
Gates JR: Roman AJ(eds): *Non-epileptic seizures*, Boston, Butterworth-Heinemann, 2000.
Mattson RH et al: *N Engl J Med* 327:765–771, 1992.
Temkin NR: *N Engl J Med* 323:497–502, 1990.
Treiman DM: *Adv Neurol* 34:377–384, 1983.
Treiman DM et al: *Epilepsy Res* 5(1):49–60, 1990.
Volpe JL: *Pediatrics* 84:422–428, 1989.
Wyllie E ed.: *The treatment of epilepsy, principles and practice, ed 3,* Philadelphia, Lippincott Williams & Wilkins, 2001.

Zaidat OO, Suarez JI: Neurosurgical care of the elderly, In *Geriatric neurosurgery*, Park Ridge, AANS, 1999.

EVOKED POTENTIALS

Evoked potentials (EPs) are recordable changes in the electrical activity of the nervous system in response to an external stimulus. They are an adjunct to the history and physical exam and may provide corroborative evidence of disease of the nervous system. EPs utilize the functional integrity of the nervous system to provide information about the anatomical location of lesions. They may detect the presence of lesions that are not clinically apparent, but are of little value in providing clues to the origin or cause of the lesions.

The clinically useful EPs are derived from stimulation of one of the modalities of the sensory system—visual (VEP), brainstem auditory (BAEP), and somatosensory (SEP)— and are recorded from electrodes on the scalp. Because of the low voltage of EPs (100 times smaller than the scalp EEG), multiple stimulations with averaging and filtering are necessary to separate the signal from background noise. The actual signal recorded may be either "near-field" (the electrode is placed *near* the generator of the signal in the cortex, for example, P100 wave of the VEP generated by the occipital cortex) or "far-field" (the electrode is placed *far* from the generator of the signal, which is volume conducted through the tissues of the body to the recording electrodes on the scalp, for example, P11 wave of the SEP generated by the dorsal root entry zone). In general, the latency from stimulus to recorded potential is more important than signal amplitude. The potentials are usually designated by the letter "P" or "N" followed by a number. "P100" is a wave of *positive* deflection occurring at a latency of 100 ms. "N20" is a wave of *negative* deflection occurring at a latency of 20 ms. By convention, "positive" is a downward and "negative" an upward needle deflection. It should be remembered that *absolute latencies and standard deviations are quite laboratory specific* (Figure 14).

Electroretinograms (ERGs) are derived from stimulation of the retina with light while recording electrical activity directly from the cornea. When combined with VEPs, ERGs can be useful in prognosis for recovery of visual function and differentiation of retinal from optic nerve disease.

Motor-evoked potentials (MEP) are derived from stimulating the CNS motor system with magnetically induced or directly applied electrical current. Recordings are made from electrodes placed over muscles. MEPs have yet to gain significant clinical use and will not be discussed further.

Visual-evoked potentials are primarily used to detect *anterochiasmatic* lesions of the visual system. Their usefulness in retrochiasmatic lesions is minimal. The most useful VEPs are generated by checkerboard pattern-reversal stimuli that evoke large, reproducible potentials. Check sizes sub-tending greater than 40 degrees of arc preferentially stimulate retinal

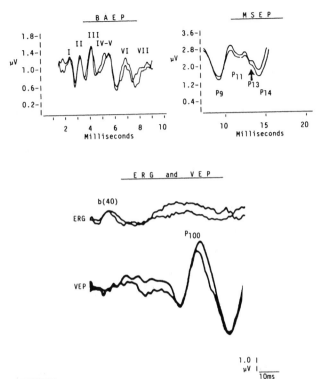

FIGURE 14

Normal evoked potentials.

luminance channels. Those less than 30 degrees stimulate contrast and spatial frequency detectors, and those less than 15 degrees mainly stimulate the fovea. *P100* is the most useful and reproducible wave. It is generated by the striate cortex as a near-field potential and recorded from electrodes placed over the occipital cortex. A significant prolongation of latency between eyes with alternate *full-field monocular* stimulation is evidence for anterochiasmatic disease on the side with prolonged latency. P100 may be bilaterally absent or prolonged with chiasmatic lesions. Refractive errors and macular disease can affect both the latency and amplitude of VEPs (see also Electroretinograms below).

Brainstem auditory-evoked potentials detect lesions of the auditory system and mid-upper brainstem. Click stimuli of 50 to 100 μs square-wave pulses to headphones or ear-insert transducers are used to elicit seven recordable potentials at the scalp. Waves I through VII occur within 10 ms after stimulation and are generated by propogating action potentials within the eighth cranial nerve (CN) and central auditory pathways. They are volume conducted to the scalp and recorded there as far-field potentials. The specific generators of the waves are controversial, but most authorities agree with the following schema: I—distal CN VIII; II—proximal CN VIII; III—bilateral superior olivary complex; IV—ascending auditory fibers in the rostral pons; V—inferior colliculus; VI—medial geniculate nucleus; VII—distal auditory radiations. Waves VI and VII are often unobtainable or inconsistent and are clinically useless. Waves II and IV may be buried in, or fused to other waves, and are not as important as waves I, III, and V. Absolute latencies are not as important as the I-III-V interpeak latencies (IPLs).

Commonly recognized abnormal BAEP patterns include the following:

1. *Absence of all waves:* Peripheral hearing loss, excessive background noise, technical error (rarely in Friedreich's ataxia, distal CN VIII lesions, or system atrophies).
2. *Wave I only (or increased I-III IPL):* Lesions of the proximal acoustic nerve or pontomedullary junction near the root entry zone (peripheral demyelination or inflammation, cerebello-pontine [CP] angle tumors, pontine glioma, MS, leukodystrophies, neonatal anoxia, or brainstem infarct).
3. *Waves I-III only (or increased III-V IPL):* Lesions sparing the pontomedullary junction but affecting the pons to low midbrain (most commonly seen with MS, any disorder of pontine tegmentum, or large extrinsic masses compressing the brainstem—especially CP angle tumors opposite the stimulated ear).
4. *Increased I-III, III-V, and I-V IPL:* Diffuse or multifocal disease such as demyelination, brainstem glioma, and especially hypothermia. (*NOTE:* BAEPs are extremely stable over wide ranges of metabolic derangement. Diffuse prolongation of IPLs should not be explained by metabolic abnormality.)

Somatosensory-evoked potentials are obtained from electrical stimulation of the median nerve at the wrist (MSEP) or the posterior tibial nerve at the ankle (PTSEP). Analysis of SEPs can give information about the integrity of the sensory component of peripheral nerves, spinal cord, brainstem, and to a lesser extent, the cortex. Recordings of far-field potentials are made over the scalp, and both near- and far-field potentials may be obtained at other points along the proximally propogating action potential.

MSEP: Four clinically useful "early" components of MSEPs and their presumed generators have been identified and are consistent and reproducible regardless of position of scalp electrodes. *P9* originates from the distal brachial plexus, *P11* from the dorsal root entry zone, *P13* from the dorsal columns of the cervical cord, and *P14* from the medial lemniscus of the brainstem. It can be seen that absence of a component or increased IPL provides evidence of a lesion along the course of propogation. Other "late" components (approximately N19, P23, N32, P40, and N60) have been identified and probably correspond to thalamic or suprathalamic generators. They are prolonged with decreasing levels of arousal and are not reproducible from person to person, or from the same person at different times or with changes of state. They also vary with different recording montages. Their usefulness is seen only when simultaneous bilateral stimulation produces asymmetries.

PTSEP: This is the most "laboratory specific" EP, with widely differing waveform designations and terminology. *PV* (propogated volley) is the designation given to the near-field potential recorded over the lower spine, which roughly corresponds to the cauda equina and lower gracile tract. It increases in latency with more proximal recording sites. *N22* is probably generated by axon collaterals in the dorsal columns near the thoracolumbar junction. Later components can be recorded from the scalp and represent more rostral brainstem, thalamic, and cortical generators. Their usefulness is proportional to the technique and reliability of the given laboratory. As with MSEPs, PTSEPs can give localizing information pertaining to lesions along the course of propogation.

Electroretinograms: Two types of ERGs are in common use. Flash ERGs are useful for detecting retinal lesions and will not be discussed. Pattern ERGs (P-ERGs) utilize a checkerboard pattern-reversal stimulus. When a small enough check size is used (less than 2.4 degrees of arc), the major positive wave recorded from the cornea (b-wave) represents retinal ganglion cell function. The latency of "b" is about 40 ms and is prolonged or abolished by disease processes in or distal to the ganglia. When "b" is subtracted from the simultaneously recorded P100 of the VEP, retinocortical time (RCT) can be determined (RCT = P100 − b). RCT is a more accurate reflection of optic nerve integrity proximal to the retinal ganglia and is independent of macular disease.

Three abnormal patterns of P-ERG/VEP have been identified.

1. *Normal P-ERG, delayed VEP, and RCT:* Demyelination of the optic nerve.
2. *Normal P-ERG, absent VEP:* Acute total block of optic nerve fibers.
3. *Absent P-ERG, absent VEP:* Severe macular disease or long-standing severe optic nerve disease with retrograde degeneration of retinal ganglion cells.

There is also evidence that decreased amplitude of P-ERGs in recent optic neuritis has a poor prognosis for visual recovery, and progressive loss of P-ERG amplitude correlates with the development of optic nerve atrophy.

Evoked potentials and multiple sclerosis: EPs are most useful in the evaluation of MS (1) to demonstrate sensory abnormalities when the history or exam is equivocal and (2) to demonstrate clinically inapparent lesions when demyelination is suspected in other areas of the nervous system. Less important uses are (3) to define the distribution of the disease process and (4) to monitor changes in a patient's status. *When the diagnosis of MS is clinically definite, EPs will add little additional information.*

E

EVOKED POTENTIALS

Abnormal VEPs are present in about 95% of cases of optic neuritis, regardless of how remote and regardless of whether vision has returned. About 50% of MS patients has abnormal VEPs even without clinical evidence of optic nerve involvement. Whereas about 35% of patients with progressive myelopathy have abnormal VEPs, only about 10% show abnormality after a single episode of transverse myelitis.

Forty-six percent of patients with MS have abnormal BAEPs, regardless of clinical classification. Thirty-eight percent of patients without clinical findings of brainstem involvement show abnormalities. The most common abnormalities are decreased or absent wave V or increased III-V IPL.

Of 1000 MS patients with varying classifications, 58% had abnormal MSEPs and 76% had abnormal PTSEPs.

The differential sensitivity of EPs in detecting white matter lesions in MS is related to the length of fiber tract being tested (i.e., the order of sensitivity is SEP greater than VEP and BAEP). *As the degree of clinical certainty of the diagnosis increases from possible to probable to definite, the detection rate of lesions will be greater but the usefulness of the information obtained will be less.*

Evoked potentials and other neurologic diseases: Many attempts have been made to use EPs as prognostic indicators of disease and trauma. In general, results are conflicting and no better than following clinical signs and symptoms. There is currently no definite role for EPs in the evaluation of brain death or recovery from coma. Intraoperatively, SEPs (during spinal cord surgery) and BAEPs (during posterior fossa surgery) may provide an early indication of compromise of neural tissue. In cervical spondylosis, PTSEPs may eventually help predict which patients are more likely to develop a significant cord deficit so that early surgical intervention can be considered. Flash VEPs have been used by some centers to monitor changes in intracranial pressure, but this is controversial.

REFERENCE

Gilmore R, ed: *Neurologic clinics,* Philadelphia, WB Saunders, 1988.

EYE MUSCLES

Because of their insertional properties, the six extraocular muscles affect eye movements in the three planes relative to primary position (see Table 32). In testing muscle strength, the optical axis is aligned with a muscle's main vector. The superior and inferior rectus muscles insert on the anterior globe at 23 degrees temporal to the primary position. Therefore these muscles function solely in the vertical plane only when the eye is abducted 23 degrees. The oblique muscles insert on the posterior globe at 51 degrees nasal to the primary position. Thus adduction maximizes the depressor effect of the superior oblique, whereas abduction maximizes intorsion (see Figure 15).

Diplopia testing in paralytic strabismus begins with measurement of visual acuity, confrontation visual fields, and observation of any abnormal

TABLE 32
ACTIONS OF EYE MUSCLES IN PRIMARY POSITION

Muscle	Primary Action	Secondary Action	Tertiary Action
Lateral rectus	Abduction		
Medial rectus	Adduction		
Superior rectus	Elevation	Intorsion	Adduction
Inferior rectus	Depression	Extorsion	Adduction
Superior oblique	Intorsion	Depression	Abduction
Inferior oblique	Extorsion	Elevation	Abduction

head posture. *Head tilt occurs in the direction of action of the weak muscle.* Range of motion in each eye is tested in the nine cardinal positions of gaze with the opposite eye covered (ductions) and with both eyes viewing (versions). *Misalignment can be seen in the corneal reflection of a penlight* and can be tested in all directions of gaze (Hirschberg's test).

Subjective diplopia testing relies on the principles that the disparate images are maximally separated in the main field of action of the paretic muscle and that *the more peripheral image belongs to the paretic eye* (see Figure 16). The Maddox rod tests primarily for phoria because it

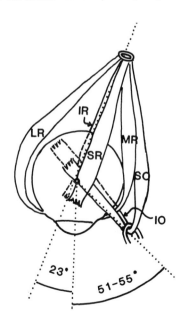

FIGURE 15
Insertion of ocular muscles of the globe. LR = lateral rectus; MR = medial rectus; SR = superior rectus; IR = inferior rectus; SO = superior oblique; IO = inferior oblique.

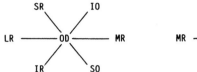
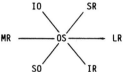

FIGURE 16

Main field of action of individual eye muscles.

disrupts fusion; therefore only the noncomitant deviations (unequal in different fields of gaze) should be considered abnormal. The paretic eye and the position of gaze producing the maximum separation of the images can be determined; the paretic muscle can be identified.

Objective tests include the cover-uncover test for tropia and the alternate cover test for phoria, which are performed in the primary position and in each cardinal position. Deviation of the nonparetic eye when covered (secondary deviation) is always greater than the deviation of the paretic eye when covered (primary deviation).

REFERENCE

Leigh RJ, Zee DS: *The neurology of eye movements*, ed 3, New York, Oxford University Press, 1999.

FACIAL NERVE

The *course of the facial nerve* (cranial nerve [CN] VII) is depicted in Figure 17. The numbers in the figure refer to the following *locations of the lesions*:

1. Peripheral to chorda tympani in facial canal or outside stylomastoid foramen. Peripheral upper and lower facial weakness (motor aspects of CN VII) only. Usually related to trauma.
2. Facial canal (mastoid), involving chorda tympani. In addition to upper and lower facial weakness, patients have loss of taste over the anterior two thirds of tongue and decreased salivation.
3. Facial canal, involving the stapedius nerve. As in 1 and 2, plus hyperacusis.
4. Geniculate ganglion. Usually associated with pain in the ear. May have decreased lacrimation.
5. Internal auditory meatus. Complete CN VII (facial weakness; decreased taste, salivation, and lacrimation) plus CN VIII dysfunction (deafness and/or vestibular symptoms).

F

FACIAL NERVE

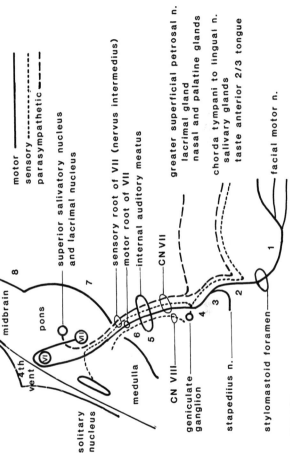

FIGURE 17
Facial nerve.

motor ——————
sensory ------------
parasympathetic ◆━━◆━━◆

midbrain
pons
4th vent
medulla
solitary nucleus

superior salivatory nucleus and lacrimal nucleus

sensory root of VII (nervus intermedius)
motor root of VII
internal auditory meatus
CN VII

greater superficial petrosal n.
lacrimal gland
nasal and palatine glands

chorda tympani to lingual n.
salivary glands
taste anterior 2/3 tongue

facial motor n.

CN VIII
geniculate ganglion
stapedius n.
stylomastoid foramen

6. Extrapontine, subarachnoid. May have other cranial nerve involvement. Hemifacial spasm is more commonly associated with more proximal lesions of CN VII.
7. Pontine (nuclear or infranuclear). Millard-Gubler, Foville's, and Brissaud's syndromes (see Ischemia).
8. Supranuclear. Lesions may occur anywhere from mid-pons to motor cortex and are usually associated with other findings such as hemiparesis, hemisensory deficit, language disturbance, or homonymous hemianopia, depending on location. Taste, salivation, and lacrimation are not involved. Lower facial weakness is much more prominent than upper because of bilateral input to the portions of the facial nucleus controlling the upper face; input for the lower face is from contralateral cortex. Mild weakness may appear only as slight drooping of the angle of the mouth, slight widening of the palpebral fissure, or flattening of the nasolabial fold.

Causes of facial nerve palsies are many, although "idiopathic" Bell's palsy (often related to herpes simplex) is most common. Other treatable and potentially serious causes should be excluded by careful history, examination, and where indicated, neuroradiologic and electrodiagnostic studies.

Bell's palsy is attributed to swelling of the nerve or nerve sheath in the facial canal. CN VII findings are variable, depending on the site and extent of lesion. Recovery is spontaneous and complete in 90% of cases. Electromyographic evidence of denervation indicates a worse prognosis for complete recovery. Partial or incomplete recovery may be associated with contractures, synkinetic motor movements (e.g., angle of mouth and lids), excessive tearing with salivary gland stimulation ("crocodile tears"), or gustatory sweating. Ramsay-Hunt syndrome refers to herpes zoster of the geniculate ganglion; herpetic lesions are visible on the tympanic membrane, external auditory canal, and pinna.

Other causes of peripheral facial weakness include trauma (facial, skull fracture), surgery (middle ear, mastoids, cranial nerve V), neoplasms (schwannoma, neurofibroma, nasopharyngeal carcinoma, leukemia, lymphoma, hemangioma, glomus tumors, cholesteatoma, parotid tumors), and infections involving the subarachnoid space, petrous portion of the temporal bone, middle ear, mastoid, parotid, or the facial nerve itself. Involvement may result from granulomatous infiltration of the meninges or, as in the case of sarcoidosis, with parotid gland swelling. Facial weakness may be congenital, as in the Möbius' syndrome, with greater upper than lower facial diplegia, paralysis of abduction of the eye, ptosis, and, occasionally, abnormal musculature of the tongue, sternocleidomastoid, and muscles of mastication. Recurrent facial paralysis and facial swelling (Melkersson's syndrome) occurs rarely and may be associated with a furrowed tongue (Melkersson-Rosenthal syndrome). The nerve itself may be involved in Guillain-Barré syndrome, acute intermittent porphyria, and lead poisoning. Facial weakness may also be seen in myasthenia gravis and various myopathies. Rarer causes include osteopetrosis, thiamine deficiency, and hemorrhage into the facial canal. Bilateral facial paralysis can also be seen with brainstem diseases, meningitis, or facioscapulohumeral muscular dystrophy.

Pontine involvement is most commonly vascular but may result from infection, hemorrhage, trauma, neoplasm, or demyelinating disease. Facial myokymia may occur with pontine lesions. *Supranuclear* causes are many and include vascular, neoplastic, traumatic, and infectious causes.

Blepharospasm is bilateral, episodic, involuntary contractions of orbicularis oculi muscles of undetermined origin. When lower facial muscles are involved, blepharospasm may be part of Meige's disease (see Dystonia).

Hemifacial spasm is painless unilateral facial spasms, either repetitive or lasting up to several minutes. It is frequently exacerbated by alkalosis. Differential diagnosis includes focal seizures. An aberrant vascular loop compressing the facial nerve as it exits the pons is often the cause. Treatment is carbamazepine, botulinum toxin, or surgical decompression.

Facial myokymia is often benign and self-limited. Persistent myokymia may be seen in multiple sclerosis or brainstem neoplasm or after stroke.

Treatment of facial nerve disorders is aimed at the primary cause. Corneal exposure should be prevented with lubricating ointment but may also require tarsorrhaphy. Electrical physiotherapy may be detrimental and should not be used. Corticosteroid treatment within the first 2 days of "idiopathic" Bell's palsy may prevent the progression to complete denervation. Prednisone, 1 mg/kg, is given in divided doses for 5 to 6 days and tapered over 5 days if paralysis is incomplete, but continued for another 10 days and tapered over the subsequent 5 days if paralysis is complete. Acyclovir 800 mg PO five times a day may be combined with prednisone.

FONTANEL

The anterior fontanel is an interosseous space located at the juncture of the sagittal and coronal sutures; the posterior fontanel is located at the juncture of the sagittal and lambdoidal sutures. At birth both fontanels are open. The posterior fontanel becomes fused in the first few months of life. By age 7 months, the anterior fontanel is fibrous; by age 2 years, it is palpable as a midsagittal depression. The anterior fontanel may be quite large at birth; this has little significance unless associated with palpably split sutures. If the infant has been delivered vaginally, the cranial bones may override each other and the fontanel may be difficult to palpate. When the infant cries, the fontanel may be tense and bulging. At other times it should be soft and flat and may pulsate. A "full" or "tense" fontanel when the infant is quiet is a sign of increased intracranial pressure. Causes of delayed closure of the anterior fontanel (persistently large) include prematurity, malnutrition, increased intracranial pressure, chromosomal abnormalities (trisomies 13, 18, and 21), metabolic disorders (hypothyroidism, rickets and hypophosphatasia), and primary bone disorders (achondroplasia, cleidocranial dysostosis, and osteogenesis imperfecta).

FRONTAL LOBE

The frontal lobe consists of the motor, premotor, and prefrontal areas. The motor cortex (Brodmann's area 4) also contains giant pyramidal (Betz) cells. "Motor homunculus" is the somatotopic representation of the contralateral body. The function of this region is to control the voluntary, skilled movement; Betz cells contribute 30% of the corticospinal tract (pyramidal tract) and corticobulbar tract. The premotor (Brodmann's area 6) also includes the supplementary motor cortex (SMA). The main function of the SMA is programming, preparation of movement, and control of posture. The premotor cortex also includes the frontal eye field area (Brodmann's area 8) and Broca's area (Brodmann's areas 44 and 45). The prefrontal areas lie anterior to the premotor area with extensive connections to parietal, temporal, and occipital cortices. These areas help coordinate intellect, judgment, and planning of behavior. Partial seizures, contralateral hemiplegia, and neurobehavioral syndromes may arise from different lesions of the frontal lobe. Aphasia is associated with dominant frontal lobe lesion. Three behavioral syndromes have been described with prefrontal lesions. These syndromes may exist in pure or mixed forms:

1. *Orbitofrontal:* Disinhibition, impulsiveness, emotional lability, euphoria, poor judgment, and distractibility.
2. *Frontal convexity syndrome:* Apathy, psychomotor retardation, poor word-list generation, motor perseveration and impersistence, and inability to execute multistep behaviors.
3. *Medial frontal syndrome*: Paucity of spontaneous movement, sparse verbal output, lower extremity weakness, and incontinence.

G

GAIT DISORDERS

Gait depends both on maintenance of equilibrium and on mechanisms of locomotion. Classification of gait disorders has traditionally been based on visual recognition of typical gaits such as those seen in spasticity, parkinsonism, chorea, ataxia, and hysteria. A better classification is based on the level of dysfunction. Lowest-level gait disorders arise because of musculoskeletal, peripheral nervous system, vestibular, or sensory dysfunction. Middle-level gait disorders encompass hemiplegic, paraparetic, cerebellar ataxic, parkinsonian, choreic, and dystonic gaits. Highest-level gait disorders are due to difficulties in frontal planning and execution and include cautious gait, frontal and subcortical dysequilibrium, gait ignition failure (gait apraxia), and frontal gait disorders. Diagnosis of gait disorders is based on history and associated neurologic findings. Isolated gait disorders in the elderly are frequently due to treatable disorders such as Parkinson's disease, cervical myelopathy, or normal-pressure hydrocephalus.

REFERENCE

Nutt JG, Marsden CD, Thompson PD: *Neurology* 43:268–279, 1993.

GAZE PALSY

Horizontal gaze palsies: A unilateral gaze (for both saccadic and pursuit movements) palsy may indicate a contralateral cerebral hemispheric (frontoparietal), contralateral midbrain, or ipsilateral pontine lesion. Except when the pontine lesion is at the level of the abducens nucleus, either involving the nucleus itself or the paramedian pontine reticular formation, the eyes can be driven toward the side of the palsy with cold caloric stimulation of the ipsilateral ear or oculocephalic maneuvers. Hemispheric lesions characteristically produce transient defects; brainstem lesions may be associated with enduring defects. An acute cerebellar hemispheric lesion can result in an ipsilateral gaze palsy that can be overcome with calorics. Unilateral saccadic palsy with intact pursuit is unusual and indicates an acute frontal lesion. Unilateral impaired pursuit with normal saccades is usually due to an ipsilateral deep posterior hemispheric lesion with a contralateral hemianopia.

Vertical gaze palsies: The rostral interstitial nucleus of the medial longitudinal fasciculus (riMLF) in the upper midbrain contains the cells that generate vertical eye movements. A medially placed lesion will result in both an up-gaze and down-gaze palsy. An isolated down-gaze palsy is due to bilateral or lateral midbrain lesion. Isolated up-gaze palsies occur with lesions of the posterior commissure, bilateral pretectal regions, and large unilateral midbrain tegmental lesions. In the dorsal midbrain (Parinaud's) syndrome the paralysis of upward gaze is usually associated with convergence-retraction nystagmus, lid retraction, and light-near dissociation of the pupils. An acute bilateral pontine lesion at the level of the abducens nucleus may result in a transient up-gaze paralysis in addition to bilateral horizontal gaze palsy.

Conjugate eye deviations: Horizontal deviations are associated with acute gaze palsies as described above and with irritative cerebral foci (seizure or intracerebral hemorrhage), which usually drive the eyes to the side opposite the lesion. Ipsiversive eye and head movements, however, are reported with focal seizures. Tonic upward deviations occur in the oculogyric crisis of postencephalitic parkinsonism and, more commonly, as an idiosyncratic reaction to phenothiazines. They may also occur in coma, usually as a result of anoxic encephalopathy. Downward deviations may occur transiently in normal neonates but also in infantile hydrocephalus and in adults with metabolic encephalopathy, bilateral thalamic infarction, or hemorrhage.

GERSTMANN'S SYNDROME

A clinical tetrad of agraphia, acalculia, right-left disorientation, and "finger agnosia." Finger agnosia may manifest as bilateral difficulties in finger naming, moving fingers to command, matching of fingers to demonstration, or recognizing stimuli ("wiggle the finger that I touch"). When all features are present, a dominant inferior parietal or posterior perisylvian lesion is highly likely. Aphasia, alexia, or constructional apraxia almost always accompanies the syndrome. Developmental Gerstmann's syndrome occurs in children with or without dyslexia. Verbal IQ among such children is often significantly higher than performance IQ.

REFERENCES

Devinsky O: *Behavioral neurology*: 100 maxims, New York, Oxford University Press, St. Louis, Mosby, 1992.
Mesulam MM: *Principal of behavioral and cognitive neurology*, New York, Oxford University Press, 2000.

GLOSSOPHARYNGEAL NEURALGIA

This has similar etiology and pathogenesis as trigeminal neuralgia. Clinical features also are similar, although distribution is different and the pain may be more variable with longer duration and is associated with autonomic dysfunction (salivation, lacrimation, bradycardia, and syncope). Pain distribution is to the throat, posterior one third of the tongue, tonsillar pillars, eustachian tube, and ear. Trigger points are variable, most commonly associated with swallowing, chewing, speaking, laughing, coughing, or touching particular areas in the distribution of the glossopharyngeal nerve and upper sensory fibers of the vagus nerve. Onset is after age 40, with males and females affected equally.

The *differential diagnosis* includes underlying causes such as oropharyngeal carcinoma, paratonsillar abscess, enlarged styloid process, or enlarged tortuous vertebral or posterior inferior cerebellar arteries, and SUNCT syndrome (short-lasting, unilateral, neuralgiform headache attacks with conjunctival injection and tearing). Evaluation for glossopharyngeal neuralgia should include a thorough ear, nose, and throat exam.

Treatment is aimed at underlying causes of "symptomatic" neuralgias. Otherwise, carbamazepine or phenytoin or both may be used, although the response to these is less than 50%. Surgical therapy has included microsurgical decompression of the glossopharyngeal and vagal root entry zones and section of the glossopharyngeal nerve.

REFERENCES

Kobata H et al: *Neurosurgery* 43:1351–1361, 1998.
Tenser RB: *Neurology* 51:17–19, 1998.

GLUCOSE

In contrast to other tissues, the brain normally derives its energy from carbohydrates only. A significant drop in blood sugar will diminish oxygen utilization and intracellular energy production. Typical constellation of signs and symptoms resulting from hypo- or hyperglycemia are described below.

1. *Hypoglycemia:* Symptoms arise from neuroglycopenia and endogenous release of catecholamines. Mild hypoglycemia produces hunger, weakness, dizziness, blurred vision, anxiety, tremor, tachycardia, pallor, diaphoresis, headache, and mild confusion. With more severe hypoglycemia, the preceding symptoms are followed by seizures (glucose <30 mg/100 ml) with progression to coma, pupillary dilation, hypotonia, and extensor posturing (glucose <10 mg/100 ml). The presence of hyperventilation may lead to paraesthesias. *Focal findings may mimic cerebrovascular disease.* Symptoms, signs, and residual neurologic deficit depend on the rate of onset, duration, and severity of hypoglycemia. Patients with chronic hypoglycemia may have no sympathetic symptoms but present with cognitive or behavioral disturbances. Repeated severe attacks of hypoglycemia may result in dementia because of damage to hippocampal neurons. The degree of EEG slowing correlates well with the severity of hypoglycemia, but *enhanced response to hyperventilation appears first*. Epileptiform discharges are rare even if hypoglycemic convulsions occur.

2. *Hyperglycemia:*

A. Diabetic ketoacidosis is the most common cerebral complication of diabetes and is frequently accompanied by stupor or coma. Muscle cramps, dysesthesias, and diffuse abdominal pain may occur. The neurologic changes correlate best with serum osmolarity, although dehydration, acidosis, and associated electrolyte disorders contribute. *The treatment of diabetic ketoacidosis may lead to fatal cerebral edema if blood osmolarity is rapidly lowered relative to brain osmolarity*. Treatment may also cause hypophosphatemia, hypokalemia, and hypoglycemia. In diabetic ketoacidosis, generalized slowing on EEG parallels declining consciousness.

B. Hyperglycemic nonketotic states result in CNS complications due to extracellular hyperosmolarity. Neurologic manifestations are variable and include hallucinations, depression, apathy, irritability, seizures (typically transient focal or epilepsia partialis continua), flaccidity, diminished deep tendon reflexes, tonic spasms, myoclonus, meningeal signs, nystagmus, tonic eye deviations, and reversible loss of vestibular caloric responses. As the blood glucose rises above 600 mg/dl, coma may develop. Studies indicate that hyperglycemia can lead to poor outcome in stroke patients during the acute phase, and tight control of blood sugar is recommended. Seizures generally improve within 24 hours of rehydration and correction of hyperglycemia. The EEG may show corresponding focal abnormalities, including periodic lateralized epileptiform discharges.

In both ketotic and nonketotic hyperglycemia, care should be placed in recognizing and treating the underlying stressor, which may include stroke, myocardial infarction, infection, or other acute medical illnesses.

3. *Hypoglycorrhachia*, low CSF glucose, is usually associated with infection, either bacterial or chronic meningitis. It may also be seen in meningeal carcinomatosis. Persistent low CSF glucose with normal serum

G

GLUCOSE

glucose levels in a patient with seizures and developmental delay may be a result of a genetic defect in glucose transport across the blood-brain barrier. These long-term neurologic sequelae may be prevented by a ketogenic diet.

REFERENCES

De Vivo et al: *N Engl J Med,* 325:703–709, 1991.
Jorgenson HS et al: *Stroke* 25:1977–1984, 1994.

GRAVES' OPHTHALMOPATHY

Graves' ophthalmopathy refers to any thyroid-associated ophthalmopathy. Approximately 50% of patients with Graves' disease will manifest ophthal-mopathy. The mean presenting age of thyroid ophthalmopathy is 43 years, ranging between 8 and 88 years. Cigarette smoking is a well-established risk factor for more severe ophthalmopathy; the risk is proportional to the amount of cigarette consumption. Alterations in cellular immunity (CD4/CD8 T-lymphocytes ratio) are thought to initiate the orbital changes associated with thyroid ophthalmopathy. Activated CD4 T-helper lympho-cytes may bind to orbital fibroblasts that express thyroid-type receptors and antigens, subsequently producing edema and fibrosis. Also, loss of CD8 T-suppressor cells may contribute to the inflammatory process, plasma cell proliferation, and production of autoantibodies specific for extraocular tissues.

Clinical features: Dryness, "gritty" sensation, lacrimation, photophobia, blurring of vision, deep orbital pressure or diplopia. Diplopia is due to fibrosis of ocular muscles that do not extend fully when their antagonist contracts. Fibrosis of the inferior rectus, the most frequently affected muscle, causes diplopia on upgaze. Other findings on examination are periorbital and lid edema, lid retraction, lid lag, conjunctival chemosis and injection, and corneal exposure ranging from minor lagophthalmos to com-plete decompensation and corneal perforation. Some patients have com-pressive optic neuropathy with decreased visual acuity, optic disc changes, visual loss, dulling of color perception, and visual field defects. *Diagnostic evaluation* of thyroid eye disease includes thyroid function tests, serum thyrotropin receptor antibody, serum antimicrosomal and antithyroglobulin antibodies. Enlarged extraocular muscles can be demonstrated by ultra-sonography, CT, or MRI.

Treatment: Most cases of thyroid ophthalmoplegia resolve spontaneously. The therapeutic intervention is separated into acute and chronic phases. Acute intervention is prompted by the development of the vision-threatening conditions of optic neuropathy and corneal exposure. Compressive optic neuropathy is usually treated with high-dose corticosteroids and, less com-monly, emergent surgical decompression. Orbital radiation therapy is proven to be safe and effective in acute ophthalmopathy; high-dose IVIg is equal in efficacy to systemic corticosteroids. In preexisting ophthalmopathy, 67% of people who received radioiodine followed by a 3-month course of oral prednisone showed improvement. In minor corneal exposure, conservative measures such as lubrication and taping of the lids or use of a moisture chamber while sleeping are often sufficient. In more severe cases, tarsorrhaphy may be necessary and the use of botulinum toxin has been suggested.

REFERENCE

Zobian J, Mans M: *Curr Opine Ophthalmula* 9:105–110, 1998.

HALLUCINATIONS

The DSM IV-R defines hallucinations as a "sensory precept without external stimulation of the relevant sensory organ." Some distinguish true hallucinations (experiences perceived as real and outside the body) from pseudohallucinations (perceived as occurring within the body or known to be unreal). Phenomona include lilliputian (small animals or people), brobdingnagian (giants), and autoscopic (seeing one's self from outside) characteristics, as well as palinopsia, voices, palinacusis, crawling sensations, shooting pains, smells, and other features.

I. Differential diagnosis of visual hallucinations.
   A. Ocular disorders: Associated with reduced vision. These are usually formed, bright, colored images. *Charles Bonnet syndrome* is isolated visual hallucinations, usually of ocular cause. These include enucleation; cataracts; macular, choroidal, and retinal disease; vitreous traction.
   B. CNS disorders: May be due to lesions anywhere along the optic pathways and visual association cortices. Also seen with midbrain disease ("peduncular hallucinosis"; complex forms, usually with other brainstem signs), dementias, epilepsy, migraine, and narcolepsy. Hypnagogic hallucinations occur just before falling asleep, and hypnopompic hallucinations occur on awakening.
   C. Medical disorders: Seen in 40% to 75% of delirious patients; usually brief, nocturnal, and emotionally charged. Causes include alcohol and drug withdrawal, hallucinogens, sympathomimetics, and metabolic encephalopathies.
   D. Psychiatric disorders: Schizophrenia, mania or depression, and hysteria.
   E. Normal individuals: Dreams, hypnagogic hallucinations, hypnosis, childhood (imaginary companion), sensory deprivation, sleep deprivation, intense emotional experiences.
II. Differential diagnosis of auditory hallucinations.
   A. Diseases of the ears or peripheral auditory nerves.
   B. CNS diseases: Epilepsy, neoplasms, and occasionally, vascular lesions.

    C. Toxic or metabolic: Alcoholic hallucinosis, encephalopathies.

    D. Psychiatric: Schizophrenia (60% to 90% of patients), affective disorders, conversion reactions, multiple personality disorder.

III. Tactile, somatic, and phantom limb hallucinations. Phantom limb is the sensation of persistent presence of an amputated extremity and is found in almost all amputees; usually described as the phantom limb being numb or tingling, of normal size, correctly aligned, with peripheral areas more prominent, and recedes gradually.

    Tactile hallucinations occur commonly in patients with schizophrenia (15% to 50%) and affective disorder (25%). Formication (the sensation of insects crawling) is found in alcohol and drug withdrawal (especially sympathomimetics) and dementias.

IV. Olfactory and gustatory hallucinations. Medial temporal lobe lesions and complex partial seizures ("uncinate fits") may produce olfactory hallucinations. They may also occur in migraine, dementias, toxic and metabolic conditions, depression, and Briquet's syndrome (20% to 25% of patients). Gustatory hallucinations may be seen in manic-depressive illness, schizophrenia, Briquet's syndrome, and partial seizures.

REFERENCE

Trimble MR, Cummings JL (eds): *Contemporary behavioral neurology*, Boston, Butterworth-Heinemann, 1997.

HEADACHE

Headache disorders are extremely common. The lifetime prevalences of headache (any kind), migraine, and tension-type headache have been estimated as 93%, 8%, and 69% for men and 99%, 25%, and 88% for women. The prevalence for tension-type headache decreases with increasing age, whereas migraine shows no correlation to age.

CLASSIFICATION

The full classification by the International Headache Society can be found in *Cephalalgia*, 1988.

1. *Migraine*. Migraine is characterized by unilateral, pulsating, moderate to severe headache, often increasing with physical activity and helped by sleep. It is often accompanied by nausea or vomiting, photophobia, and phonophobia. Migraine may be preceded or accompanied by auras, most commonly visual fortification spectra, scintillating scotomas, or flashes of light (photopsias). Migraine subtypes include those with aura (classic, complicated, ophthalmic, hemiparesthetic, hemiplegic, or aphasic) and without aura (common migraine), ophthalmoplegic migraine (most commonly complete oculomotor palsy), retinal migraine, basilar migraine, and childhood periodic syndromes (migraine equiva-

lents), including acute confusional states, benign positional vertigo, cyclic vomiting, "Alice in Wonderland" syndrome, paroxysmal leg pains, and alternating hemiplegia of childhood. Occasional migraines may be pure "acephalgic" auras without headache, but these may require investigation to rule out other intracranial processes. Complications of migraine include status migrainosus and migraine stroke.

2. *Cluster headaches*. Predominantly affect men in a ratio of 4.5 to 6.7:1; may occur at any age, but most often occur in the late twenties. Periodicity is the main feature of cluster headaches; the average cluster period lasts 2 to 3 months and recurs every year or two. Cluster headaches are nocturnal in more than 50% of patients and in many patients are characterized by a circadian regularity. They are often precipitated by alcohol use (during the cluster). Cluster headaches can be episodic or chronic.

There is no associated aura. The pain reaches its peak 10 to 15 minutes after onset and generally lasts for 45 to 60 minutes, occurring at a frequency of 1 to 3 per day. The pain is usually felt in the trigeminal nerve distribution and is excruciating, penetrating, and nonthrobbing. Signs associated with cluster headache are conjunctival injection, lacrimation, nasal congestion, rhinorrhea, forehead and facial sweating, miosis, ptosis, and eyelid swelling. Patients may pace due to pain.

Symptomatic cluster headache treatment includes 100% O_2 or ergots and triptans, which are very effective. Prophylactic treatment consists of lithium, the effectiveness of which is known within a week, calcium channel blockers, methysergide, corticosteroids, and ergotamine. The prophylactic treatment of choice is a combination of ergotamine and verapamil. The most effective treatment for chronic cluster headache is a combination of lithium and verapamil, to which ergotamine can be added for resistant headaches. If these fail, a 2-week tapering course of corticosteroids may break the cycle.

3. *Chronic paroxysmal hemicrania*. A type of cluster headache in which there is severe unilateral orbital or supraorbital pain, or both, always on the same side. Headaches last from 2 to 10 minutes and occur daily up to 15 times a day. This type of headache also has the same associated signs as cluster headache. A diagnostic-therapeutic test for chronic paroxysmal hemicrania is that attacks show an absolute, specific responsiveness to indomethacin (150 mg or less).

4. *Tension-type headaches*. These headaches are episodic but may transform into the chronic variety. The headaches are diffuse, bilateral, pressing or "tightening" in quality, and mild to moderate in severity. Pain often involves the posterior aspects of the head and neck. Photophobia, phonophobia, or mild nausea may occur rarely. Vomiting is not a feature of chronic tension-type headache.

5. *Drug-induced headache*. When used frequently and in excessive quantities, symptomatic medications used for acute relief of headaches may perpetuate headaches. Two main forms of drug-induced headache occur:

analgesic-rebound headache and ergotamine-rebound headache. The features of a drug-induced headache are a self-sustaining, rhythmic, headache-medication cycle characterized by daily or near-daily headache and a predictable use of pain medication as the only means of relief. Distinguishing drug-induced headache from a primary headache disorder such as tension or migraine is difficult, since migraine patients may manifest some features of migraine without the typical pattern of the attacks. Migraines may also transform in a chronic daily headache pattern. Other accompanying symptoms include asthenia, nausea, restlessness, irritability, memory problems, difficulty with concentration, behavior problems, sleep abnormalities, and tolerance to symptomatic medications. After the initial withdrawal period, there is often improvement in symptoms, as well as a reduction in the frequency and severity of headache. The use of excessive amounts of daily symptomatic medications nullifies the beneficial effects of concomitant prophylactic medications.

6. *Headache associated with other medical conditions.* Headache may be a symptom of local cranial disease (sinusitis, otitis, dental conditions), upper cervical spine conditions (see Craniocervical Junction), or systemic diseases. Acute severe headache raises the possibility of life-threatening conditions such as subarachnoid hemorrhage or meningitis. Headache is a cardinal feature of pseudotumor cerebri and temporal arteritis. Brain tumor headache is not always localized and often simulates tension or migraine. The classic pattern of headaches that are worse on awakening is often not present. Headache is present in 25% of strokes but is not a reliable localizing finding. Headache is common after head trauma and may be indistinguishable from migraine or tension headache.

7. *Medication-related headaches.* Nitrates, caffeine, alcohol, ergotamine, analgesic abuse.

HEADACHE THERAPY

Three components of a systematic approach to treating headache are psychologic, physical, and pharmacologic. Psychologic therapy involves reassurance and counseling, as well as stress management, relaxation therapy, and biofeedback as appropriate. Physical therapy involves identifying headache triggers, such as diet, hormone variations, and stress, whose alteration may be helpful in treating selected cases. A headache calendar documenting the occurrence, severity, and duration of headaches; the type and efficacy of medication taken; and any triggering factors should be recorded by the patient. Pharmacotherapy can be divided into two approaches, symptomatic and prophylactic.

I. *Symptomatic or abortive therapy*
   A. Routine analgesics (aspirin, acetaminophen, and nonsteroidals, including ibuprofen, naproxen, indomethacin, ketorolac, and others).

B. Narcotic analgesics should be avoided but are useful for occasional, severe headaches.

C. Ergotamine preparations are available for oral, sublingual, and rectal administration and by inhalation.

1. Ergotamine 1 mg PO q 30 minutes up to 5 mg per attack.
2. Ergotamine 1 mg and caffeine 100 mg (Cafergot), 1 or 2 tabs PO q 1/2 hr up to 5 tabs per attack.
3. Ergotamine 2 mg sublingually q 30 minutes up to 3 per day.
4. Ergotamine and caffeine (Cafergot) suppository, 1 pr; may repeat in 1 hr prn.
5. Dihydroergotamine (D.H.E. 45) (see Table 33).

D. Triptans.

1. Sumatriptin 6 mg IM 20 mg nasal spray or 25–50 mg orally provides relief in up to 80% of patients with acute migraine. Failure to respond to the initial dose makes it unlikely that response will be observed after subsequent doses. Response is often seen within 1 hour and may be repeated once every 24 hours.

   Other triptans, such as rizatriptan (10 mg), zolmitriptan (2.5 and 5 mg), and naratriptan (2.5 and 5 mg) are other alternative triptans. The fastest onset of action is rizatriptan, and the one with the least side effect profile and lowest headache recurrence is naratriptan.

TABLE 33

PROTOCOL FOR SEVERE, PERSISTENT HEADACHES

I. Dihydroergotamine (D.H.E. 45) and metoclopramide protocol is tried initially. It is contraindicated in pregnancy and in Prinzmetal's angina. For patients over 60 years of age, monitor cardiac status during first two doses of D.H.E. 45. Side effects include diarrhea, leg pains, vasospasm, chest pain, and supraventricular arrhythmia.

   A. Metoclopramide 10 mg IV plus D.H.E. 45, 0.5 mg IV over 2 to 3 min.
   B. If nausea and headache are absent, continue D.H.E. 45, 0.5 mg IV q 8 hr for 3 days with metoclopramide 10 IV. Stop metoclopramide after sixth dose.
   C. If no nausea is present and headache is persistent, repeat D.H.E. 45, 0.5 mg IV in 1 hour without metoclopramide; if nausea does not recur, give D.H.E. 45 1 mg q 8 hr for 3 days with six doses of metoclopramide. If nausea recurs with the second dose of D.H.E. 45, reduce D.H.E. 45 dose to 0.75 mg.
   D. If nausea and headache persist, hold D.H.E. 45 for 8 hours, then give D.H.E. 45, 0.3 to 0.4 mg q 8 hr for 3 days, with metoclopramide for six doses.

II. Protocol for those unable to tolerate D.H.E. 45.

   A. Prednisone 80 mg per day (short, rapidly tapering dosage).
   B. Neuroleptics: Haloperidol 5 mg PO or IM, thiothixene 5 mg PO or IM, or chlorpromazine 10 to 50 mg PO or 25-mg suppository.
   C. Opiate analgesics: Meperidine 75 to 100 mg, hydromorphone 4 mg, or morphine 10 mg.

From Raskin NH: *Neurol Clin* 8:857–865, 1990.

E. Isometheptene two capsules at onset and 1 q 1 hr prn up to 5 capsules per headache.

F. Ibuprofen 400 to 800 mg PO at onset and repeat q 4 hr prn.

G. Metoclopramide 10 mg IM, IV, or PO 15 minutes before other analgesic agents has proven useful.

H. Prednisone 40 to 60 mg PO qd over a short course may break "status migrainosus."

I. Biofeedback and behavior therapy.

II. *Prophylactic treatment of migraine*

A. Avoid inciting dietary factors such as red wine, aged cheese, chicken liver, pickled herring, chocolate, tuna, sour cream and yogurt, ripe avocado and banana, smoked meats, and foods with monosodium glutamate or nitrates.

B. Conduct trial when patient is not using oral contraceptives and nitrates, if possible.

C. Prophylactic medication for those with frequent or disabling attacks includes the following.

   1. Beta blockers.

      a. Propranolol, starting at 20 mg PO bid and gradually increasing prn to 80 mg tid. Has been used in children.

      b. Others: Nadolol (80 to 240 mg); atenolol (Tenormin) (50 to 100 mg); timolol (20 to 100 mg).

   2. Methysergide 2 mg PO tid or qid. Need drug holiday every 6 months for 1 month to prevent fibrotic retroperitoneal or mediastinal changes.

   3. Naproxen sodium (550 bid).

   4. Calcium channel blockers: Nifedipine 10 mg PO tid or verapamil 80 mg PO tid, starting dose.

   5. Amitriptyline starting at 25 mg PO qhs and increasing to 50 to 100 mg qhs.

   6. Other tricyclics.

   7. Phenelzine sulfate 15 mg PO qd, qod, or bid.

   8. Ergonovine 0.2 mg PO tid up to 2 mg qd.

   9. Combination: Ergotamine, belladonna, and phenobarbital (Bellergal) 2 to 4 tabs PO qd.

  10. Cyproheptadine 2 to 4 mg PO qid.

  11. Vascular-headache diet combined with any of the above.

  12. Depakote 250 tid to therapeutic doses.

  13. Phenytoin 200 to 400 mg per day; especially useful in children.

III. *Treatment of cluster headache*

A. Treat as for migraine (ergotamine, methysergide, sumatriptin).

B. 100% O_2 by mask at 6 L per min up to 15 minutes per attack.

C. Lidocaine 4% intranasal; 15 drops ipsilateral to headache with head extended and rotated away from side of headache.

D. Prednisone 40 to 60 mg PO qd over short course; rebound headaches can occur after discontinuation.

E. Lithium carbonate 300 mg PO bid-qid titrated to lithium levels (0.6 to 1.2 mEq/L) is especially useful for chronic cluster headaches.

F. Indomethacin 25 to 50 mg PO tid for cluster headache variants and atypical migraines (exertional migraine, benign orgasmic cephalgia, chronic paroxysmal hemicrania, cough headache, and ice-pick headache).

IV. *Chronic daily headache*

A. Discontinuation of the offending medications, especially analgesics used to excess.

B. Use of pharmacotherapeutic agents in attempt to break the cycle of continuous headache.

C. Initiation of prophylactic pharmacotherapy (often valproic acid, tricyclic or beta blocker).

D. Concomitant behavioral intervention, including biofeedback therapy, individual behavioral counseling, family therapy, physical exercise, and dietary instruction.

E. Adequate instruction on ill effects of medications with special focus on analgesics.

F. Continuity of care.

REFERENCES

Cephalagia, ed 1, vol 8, suppl 7, Norwegian University Press, 1988.

Mathew NT: *Neurology* 42(suppl 2):22–31, 1992.

Mathew NT: *Neurology* 43(suppl 3):26–33, 1993.

Sculman EA, Silberstein SD: *Neurology* 42(suppl 2):16–21, 1992.

Welch KMA: *N Engl J Med* 329:1476–1483, 1993.

HEARING

Bedside testing of hearing should include examination of the external ear and the tympanic membranes. Auditory acuity can be grossly assessed by whispering into each ear while closing the other and by comparing the distance from the ear at which the patient and the examiner can hear a ticking watch or fingers rubbing together. *Tuning fork tests* are commonly used. In Weber's test a 256-Hz tuning fork is placed at the midline vertex of the skull; sound referred to an ear with decreased acuity indicates conductive hearing loss. In Rinne's test a tuning fork placed on the mastoid and one held in front of the ear are compared; if bone conduction is greater, conductive loss is implied.

Audiologic tests are used to quantitate and localize (conductive, sensorineural, cochlear, and retrocochlear) hearing loss. *Pure-tone threshold* determines auditory threshold for tones over various frequencies and intensities for both air and bone conduction. Impairment of both air and bone conduction, especially at high frequencies, indicates sensorineural hearing loss. When bone conduction is greater than air conduction, conductive hearing loss is present. Other tests of loudness function are the alternate binaural loudness balance and the short-increment sensitivity index. Bekesy audiometry, tone decay tests, speech discrimination tests, the stapedius reflex (pathway from cochlea to eighth cranial nerve to facial nerve to stapedius muscle), and brainstem auditory evoked potentials (BAEP) help distinguish retrocochlear from cochlear lesions. Rarely, cortical deafness or auditory agnosia occurs with bitemporal lesions and BAEPs are normal.

Causes of non-retrocochlear hearing loss include bacterial, viral, or fungal infections of the external, middle, or inner ear; presbycusis; otosclerosis; cholesteatoma and glomus tumor; ototoxic drugs such as aminoglycosides, aspirin, and diuretics; Meniere's disease; and trauma.

Causes of retrocochlear (eighth cranial nerve and CNS) hearing loss include the following:

1. Tumors: Acoustic neuroma, cholesteatoma, meningioma, pontine glioma.
2. Vascular: Vertebrobasilar ischemia and inferior lateral pontine infarction or basilar occlusion.
3. Demyelinating diseases.
4. Congenital malformations: Arnold-Chiari, Klippel-Feil syndromes.
5. Degenerative diseases: Hereditary ataxias, hereditary neuropathies; Refsums disease, xeroderma pigmentosum, Cockayne's syndrome, Usher's syndrome (retinitis pigmentosa and deafness), and other rare hereditary degenerative disorders.
6. Infectious: meningitis, encephalitis, syphilis.
7. Inflammatory: Vogt-Koyanagi-Harada syndrome, Behçet's syndromes; sarcoidosis.
8. Mitochondrial diseases: Kearns-Sayre syndrome.

REFERENCE

Rudge P: *Clinical neuro-otology*, New York, Churchill-Livingstone, 1983.

HERNIATION

Herniation is defined as displacement of the cerebral or cerebellar structures from their normal compartments due to pressure differences. Most commonly, increased pressure is due to a focal lesion (e.g., tumor with cerebral edema, extra/intra-axial hemorrhage, infarct, abscess). Diffuse elevations of ICP, as in pseudotumor cerebri, rarely produce herniation.

Herniation syndromes:

1. *Central (transtentorial) herniation*—diencephalon is forced down through the tentorial incisura; seen in frontal, parietal, or occipital masses.
2. *Uncal (lateral) herniation*—usually rapid (acute), often from temporal lobe mass, pushing uncus and hippocampal gyrus over the edge of tentorium, entrapping the oculomotor nerve, and later directly compressing midbrain. Pupil dilation often appears before impaired consciousness. May pinch off posterior cerebral arteries (as with central herniation).

3. *Cingulate (subfalcine) herniation*—cingulate gyrus herniates under falx, often asymptomatic and preceding central/transtentorial herniation, can lead to bifrontal infarctions when anterior cerebral arteries become compromised.
4. *Upward cerebellar herniation*—cerebellar vermis herniates upward above the transtentorial notch compressing the midbrain; with sylvian aqueduct compression it can cause hydrocephalus and occlusion of superior cerebellar arteries leading to cerebellar infarctions. Can occasionally be seen with posterior fossa masses and may be exacerbated by ventriculostomy.
5. *Tonsillar herniation*—cerebellar tonsils herniate downward through the foramen magnum, compressing medullary respirator center, which may be fatal. In rare cases may be precipitated by lumbar puncture.

These syndromes are accompanied by characteristic clinical signs that correspond to the anatomical structures involved (see Table 34). There is a rostral-caudal progression of clinical signs seen with both central and lateral transtentorial herniation, indicating worsening herniation (see Table 35). This begins with diencephalic involvement, followed by mesencephalic, pontine, and finally medullary involvement. Two infrequent exceptions to this orderly progression, in which signs skip from the hemispheres or diencephalon to

H

HERNIATION

TABLE 34

HERNIATION SYNDROMES

Syndromes	Anatomy	Signs
Central transtentorial herniation: Caudal displacement of diencephalon through tentorial notch	Reticular formation or diencephalon initially, then rostral-caudal progression	Altered consciousness
Lateral transtentorial herniation (uncal)	Ipsilateral CN III	Ipsilateral pupil dilation, then external ophthalmoplegia
	Ipsilateral posterior cerebral artery	Contralateral homonymous hemianopsia
	Contralateral cerebral peduncle (false localizing); then follows rostral-caudal progression but may skip diencephalic stage	Ipsilateral hemiparesis
Cerebellar tonsillar herniation	Medullary respiratory center	Respiratory arrest
Cingulate herniation under falx cerebri	Anterior cerebral artery	Leg weakness

TABLE 35

ROSTRAL-CAUDAL PROGRESSION OF TRANSTENTORIAL HERNIATION

	Diencephalon	Midbrain–Upper Pons	Low Pons–Upper Medulla	Medulla
Consciousness, systemic	Agitated or drowsy to coma, diabetes insipidis	Hypothermia or hyperthermia, comatose	Comatose	Fluctuating pulse, blood pressure falls Coma
Breathing	Yawns, pauses, Cheyne-Stokes respirations	Central hyperventilation	Tachypnea (20–40 breaths per min) shallow	Slow and irregular or hyperapnea alternating with apnea, then breathing stops
Pupils	Small (1–3 mm) reaction, small but brisk	Irregular, midposition, (3–5 mm), fixed	Small midposition fixed	Dilated, fixed
Eye movements	Roving, VOR weak or brisk, fast-phase caloric response lost, loss of vertical movement	Intact VOR, may be dysconjugate response	No VOR, no caloric response	No VOR, no caloric response
Motor	Preexisting hemiplegia worsens, decorticate posturing to noxious stimuli, plantars extensor	Bilateral decerebrate posturing to noxious stimuli	Flaccid flexor response in LEs to noxious stimuli	Flaccid, no deep tendon reflexes

VOR = Vestibulo-ocular reflex; LE = Lower extremity.

the medulla, bypassing the rostral brainstem, are as follows: (1) acute cerebral hemorrhage with extravasation into the ventricles, compressing the medullary respiratory center in the floor of the fourth ventricle, and (2) when lumbar puncture is performed on patients with incipient transtentorial herniation, it may induce enough of a pressure change to produce tonsillar herniation.

For treatment of herniation, see Intracranial Pressure.

REFERENCES

Greenberg MS: *Handbook of neurosurgery*, Lakeland, FL, ed 5, Greenberg Graphics, 2001.
Plum F, Posner JB: *The diagnosis of stupor and coma*, Philadelphia, FA Davis, 1982.

HICCUPS (*Singultus, Hiccoughs*)

A reflex myoclonic contraction of the diaphragm with a forceful inspiration, associated with laryngeal spasm and closure of the glottis, producing a characteristic sound. It is mediated by the phrenic (afferent), vagus, and thoracic nerves (efferent). Gastrointestinal, pulmonary, and cardiovascular signs and symptoms may be present. Carcinoma, achalasia, and hiatal hernia are common pathologic causes. Other pathologic causes include intrathoracic distention, pulmonary or pleural irritation, pericarditis, mediastinitis and mediastinal mass, intrathoracic abscess or tumor, and aortic aneurysms. There are several CNS causes as well, including metabolic (acetonemia, uremia), drugs (sulfonamides), infection (encephalitis), hypothalamic disease (also associated with yawning), tumors of the fourth ventricle, and cerebrovascular disease (vertebrobasilar insufficiency). Chronic idiopathic and psychogenic hiccups are common as well.

Treatment in most cases is not required, because hiccups tend to be self-limited. If intractable, there is likely to be an underlying cause. Drug therapies for intractable hiccups include phenothiazines (prochlorperazine, chlorpromazine), valproic acid, phenytoin, carbamazepine, benzodiazepines (clonazepam, diazepam), and baclofen. Surgical sectioning of the phrenic nerve or selective vagotomy is occasionally required; more recently acupuncture and sertraline have been used.

REFERENCES

Macdonald J: *BMJ* 319:976, 1999.
Moretti R et al: *Eur J Neurol* 6:617, 1999.

HORNER'S SYNDROME

Horner's syndrome (oculosympathetic paresis) is due to disruption at any point along the course of the sympathetic pathway from the hypothalamus to the orbit (Figure 18). Signs are miosis (resulting from iris dilator weakness) most evident in dim illumination, ptosis (weakness of Müller's

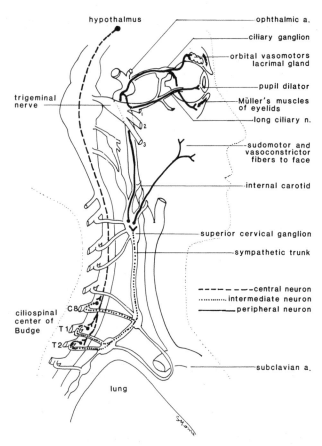

hypothalamus
ophthalmic a.
ciliary ganglion
orbital vasomotors
lacrimal gland
pupil dilator
Müller's muscles
of eyelids
long ciliary n.
trigeminal
nerve
sudomotor and
vasoconstrictor
fibers to face
internal carotid
superior cervical ganglion
sympathetic trunk
— — — — — — central neuron
.... intermediate neuron
————— peripheral neuron
ciliospinal
center of
Budge
C8
T1
T2
subclavian a.
lung

FIGURE 18

Oculosympathetic pathways.

muscle), and anhidrosis. Heterochromia of the iris occurs in congenital Horner's syndrome.

The cause of Horner's syndrome can be determined in about 60% of cases. Lesions of the first-order neuron (central) are myriad and may be due to stroke, tumor, hemorrhage, and demyelinating disease. Second-order neuron (preganglionic) causes include apical lung tumor, tuberculosis, radical neck dissection, trauma, and neck masses. Third-order neuron (postganglionic) lesions include internal carotid aneurysms, carotid dissection, cluster headaches, and migraine and do not have anhidrosis.

Cocaine eyedrops (4% to 10%) are used to differentiate Horner's syndrome from simple anisocoria on a pharmacologic basis. By preventing norepinephrine reuptake at sympathetic nerve endings, the eyedrops cause normal pupils to dilate. Lesions of any part of the sympathetic pathway cause failure or pupillary dilation because of lack of norepinephrine at the nerve terminal.

Evaluation for central and preganglionic lesions should include careful neck palpation, apical lordotic chest x-ray views, and possibly CT of the neck and chest. New-onset postganglionic Horner's syndrome suggests carotid artery disease. Isolated postganglionic Horner's syndrome is generally benign.

REFERENCE

Loewenfield IE: *The pupil anatomy, physiology and clinical applications*, vol 1, Ames, IA, Iowa State University Press, 1993.

HUNTINGTON'S DISEASE

Huntington's disease (HD) is an autosomal-dominant neurodegenerative disease characterized by progressive choreoathetosis, psychological or behavioral changes, and dementia. Although chorea is generally thought to be the first sign of HD, behavioral changes may occur a decade or more before the movement disorder, with depression the most common symptom. Patients may become erratic, irritable, impulsive, and emotionally labile.

The reported mean age of onset ranges from 35 to 42 years, with an average duration from onset to death of 17 years. Three percent of patients develop signs and symptoms before the age of 15, with rigidity, myoclonus, dystonia, and seizures more evident than chorea; in these cases, the course is rapid and there is often paternal transmission.

Neuropathology reveals neuronal loss that is more severe in the caudate and putamen, along with a glial response. Several neurotransmitter systems are altered, with abnormally increased or decreased levels of neurotransmitters, biosynthetic enzymes, and receptor-binding sites.

Genetic testing has been based on linkage analysis of affected families. The gene has now been identified and the disease state correlated with excess copies of a trinucleotide CAG repeat.

CT and MRI reveal atrophy of the caudate nucleus and cortex. PET studies have revealed relative hypometabolism in the striatum of some patients at risk for the disease.

Treatment is aimed at reducing the movement disorder when it is disabling or embarrassing. Haldol is quite effective at doses of 1 to 40 mg per day but may cause dyskinetic movements if usage is prolonged.

REFERENCES

Gutekunst CA et al: *Curr Opin Neurol* 13(4):445–450, 2000.
Huntington Disease Collaborative Research Group: *Cell* 72:971–983, 1993.

HYDROCEPHALUS

Hydrocephalus (HCP) is characterized by an increase in volume of cerebrospinal fluid (CSF) associated with dilatation of the ventricles. Three mechanisms can cause HCP: (1) obstruction of CSF pathways, (2) defective absorption of CSF, and (3) oversecretion of CSF (rare, but seen with choroid plexus papilloma).

I. *Noncommunicating hydrocephalus* is due to intraventricular obstruction of the foramen of Monro, the third ventricle, the aqueduct, or the foramina of Luschka or Magendie. Aqueductal stenosis, cysts, intra- and extraventricular tumors, inflammation, and congenital malformations are some of the causes.

II. *Communicating hydrocephalus* is most often due to obstruction of CSF pathways in the subarachnoid space, arachnoid villi, or draining veins. *Causes* include inflammation of the leptomeninges from prior infection or hemorrhage, tumors, posttraumatic obstruction, and congenital malformations (most commonly Arnold-Chiari malformation).

III. *Normal pressure hydrocephalus* (NPH) is a syndrome of communicating hydrocephalus without evidence of intracranial hypertension. Clinically, it is characterized by the triad of (1) gait disturbance characterized by slow velocity short steps with low height, (2) dementia, and (3) urinary incontinence. Diagnosis is based on history and supported by imaging and normal opening CSF pressure. Treatment is surgical shunting. *The most favorable responses occur in nondemented patients*.

IV. *Hydrocephalus ex vacuo* describes the phenomenon of an increase in volume of cerebrospinal fluid under normal pressure in compensation for loss of brain mass (cerebral atrophy).

Clinical presentation will vary depending on age and whether the HCP is acute or chronic. In an infant, the most common symptoms are irritability, poor feeding, and lethargy. On exam, there may be bulging, tense fontanelle, separation of sutures, increased head circumference, frontal bossing, globular but symmetric head shape, "setting sun" sign due to paralysis of upward gaze, and loss of developmental milestones. In older children (>6 years of age) and adults, the most common symptoms are headache and emesis that are worse in the morning, diplopia, loss of gross and fine motor coordination usually manifested as a gait abnormality, CN VI palsy, absent retinal pulsation, and papilledema.

Diagnosis is made by CT or MRI (see Figure 19). A small or normal fourth ventricle usually implies obstruction proximal to it. A dilated fourth ventricle implies obstruction distally, either at the outflow of the foramina of the fourth ventricle or in the subarachnoid space. In the infant with an open anterior fontanelle, ultrasonography is useful for assessing ventricular size and presence of blood. CSF examination may be helpful in diagnosing the etiology of HCP, but LP is contraindicated when imaging studies show evidence of mass effect, midline shift, effacement of cortical sulci, or effacement of the suprachiasmatic, basilar, quadrigeminal, or cerebellar cisterns.

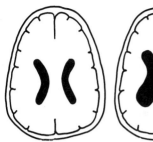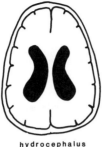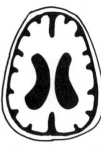

normal   hydrocephalus   atrophy (ex vacuo)

FIGURE 19

MR or CT appearance of normal and enlarged ventricles.

H

HYPERVENTILATION

Treatment of HCP is mainly extraventricular shunting. Improvement with LPs in NPH may be diagnostic in some cases and also has some predictive value in assessing shunt responsivity. The most common symptom to improve is incontinence and then gait disturbance. Dementia is less likely to respond. Pharmacological treatment of CSF overproduction includes carbonic anhydrase inhibitors, such as acetazolamide and furosemide.

REFERENCES

Fishman RA: *Cerebrospinal fluid in diseases of the nervous system*, Philadelphia, WB Saunders, 1992.
Greenberg MS: *Handbook of neurosurgery*, Lakeland, FL, ed 5, Greenberg Graphics, 2001.

HYPERVENTILATION

Inspiratory patterns reflect many factors and may provide localizing information.

Involuntary hyperventilation resulting from autonomic hyperactivity of brainstem respiratory centers is rare; hypoxemia, acid-base disorders, CSF acidosis, pulmonary disease, drug effects, and voluntary hyperventilation are more common causes.

Voluntary hyperventilation is usually related to anxiety. Symptoms include chest pain, palpitations, dyspnea, lightheadedness, perioral and fingertip numbness or parathesias, cramps, GI distress, insomnia, a feeling of fright, and occasionally syncope. Arterial blood gas levels should show a respiratory alkalosis during an attack. Reproduction of symptoms by hyperventilation is diagnostic.

Posthyperventilation apnea is characterized by an exaggerated apneic response to lowered $PaCO_2$ seen with bilateral hemispheric dysfunction. The diagnosis is made when more than 12 seconds of apnea follows 20 to 30 seconds of voluntary hyperventilation (normal response, less than 10 seconds of apnea).

Cheyne-Stokes breathing, central neurogenic hyperventilation, and *apneustic* and *ataxic respirations* may occur during coma (see Coma for a discussion of these entities).

REFERENCE

Colice GL: *Neurologic disorders and respiration, Clin Chest Med* 10(4):521–543, 1989.

HYPOTONIC INFANT

Hypotonia in infancy can be caused by lesions at any level of the nervous system. The history and examination help determine the site of dysfunction and identify the cause of the hypotonia. Family history of disease is present in some cases (see Table 36).

TABLE 36
DIFFERENTIAL DIAGNOSIS OF THE HYPOTONIC INFANT

I. CNS disease.
  A. Perinatal hypoxia-ischemia.
  B. Congenital infection.
  C. Encephalitis, meningitis.
  D. Trauma.
  E. Hydrocephalus.
  F. Tumors.
  G. Trisomies 21 and 13.
  H. Aminoacidopathy.
  I. Storage diseases.
  J. Werdnig-Hoffmann syndrome.
  K. Poliomyelitis.
  L. Leigh disease.
  M. Prader-Willi syndrome.
II. Neuropathy.
  A. Guillain-Barré syndrome.
  B. Infantile neuropathy.
III. Neuromuscular junction.
  A. Myastenia gravis.
  B. Infantile botulism.
IV. Muscle disease.
  A. Congenital myopathies.
  B. Myotonic dystrophy
  C. Carnitine deficiency.
V. Nonneurologic.
  A. Ehlers-Danlos syndrome.
  B. Sepsis.
  C. Dehydration.
  D. Hypothyroidism.
  E. Hypothermia.
  F. Rickets.

In a classic case, a hypotonic ("floppy") infant assumes a frog-leg posture (hips abducted and externally rotated and the entire length of the limbs in contact with the flat surface). There is decreased resistance to passive movement and marked head lag with hand traction in the supine position. In ventral suspension, neck extension is absent, and elbow and knee flexion is minimal.

Increased reflexes indicate a CNS lesion. If they are normal, a myopathy has to be ruled out. Neuropathy causes decreased reflexes. Decreased alertness, poor response to external stimuli, and poor suck or grasp reflex suggest CNS disease. Muscle fasciculations occur with neuropathy and anterior horn cell disease. Hypotonia with weakness suggests anterior horn cell or peripheral nervous system disease.

Beyond the neonatal period hypotonic infants frequently come to medical attention with delay in achieving motor milestones. Assessment of nonmotor-dependent activity such as social response, smiling, and vocalization is important in determining associated intellectual delay. Mental retardation in association with hypotonia suggests a CNS origin.

Benign congenital hypotonia is a diagnosis of exclusion, with a generally good prognosis, although some affected children remain clumsy throughout development.

REFERENCE

Berg BO (ed): *Principles of child neurology*, New York, McGraw Hill, 1996.

I

IMMUNIZATION

When neurologic complications are identical to naturally occurring disease, it is impossible to determine in a specific case whether the disorder and the immunization are related or coincidental. Therefore analytic population-based studies of adverse reactions are required to analyze immunization-related syndromes.

The following types of vaccines are available:

I. *Killed organisms*: Influenza, pertussis, and rabies vaccines are associated with toxic or allergic reactions involving the nervous system: *Haemophilus influenzae* type b and hepatitis B vaccines have no neurologic complications.

   A. *Influenza*: Neurologic complications were rarely noted before 1976, when an increased incidence of Guillain-Barré syndrome occurred in the adult population following immunization against swine flu, but such an increase has not occurred with subsequent vaccine programs. Patients with a history of Guillain-Barré syndrome should not receive influenza vaccination.

B. *Pertussis*: Simple febrile seizures may be a consequence of pertussis immunization if the fever has no other cause and both fever and seizures occur within 24 hours of administration. There is also a causal relationship between diptheria-pertussis-tetanus (DPT) vaccine and shock-like states or acute encephalopathy (defined in controlled studies as encephalopathy, encephalitis, or encephalomyelitis). The risk of acute encephalopathy is 0.0 to 10.5 per million immunizations. There is insufficient evidence to indicate a causal relationship between DPT vaccine and permanent neurologic damage, aseptic meningitis, learning disabilities, and attention-deficit disorder. There is evidence, however, that DPT vaccine has no causal relationship to infantile spasms, hypsarrythmia, Reye's syndrome, or Sudden Infant Death Syndrome.

C. *Rabies*: Whole-virus vaccines that contain myelin basic protein are associated with encephalomyelitis and polyneuritis within 2 weeks after immunization.

II. *Live-attenuated viruses*: Measles, mumps, rubella, poliomyelitis, and varicella vaccines produce their natural diseases and expected complications of the natural disease.

A. *Measles*: Ordinarily combined with mumps and rubella (measles, mumps, and rubella [MMR] vaccine). Except for febrile seizures in children who are genetically predisposed, neurologic complications are uncommon. The risk of encephalopathy is small compared to the 1-per-1000 risk of encephalopathy from natural measles.

B. *Rubella*: Transient arthralgias may develop in up to 40% of patients. No causal evidence exists for association with polyneuritis or other neuropathies.

C. *Poliomyelitis*: Paralytic poliomyelitis is the only known complication of oral polio vaccine (OPV) and almost always occurs after initial immunization. Approximately one-third of cases have occurred in OPV recipients, one half in contacts of recipients, and the remainder in immunodeficient recipients or contacts.

D. *Varicella*: No neurologic complications have been reported.

III. *Toxoids*: May produce rare allergic reactions. The only contraindication is a history of neurologic or severe hypersensitivity reaction following a previous dose. Tetanus and diphtheria are often given together, making it difficult to attribute adverse reactions to one without the other. Demyelinating neuropathy with complete recovery occurs in rare instances.

REFERENCES

Aminoff MJ: *Neurology and general medicine*, ed 3, New York, Churchill Livingstone, 2001.

Howson CP, Howe CJ, Fineberg HV, eds: *Adverse effects of pertussis and rubella vaccines*, Institute of Medicine, Washington, DC, National Academy, 1991.

IMPOTENCE

Penile erection is mediated by the cavernous nerves from S2-4 roots and dependent on the integrity of both the paired cavernosal arteries (which supply the corpora cavernosa) and the subtunical veins (which drain it). Nitric oxide release from cavernous nerves and vascular endothelium promotes formation of cGMP, which stimulates smooth muscle relaxation, allowing increased arterial flow into the corpora cavernosa and resultant compression of outflow veins—facilitating rigidity. Sympathetic input from T11-L2 constricts arterioles, reducing inflow and permitting venous drainage; this promotes detumescence and explains how sympathetic overactivity produces psychogenic impotence.

Erectile dysfunction may affect up to 30 million U.S. men, and the prevalence and severity increase with age, tripling in incidence from the 20s to the 50s. Organic etiology may be found in more than 80% of cases lasting more than a year. Organic causes are as follows: (1) neurologic: MS, spinal cord injury, pelvic nerve trauma (prostatectomy, pelvic injury, radiation); (2) arterial: atherosclerosis, trauma; (3) venous: diabetes, Peyronie's disease, normal aging; and (4) endocrine: low testosterone (primary or secondary), high prolactin. Drugs affecting any of these systems can exacerbate the problem, and the same vascular risk factors implicated in coronary and cerebrovascular disease (diabetes, hypertension, hyperlipidemia, smoking) increase the risk of erectile dysfunction.

Diagnosis is greatly eased if the patient reports achieving even very occasional firm, persistent erections (nocturnal, morning, with masturbation)—this removes concern for a vascular basis and suggests a psychogenic etiology. Sphincter or sensory dysfunction suggest a neurologic basis; difficulty maintaining erection suggests venous insufficiency; delay in achieving erection suggests arterial insufficiency; and painful erection suggests Peyronie's disease or priapism. Examiners should look for evidence of feminization (suggesting a hormonal basis) or peripheral vascular disease, abnormalities of the external genitalia, and adequacy of anal sphincter tone and the bulbocavernosus reflex. Serum prolactin, testosterone, fasting glucose, and lipid panel should be evaluated. Additional workup may include penile-brachial index, penile ultrasonography, cavernosometry, and pelvic arteriogram.

Treatment: Sildenafil, an oral agent introduced in 1998, has become first-line therapy for erectile dysfunction, with an overall efficacy of around 50%. It works by inhibiting the phosphodiesterase specific to the corpora cavernosa, thereby increasing cGMP. It is particularly effective in psychogenic cases and less severe organic dysfunction (including diabetes) and is also effective to a lesser extent in cases of severe organic dysfunction including spinal cord injury. Sildenafil is absolutely contraindicated in patients taking nitrates, as the associated hypotension has been associated with myocardial infarction and stroke.

Other therapies include alprostadil penile injection (estimated efficacy for organic disorders is 80%), alprostadil intraurethral pellet (much less efficacious), and penile prosthesis (requiring surgery but effective and reliable). Testosterone supplements may help, particularly in cases of decreased libido. Yohimbine is a mixed alpha(1)-alpha(2) adrenergic receptor antagonist that works by a dual mechanism; it facilitates sexual arousal by acting on alpha(2) adrenergic receptors in the central nervous system and blocks adrenergic influences at the peripheral level.

REFERENCE

Morgentaler A: *Lancet* 354:1713–1718, 1999.

INTRACRANIAL PRESSURE (ICP)

Basic concepts of ICP: Normal values of intracranial pressure range from 5 to 15 mmHg (torr), which equals 65 to 200 mm CSF or H_2O (conversion: 1 torr = 13.6 mm H_2O). Factors that determine the level of ICP are the volume of intracranial contents, and arterial and venous pressures. After the cranial sutures fuse, the skull becomes an inelastic, closed container with fixed total intracranial volume consisting of three components: brain, CSF, and blood. The *Monroe-Kellie doctrine* states that the sum of intracranial brain tissue, CSF, and blood volumes is constant, therefore an increase in the volume of one must be compensated by an equal decrease in another compartment. Slow increases in the volume of one compartment can be compensated by decreases in the others, but a rapid rise in ICP is not well tolerated and increases the risk of herniation or the occurrence of global ischemia and is a neurologic emergency. Cerebral perfusion pressure (CPP) is critical to maintain adequate cerebral blood flow (CBF) and is calculated as a difference between mean arterial pressure (MAP) and ICP (CPP = MAP − ICP). CPP less than 50 mmHg is detrimental to brain function and survival. Following any major cerebral injury, ICP should be maintained as close to normal as possible, to provide a margin of safety. Continuous ICP monitoring provides useful information about "pressure waves" and may be used to guide treatment. Plateau waves, consisting of episodic surges in ICP sometimes exceeding 450 mm H_2O, can occur several times an hour, especially with pain and iatrogenic maneuvers such as suctioning, and are associated with increased risk of herniation.

Clinical presentation of increased ICP depends on the underlying process, compartmentalized or diffuse, and whether it is acute or chronic. Manifestations of headache, papilledema, diplopia, or focal signs may occur. *Cushing's triad of bradycardia, hypertension, and slowing of respiration* may occur, as may cardiac arrhythmias such as atrial fibrillation, nodal and ventricular bradycardia, large T waves, prolonged Q-T intervals, and changes in ST segments.

Causes of increased ICP: Space-occupying lesions, cerebral edema, trauma, intra/extra-axial hemorrhages, infections, venous sinus thrombosis, and pseudotumor cerebri. An acute rise in blood pressure beyond the autoregulatory curve causes an elevated ICP as seen in hypertensive encephalopathy; chronic hypertension does not cause a change in ICP. Processes that increase venous pressures cause increases in ICP, i.e., jugular compression (as reflected by *Queckenstedt's test* during LP), superior vena cava obstruction, congestive heart failure (CHF), or Valsalva maneuvers. Postural effects alter the pressures in the intracranial venous sinuses, which in turn alter the CSF pressure.

Treatment:

A. *General measures:* Head elevation to 30 to 45 degrees above horizontal, equal fluid balance, fever control (hyperthermia markedly increases CBF as a reflection of increased cerebral energy metabolism), and avoiding hypotonic IV solutions. Anticonvulsants are sometimes given to prevent rises in ICP with seizures.

B. *Active measures:* (1) Hyperventilation results in cerebral vasoconstriction and rapidly decreases ICP. The PCO_2 should be maintained between 25 and 30 mmHg. (2) Mannitol is given as a 20% IV solution, 0.5 to 1 g/kg over 15 minutes, and repeated at 4- to 6-hr intervals. Mannitol is best used when ICP can be directly monitored; otherwise, it should be titrated to produce a serum osmolality of 315 to 320 osmol/l. After 3 to 4 hours, brain and plasma osmolalities equilibrate, requiring increasingly higher plasma osmolalities for the same effect. Urine output should be monitored. Side effects include renal failure, CHF, and pseudohyponatremia. (3) Furosemide (10 to 20 mg IV q 6 hr) and (4) dexamethasone 0.25 to 0.5 mg/kg IV q 6 hr) are also useful. Glucocorticoids are useful in controlling brain edema associated with brain tumors and meningitis, but are of uncertain value in other forms of cerebral edema. (5) Hypothermia (27 to 36°C) decreases ICP by 50%, but peak effect takes several hours, and it may also decrease cerebral perfusion. (6) Barbiturate coma with burst suppression can decrease ICP and is a last resort medical therapy; complications include further sedation of comatose patients and hypotension, often requiring vasopressors to maintain blood pressure. (7) Hypertonic saline can be used as a potential measure in lessening the ICP, particularly in diffuse cerebral edema and head trauma patients.

Surgical treatment includes monitoring by subdural, subarachnoid or ventricular pressure transducers, which may provide accurate information regarding efficacy of intervention. Surgical therapy by ventricular shunting offers immediate reduction in ICP, especially in cases with hydrocephalus. Hemicraniectomy has been used after massive middle cerebral stroke and appears to be promising.

Intracranial hypotension: Decreased ICP may occur in the setting of CSF leakage, either spontaneously through openings in the dura to sinuses or mastoid, after lumbar puncture or neurosurgery, or through overshunting. Postural headache, similar to that observed after lumbar puncture, is a frequent symptom. Diagnosis is confirmed by demonstration of CSF leak on cisternogram or other evidence of CSF leak (positive glucose test in pharyngeal secretions). MRI may show meningeal enhancement.

Spontaneous remission may occur, and treatment depends on etiology; occasionally dural graft may be necessary.

REFERENCES

Fishman RA: *Cerebrospinal fluid in diseases of the nervous system*, ed 2, Philadelphia, WB Saunders, 1992.
Greenberg MS: *Handbook of neurosurgery*, Lakeland, FL, ed 5, Greenberg Graphics, 2001.
Qureshi AI, Suarez JI et al: *Crit Care Med* 26:440–446, 1998.

ISCHEMIA

A thorough medical evaluation is required for the diagnosis and management of cerebrovascular injury. The history should include age, race, family history, handedness, comorbidities, medications, time of onset, and prior pattern of neurologic deficits. History, physical examination, and imaging studies determine risk factors, localize lesions, delineate underlying pathophysiologic conditions, and guide treatment. In the United States, stroke of all types ranks third as a cause of death, second only to heart disease and cancer.

STROKE CLASSIFICATION

Cerebral ischemic events are classified by anatomic location, size of blood vessels (small and large vessel disease), duration of deficit, and mechanism (cardioembolic, atherosclerotic, lacunar).

A. *Transient ischemic attacks* (TIAs) and reversible neurologic deficits (not used as often any more) have duration lasting up to 24 hours and 3 weeks, respectively. Typically TIAs last less than 30 minutes and commonly resolve within an hour. *Attacks lasting only a few seconds are rarely TIAs, with the exception of amaurosis fugax, which can resolve in 30 to 60 seconds*. When TIA deficits do not resolve completely after 1 to 2 hours, they are frequently associated with strokes on pathologic examination or imaging.

B. *Completed stroke* indicates that the patient has a stable neurologic deficit without evidence of progression or resolution. Completed stroke refers to the acute onset and persistence of neurologic dysfunction resulting from cerebrovascular disease (hemorrhagic or ischemic infarction).

C. *Progressing stroke.* Waxing and waning neurologic deficit with ultimate worsening.

Classification by duration is of limited value, as it does not provide detailed insight into the pathophysiologic characteristics of the injury.

Central nervous system ischemia or infarction may be described in terms of vascular anatomy (see Table 37). The cerebral vasculature is divided into *anterior* (carotids) and *posterior* (vertebrobasilar) distributions. There are many variants in cerebrovascular anatomy. In about 5% of patients, the Circle of Willis is congenitally absent. Brainstem cross-sectional anatomy that correlates with many of the syndromes described in Table 38 is shown in Figures 20–22.

TABLE 37

SIGNS AND SYMPTOMS OF ISCHEMIC VASCULAR OCCLUSION

Artery	Signs and Symptoms
Common carotid artery (CCA) or Internal Carotid Artery (ICA)	Ipsilateral eye; distal vessels; may be asymptomatic
Middle cerebral artery (MCA)	Contralateral hemiparesis (face and arm greater than leg); horizontal gaze palsy; hemisensory deficits; homonymous hemianopsia; language and cognitive deficits (aphasia, apraxia, agnosia, neglect)
Anterior cerebral artery (ACA)	Contralateral hemiparesis (leg greater than arm and face); contralateral grasp reflex and gegenhalten; abulia; gait disorders; perseveration; urinary incontinence; may produce bilateral signs caused by involvement of a single vessel of common origin
Posterior cerebral artery (PCA)	Contralateral homonymous hemianopsia (or quadrantanopsia); may produce memory loss, dyslexia without dysgraphia, color anomia, hemisensory deficits, and mild hemiparesis; may be supplied by the anterior circulation
Cerebellar infarction	Dizziness, nausea, vomiting, nystagmus, ataxia *Recognition is important to detect brainstem compression caused by swelling;* neurosurgical decompression may be lifesaving.

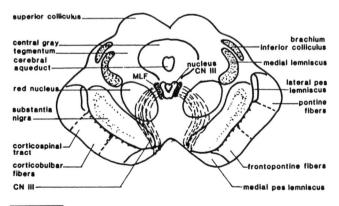

FIGURE 20

Midbrain cross-section. MLF, Medial longitudinal fasciculus.

TABLE 38

BRAINSTEM SYNDROMES

Syndrome	Localization	Clinical Features	
		Ipsilateral	Contralateral
Benedikt's	Midbrain tegmentum, red nucleus, cranial nerve (CN) III, cerebral peduncle	CN III palsy	Hemiataxia, tremor, hemiparesis, hyperkinesia
Claude's	Paramedian midbrain tegmentum, red nucleus, ND III, superior cerebellar peduncle	CN III palsy	Hemiataxia, tremor, hemiparesis
Weber's syndrome	Ventral midbrain, CN III, cerebral peduncle	CN III palsy	Hemiparesis
Parinaud's	Dorso rostral midbrain, posterior commissure and its interstitial nucleus		Paralysis of upward gaze and accommodation, light-near dissociation of pupil lid retraction, convergence-retraction nystagmus
Nothnagel's	Dorsal midbrain, brachium conjunctivum, CN III nucleus, medial longitudinal fasciculus	Ataxia, CN III palsy, vertical gaze palsy	
Raymond-Cestan	Medial mid-pons (paramedian branch, mid-basilar artery), middle cerebellar peduncle, corticobulbartract, corticospinal tract, variable medial lemniscus	Ataxia	Hemiparesis (face, arm, and leg), variable sensory, variable oculomotor
	Lateral mid-pons (short circumferential artery, middle cerebellar peduncle, CN V	Ataxia, paralysis of muscles of mastication, facial hemihypesthesia	
One and a half	Paramedian pontine reticular formation or CN VI nucleus, medial longitudinal fasciculus	Horizontal gaze palsy	Internuclear ophthalmoplegia
Foville's	Paramedian pontine reticular formation, CN VI, and VII, corticospinal tract	Horizontal gaze palsy, CN VII palsy	Hemiparesis, hemisensory loss, internuclear ophthalmoplegia

Syndrome	Structures involved	Ipsilateral/cranial signs	Contralateral/body signs
Millard-Gubler	Ventral paramedian pons, CN VI and VII fascicles, corticospinal tract	CN VI palsy, facial palsy	Hemiparesis
Raymond's	Ventral pons, CN VI fascicles and corticospinal tract	CN VI palsy	Hemiparesis
Babinski-Nageotte	Dorsolateral pontomedullary junction	Ataxia, hemihypesthesia in face, Horner's	Hemiparesis, hemihypesthesia in body, vertigo, vomiting, nystagmus
Wallenberg's	Dorsolateral medulla, vestibular nucleus, restiform body, CN V nucleus and spinal tract, CN IX and X, lateral spinothalamics, descending sympathetics	Lateropulsion; ataxia; loss of pain and temperature in face; paralysis of soft palate, posterior pharynx, and vocal cord; Horner's	Loss of pain and temperature in body
Cestan-Chenais	Lateral medulla	Ataxia; paralysis of soft palate, posterior pharynx, and vocal cord; Horner's, hemihypesthesia in face	Hemiparesis, hemihypesthesia in body
Avellis'	Lateral medulla, CN IX and X, lateral spinothalamics	Paralysis of soft palate, posterior pharynx, and vocal cord	Hemiparesis, hemihypesthesia
Vernet's	Lateral medulla, CN IX, X, and XI	Paralysis of soft palate; paralysis of vocal cord, posterior pharynx, and sternocleidomastoid; decreased taste over posterior third of tongue; hemihypesthesia of pharynx	Hemiparesis

Table continued on following page

ISCHEMIA

I

TABLE 38 —cont'd
BRAINSTEM SYNDROMES

Syndrome	Localization	Clinical Features	
		Ipsilateral	Contralateral
Jackson's	Lateral medulla, CN IX, X, XI, and XII	Paralysis of soft palate, posterior pharynx, vocal cords, sternocleidomastoid, upper trapezius, and tongue	Hemiparesis, hemihypesthesia
Tapia's	Lateral medulla, CN IX, X, XII (more commonly, there is extra cranial involvement)	As in Jackson's syndrome, except that sternocleidomastoid and trapezius are not involved	
Preolivary	Anterior medulla, CN XII, pyramid	Tongue atrophy or weakness	Hemiparesis

Vertebrobasilar artery (VBA) brainstem syndromes are best described in terms of neuroanatomic localization. Eponymic descriptions in the literature vary.

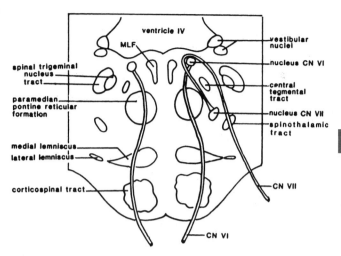

FIGURE 21

Pons cross-section. MLF, Medial longitudinal fasciculus.

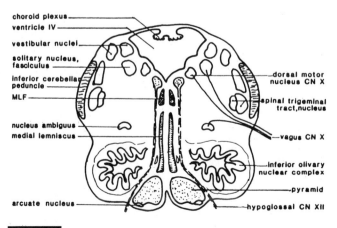

FIGURE 22

Medulla cross-section.

STROKE MECHANISM AND DIFFERENTIAL DIAGNOSIS

Identification of the ischemic mechanism is necessary for therapy selection. The characteristic clinical profile of *embolic* infarction is sudden onset of maximal neurologic deficit. Other cerebral injuries with sudden onset include intraparenchymal and subarachnoid hemorrhages, which often involve sudden headache and changes in mental status. Cerebral injury due to *small vessel disease* is often characterized by a "stuttering" course from time of onset.

TIAs may result from emboli of ulcerated carotid plaques, but imaging and pathologic studies reveal many patients with asymptomatic ulcerations. Serial arteriography in embolic infarction reveals vascular occlusion that may vanish despite persistence of neurologic deficit. In addition, recurrent TIAs correlate more with the presence of carotid stenosis and frequently manifest as border zone ("watershed") ischemic injury distal to areas of critical stenosis. *Watershed infarcts* are also seen secondary to clinically significant decrease in blood pressure.

Differential diagnosis of transient neurologic deficits includes syncope, hyper/hypoventilation syndromes, Ménière's disease, transient global amnesia (TGA), migraine, metabolic disease (hypercalcemia, hypoglycemia), psychogenic disorders, and seizures. Patients with a history of migraine may have transient neurologic deficits with or without headache. Late-life migraine may cause fleeting visual or sensory loss in the elderly. However, in this age group, careful workup is necessary to exclude vascular etiologies. For instance, isolated transient vertigo or the feeling of lightheadedness in the absence of brainstem signs may indicate labyrinthine disease or orthostatic hypotension. However, particularly in patients older than 55 years, cerebrovascular disease of the posterior circulation must be seriously considered. Transient deficits may be a manifestation of seizure; when there is involuntary motor activity or a Jacksonian-like march of symptoms, TIA is a less likely diagnosis although stroke may be heralded by a seizure.

NATURAL HISTORY AND RISK FACTORS

The recognition and reduction of risk factors is the most effective way to prevent stroke. Risk factors may be modifiable or nonmodifiable and vary with age and race. In young adults, trauma, drugs, oral contraceptives, migraine, and spontaneous arterial dissection are the most common causes of stroke. In patients 55 and older, hypertension, prior stroke or TIAs, coronary artery disease, congestive heart failure, and diabetes mellitus are important independent risk factors. Smoking, obesity, increased fibrinogen level, family history of premature death from stroke, and excessive alcohol use are also recognized as risk factors. Studies show that *atrial fibrillation (AF) is associated with a six-fold increased risk for stroke*. Of the above risk factors, AF and TIAs are most commonly associated with large vessel ischemia.

The prognosis in individuals with TIAs varies considerably. Up to one third of patients who have had a TIA will develop a disabling stroke within

5 years. Overall incidence of stroke after a TIA is 10% to 20% in the first year and thereafter 5% per year (five times the normal age-adjusted risk).

CLINICAL AND LABORATORY EVALUATION

The clinical evaluation and management during the first 72 hours of stroke onset usually determine outcome from ischemic brain injury. The National Institutes of Health Stroke Scale (NIHSS) is an effective means of measuring the total neurologic deficit (see inside back cover of this book). Careful attention should be given to supine blood pressure in both upper extremities, orthostatic blood pressure, cardiac examination, presence of carotid or cranial bruits and facial pulses, funduscopic exam, and evidence of peripheral emboli. Patients with carotid bruits have a higher incidence of TIA, stroke (2%/year on either side and 0.1% to 0.4%/year on the ipsilateral side of the bruit), myocardial infarction, and vascular death as compared to those without a bruit.

A. *Radiographic evaluation:* A CT scan should be performed on all patients to exclude the presence of hemorrhage. Unless a subarachnoid hemorrhage is suspected (10% have negative CT results), magnetic resonance imaging (MRI) is more sensitive for the detection of small strokes, particularly in the brainstem and posterior fossa. Additional techniques include MRI with diffusion (DWI) and perfusion-weighted images (PWI), as well as MRA (magnetic resonance angiography). Cerebral angiography is still considered to be the "gold standard" for studying the intracranial and extracranial vasculature when there is either an unclear or a potentially treatable condition. As a general guideline, patients with TIA in the carotid distribution should have angiography if they are considered candidates for surgery.

Transcranial Doppler is useful for noninvasive evaluation of the large cerebral arteries. It can demonstrate large vessel occlusion and help assess collateral flow in ischemic territories. Duplex carotid ultrasonography is also useful as an initial screening examination, especially for patients with carotid-distribution ischemic events. Operator dependency is ultrasonography's main disadvantage.

B. *Laboratory evaluation*: Complete evaluation includes complete blood counts, erythrocyte sedimentation rate, blood chemistries , prothrombin time (PT), and partial thromboplastin time (PTT). One may also include syphilis screening (test CSF for neurosyphilis if syphilis is highly suspected), lipid profile, urinalysis, chest x-ray, and hemoglobin electrophoresis in patients at risk for sickle cell disease (SCD). Since anticoagulation (AC) is contraindicated in established endocarditis, serial blood cultures should be obtained if there is suspicion of endocarditis (especially in patients with artificial valves or a history of intravenous drug abuse and those with congenital heart disease).

C. *Cardiac evaluation of stroke patients:* History and examination consistent with an embolic event and/or history of heart disease necessitates an evaluation of possible source for artery-to-artery embolus as well as

ISCHEMIA

I

cardioembolic sources. Cerebral and cardiac atherosclerosis share many pathogenic mechanisms and risk factors. Atherosclerotic stroke survivors are more likely to die from coronary artery disease than recurrent stroke. Evaluations identify possible cardiogenic sources of embolism and detect occult coronary artery disease (CAD). Besides intracardiac sources, proximal aortic atheroma, especially >4 mm mobile aortic plaques, is a strong risk factor for stroke. Transesophageal echocardiogram (TEE) is most useful in identifying the cardioembolic source. Holter monitoring is used when arrhythmia is implicated in stroke pathogenesis.

STROKE IN THE YOUNG EVALUATION
Additional evaluation for patients under the age of 55 and those with no clear risk factors includes cardiac evaluation as discussed earlier. Cardiac sources in young adults may include patent foramen ovale and atrial septal aneurysm. Mitral valve prolapse is not clearly correlated with increased stroke in the young. A search for causes of increased coagulability should be initiated before starting anticoagulation (antiphospholipids antibodies, anticardiolipin antibodies, heparin cofactor II deficiency, antithrombin III, protein C and S, activated protein C, factor V Leiden), antinuclear antibodies, serum viscosity, protein electrophoresis, ANA/rheumatologic profile, and serum homocystine and amino acid levels. Mitochondrial studies may be indicated in selected cases such as MELAS (mitochondrial encephalopathy with lactic acidosis and stroke). Peripheral blood sample may be diagnostic, searching for mutation, but muscle biopsy may be needed. Skin biopsy or genetic testing for notch-3 mutation in cases of suspected CADASIL (cerebral autosomal dominant arteriopathy with subcortical infarct and leukoencephalopathy) may prove to be helpful.

TREATMENT: GENERAL MEASURES
A. *Prevention of secondary complications:* Secondary complications in stroke patients (primarily deep vein thrombosis (DVT), urinary tract infection (UTI) and pneumonia) may be minimized by prophylactic measures. Venous stasis may be prevented by the use of Jobst stockings, sequential compression devices, and subcutaneous heparin (when not medically contraindicated). Both decubiti and stasis may be prevented by patient mobilization. Depressed gag reflexes or dysphagia should be carefully evaluated to avoid the risk of aspiration pneumonia. Alterations in bladder function are common after stroke and are treated as needed. Intermittent catheterization reduces the risk of infection compared to an indwelling urinary catheter.

  B. *General measures to minimize ischemia:* Once prolonged ischemia occurs, little can be done to reverse neuronal death. However, the area surrounding an ischemic injury, the so-called "ischemic penumbra," is at continued risk secondary to impaired autoregulation and perfusion. Damage to this area may be reversed and is critically influenced by management choices in the first 72 hours of stroke onset. In hypertensive patients, rapid lowering of blood pressure should be avoided. Although considerable controversy exists regarding optimal blood pressure control in the period immediately after stroke, there is greater risk in lowering blood pressure than in allowing it to remain at high levels (within 20 to 40 mmHg of baseline). Blood pressure reduction is indicated by symptoms of hypertensive crisis (e.g., acute renal failure, convulsions, or myocardial infarction). Bed rest is recommended during and immediately after a stroke to prevent postural changes in blood pressure, which coupled with impaired autoregulation may exacerbate ischemia. Although blood pressure management remains under debate, there are now clear indications for tight control of body temperature and glucose level. Avoiding lactic acidosis may prevent secondary worsening of noninfarcted tissue in the ischemic penumbra.

ANTICOAGULATION THERAPY IN ACUTE STROKE AND TIAS

There are a number of relative indications for AC therapy in the presence of acute ischemia, including the following: aortic arch mobile plaque >4 mm, ventricular aneurysm/thrombus, atrial fibrillation, atrial septal aneurysm, valvular disease/replacement, and spontaneous echocardiographic contrast that suggests low blood flow velocity. Other potential indications for AC include stenosis of a major vessel in an inoperable location, distal stump thrombus, or ulceration of an atheromatous plaque. Only one prospective trial in acute stroke used IV heparin regardless of cardiac status and no clear benefit was demonstrated. Thus, heparin use remains controversial. Heparin has been traditionally used in critical large cerebral vessel stenosis, in crescendo TIAs, and in progressing and fluctuating stroke. Since recurrent stroke is relatively uncommon, particularly in the first 7 days, physicians still have no clinical basis for early initiation and use of heparin beyond anecdotal success. Complications of heparin AC include symptomatic intracranial hemorrhage, asymptomatic hemorrhagic transformation of infarction, major and minor extracranial bleeding, thrombocytopenia, and thrombophlebitis. Contraindications for heparin use include recent surgery, trauma, seizure, recent gastrointestinal bleed, and the presence of a large, acute infarct or hemorrhage. Strokes affecting greater than two thirds of the MCA territory on the CT scan have an increased risk for hemorrhagic transformation during heparin therapy. The advent of DWI and PWI may improve the prediction of the risk of hemorrhage with heparin therapy.

ANTICOAGULATION THERAPY IN CARDIOEMBOLIC STROKE

There is good evidence that AC therapy reduces the risk of future embolization. Since the risk of stroke in patients with AF and sinus node disease is six times greater than in those without AF, patients with AF should receive AC therapy. Long-term AC therapy with warfarin requires monitoring (PT) and international normalized ratio (INR) to ensure values of 1.2 to 1.5 times the control value of PT, which translates to INR between 2 and 3. Even without a history of TIA or stroke, candidates for AC include patients with asymptomatic/symptomatic atrial fibrillation, atrial fibrillation with co-existing cardiomyopathy, mechanical prosthetic cardiac valves, symptomatic mitral valve prolapse, and intracardiac mural thrombus. When not medically contraindicated cardioversion should be considered. Short-term AC therapy is recommended in the setting of cardioversion for AF.

Many large embolic strokes (i.e., greater than two thirds of an arterial territory) occur in association with a known cardiac source (e.g., mural thrombus). A completely satisfactory course of action is difficult to select since AC therapy may worsen the neurologic deficit and morbidity/mortality outcome through hemorrhagic transformation. Unfortunately, withholding AC therapy may lead to repeated embolization. Management of such cases must be highly individualized. AC therapy provides no benefit in patients with embolism resulting from marantic endocarditis, calcific valves, or atrial myxoma. When embolic stroke is associated with prosthetic valve, AC therapy should be withheld while arteriography and contrasted CT scans are performed to exclude ruptured mycotic aneurysm.

USE OF ANTICOAGULANTS

Anticoagulation therapy is usually achieved with IV heparin administration and then maintained with oral administration of warfarin, due to transient protein C and S deficiency with initiation of warfarin.

Unlike the use of heparin in thromboembolic diseases, bolus administration is avoided with cerebral embolism because of the risk of hemorrhagic complications. The heparin infusion rate is adjusted every 4 to 6 hours until obtaining a maintenance level with activated PTT of 1.5 times the control value. Patients should be monitored for evidence of excessive anticoagulation (petechiae, microscopic hematuria, occult blood in stool, signs and symptoms of retroperitoneal bleeding). Heparin can be reversed with protamine sulfate (use 10 to 15 mg IV protamine sulfate; 1 mg neutralizes 100 USP units of heparin).

The necessity of warfarin loading is controversial. Loading may result in supratherapeutic levels. Warfarin dose is typically 2 to 10 mg/day. PT is determined daily, and the dosage is adjusted to maintain an INR of 2 to 3. Valve replacement patients require an INR of 3 to 4. Higher levels of anticoagulation are associated with a greater incidence of hemorrhagic complications. Numerous factors, including many drugs and liver disease, influence the response to warfarin. After satisfactory anticoagulation is attained with warfarin, the PT should be determined at least every 2 weeks. Excessive prolongation of PT can be corrected with vitamin K; however, vitamin K reversal significantly prolongs the time required to re-attain therapeutic AC levels with warfarin. Immediate reversal is accomplished by the use of fresh-frozen plasma.

ANTIPLATELET AGENTS

Platelets play a central role in the development of thrombi and subsequent ischemic events. In one study, the rate of infarction and death with TIAs and stroke was reduced by treatment with 1200 mg per day of aspirin. Other trials show no clear evidence that aspirin doses higher than 80 mg per day show improved benefit. In addition, lower doses are associated with decreased risk of bleeding complications. Antiplatelet agents are frequently used in small vessel, noncardioembolic infarcts; however, there is no prospective data to prove efficacy of this management. Ticlopidine (Ticlid) is an antiplatelet agent that is slightly more efficacious (at 150 mg bid) than aspirin. The use of ticlopidine necessitates initial monitoring of complete blood cell counts every other week for the first 3 months of therapy because of the risk of neutropenia. Clopidogrel (Plavix), another antiplatelet agent, is reportedly slightly more efficacious (at 75 mg qd) than aspirin and has relatively little gastrointestinal side effects. Clopidogrel-associated thrombotic thrombocytopenic purpura has been reported. Dipyridamole is another antiplatelet agent. The slow release form in combination with 25 mg aspirin bid (Aggrenox) is more efficacious than either aspirin or dipyridamole monotherapy alone.

Ancrod is an intravenous antiplatelet agent that has been shown to be slightly more effective than placebo in treating acute stroke patients.

THROMBOLYTIC THERAPY IN ACUTE STROKE

Since 1996, IV tissue plasminogen activator (tPA) has been approved in the United States for use in ischemic stroke patients within 3 hours of onset in a dose of 0.9 mg/kg (10% as a bolus and the remainder over 1 hour). The main risk with tPA administration is brain hemorrhage. Although reports reveal a ten-fold increased risk of symptomatic brain hemorrhage within the first 36 hours after tPA, patients receiving tPA were at least 30% more likely to have only minimal or no disability at 3 months.

Current recommendations include the following: (1) emergency medical support (EMS) recognition of stroke as an emergency to be able to identify more patients within the critical 3-hour window; and (2) minimal standards for stroke care facilities should include access to physician evaluation within 10 minutes, stroke expertise within 15 minutes, cranial CT scan within 25 minutes, interpretation of CT scan within 45 minutes, and intravenous tPA administration within 60 minutes of presentation. Unfortunately, only 5% of stroke victims receive tPA. Increased effort is needed to offer and administer thrombolytic therapy to qualified patients.

Direct *intra-arterial thrombolysis* (*IAT*) demonstrates a recanalization rate two to three times higher than IV thrombolysis. However, IAT requires angiographic documentation of vessel occlusion and administration within 6 hours after onset. In PROACT I and II (intra-arterial thrombolysis with Pro-Urokinase in Acute Cerebral Thromboembolism Trials) 40% of patients had slight or no neurologic disability compared to 25% of control. Recanalization rate was 67% versus 18% for controls.

Contraindication to thrombolysis includes early signs of infarction on head CT, minor/improving symptoms, seizure at onset, stroke/head trauma within 3 months, major surgery within 14 days, known intracranial hemorrhage, sustained systolic blood pressure >185 mmHg, sustained diastolic blood pressure >110 mmHg, gastrointestinal or genitourinary hemorrhage within 21 days, arterial puncture at noncompressible site within 7 days, heparin within 48 hours and elevated PTT, PT>15 seconds or INR>1.7, platelet count <100,000 ml, and serum glucose <50 mg/dl or >400 mg/dl. Also, there is a 1% to 2% incidence of anaphylactoid reactions and angioedema to tPA. Patients on angiotensin-converting enzyme may be at increased risk for angioedema with concomitant tPA therapy.

SURGICAL TREATMENT OF STROKE

A. *Carotid endarterectomy (CEA):* Carotid endarterectomy is indicated in patients with retinal or hemispheric stroke coupled with ipsilateral high-grade stenosis (70% to 90%). The rate of fatal and nonfatal stroke was reduced significantly when compared to medical therapy according to the North American Symptomatic Carotid Endarterectomy Trial (NASCET). Timing for surgery following acute stroke is most commonly 4 to 6 weeks; occasionally this may be shorter in unstable patients.

The Asymptomatic Carotid Atherosclerosis Study (ACAS) found that patients with asymptomatic carotid artery stenosis of 60% or greater reduction in diameter and whose general health makes them good candidates for elective surgery will have a reduced 5-year risk of ipsilateral stroke if carotid endarterectomy performed with less than 3% perioperative morbidity and mortality is added to aggressive management of modifiable risk factors.

B. *Hemicraniectomy:* Decompressive craniectomy may involve removal of a portion of the calvaria with durotomy or a more aggressive approach with removal of the infarcted tissue as a lifesaving procedure. This procedure can reduce the compartmentalization in the intracranial pressure and prevent brainstem herniation and death. This procedure is currently experimental. Prior to such an intervention, close monitoring is required. Placement of either intracranial pressure monitors or an intraventricular catheter is used in planning for possible surgical intervention.

C. *Bypass surgery:* Previous trials of bypass surgery were discouraging. Recent interest in bypass surgery has emerged in selected cases; those may include moyamoya disease and hemodynamic-dependent occlusion and/or stenosis in the carotid arteries with pressure-dependent neurologic deficits in patients without an alternative procedure to augment cerebral blood flow.

D. *Endovascular therapy*: stenting and angioplasty: The role of these interventions is still unclear, but they may be used in patients who are at high risk to undergo CEA or if the site of the stenosis is not amenable for surgical intervention.

E. *Neuronal tissue transplantation:* There has been an increasing interest in transplanting cultured neuronal cells at the site of the injured brain cells using stereotactic surgical guidance, aiming at restoring neurologic function.

This novel technique is still in its infancy, and it is premature to predict the real potential and outcome for this kind of intervention.

REHABILITATION

Rehabilitation decreases the long-term economic cost of stroke. Rehabilitation should be initiated 24 to 48 hours after the onset of stroke. The goals of stroke rehabilitation include restoration of lost abilities (motor and psychological), prevention of stroke-related complications, quality of life improvement, and education regarding secondary stroke prevention. New techniques in rehabilitation are on the horizon, including functional electrical stimulation and constraint-induced therapy.

RECOVERY AND PROGNOSIS

Approximately 10% of stroke survivors are without disability. Another 10% of patients are institutionalized because of markedly severe disability and inability to achieve functional independence. Factors that favor a poor prognosis include hemorrhagic stroke, impaired consciousness, heavy alcohol use, older age, male sex, hypertension, heart disease, and leg weakness. Negative predictors for functional outcome include incontinence, severe inattention, severe cognitive deficits, previous stroke, global aphasia, and complex comorbidities. The mortality rates at 1 month are 17% for patients with carotid distribution and 18% for patients with vertebrobasilar territory infarction.

Most rapid neurologic and functional recovery occurs by 3 months after a stroke. Recovery is categorized in stages, and a particular stage may be prolonged or recovery may stop at any stage. Stages include the following: (1) flaccidity, (2) spasticity, (3) synergistic movements (flexor and extensor), (4) isolated movements, (5) increased muscle strength, endurance, and coordination, and (6) return of muscle tone to pre-stroke state. Recovery from stroke may be prolonged and late functional improvements are possible.

DIFFERENTIAL DIAGNOSIS OF CEREBRAL INFARCTION

I. Cerebrovascular thrombosis associated with vascular disease.
   A. Atherosclerosis.
   B. Lipohyalinosis.
   C. Dissection.
   D. Chronic progressive subcortical encephalopathy (Binswanger's disease).
II. Cerebral embolism.
   A. Cardiac source.
      1. Valvular (mitral stenosis, prosthetic valve, infective endocarditis, marantic endocarditis, Libman-Sacks endocarditis, mitral annulus calcification, mitral valve prolapse, calcific aortic stenosis).
      2. Atrial fibrillation, sick sinus syndrome.
      3. Acute myocardial infarction, left ventricular aneurysm, or both.
      4. Left atrial myxoma.

      5. Cardiomyopathy.

      6. Acute and subacute bacterial endocarditis.

      7. Prosthetic valve dysfunction.

      8. Chagas' disease, trichinosis.

   B. Paradoxical embolism and pulmonary source.

      1. Pulmonary arteriovenous malformations (including Osler-Weber-Rendu syndrome).

      2. Atrial and ventricular septal defects with right-to-left shunts.

      3. Patent foramen ovale with right-to-left shunt.

      4. Pulmonary vein thrombosis.

      5. Pulmonary and mediastinal tumors.

   C. Artery-to-artery embolism.

      1. Cholesterol emboli.

      2. Atheroma thrombus.

      3. Complications of vascular and neck surgery.

      4. Idiopathic carotid mural thrombus, emboligenic aortitis.

      5. Emboli distal to unruptured aneurysm.

      6. Arterial dissection.

   D. Other.

      1. Fat embolism syndrome.

      2. Air embolism.

      3. Foreign body embolism (e.g., bullets, catheter tips, etc.).

III. Arteriopathies.

   A. Inflammatory.

      1. Takayasu's disease.

      2. Allergic granulomatosis (Churg-Strauss syndrome).

      3. Granulomatosis, polyarteritis nodosa, rheumatoid arthritis, Sjögren's syndrome, scleroderma, Behçet's syndromes, acute rheumatic fever, inflammatory bowel disease.

LACUNAR SYNDROMES

Lacunar infarcts are described as small, deep lesion(s) on CT or MRI usually ≤ 10 mm in diameter with density or signal consistent with infarct. Between 10% and 24% of all strokes are lacunar. There are a greater incidence of lacunes in Asians, blacks, and Hispanics than whites. Lacunar infarcts are characteristically located in the subcortical cerebrum and/or brainstem. Pathophysiology of lacunes can be categorized by four different mechanisms: (1) small vessel lipohyalinosis and fibrinoid degeneration, (2) decreased perfusion of penetrating arteries from proximal narrowing of larger vessels, (3) branch artery atheromatous occlusion, and (4) embolism.

    Patients with lacunes frequently have a history of hypertension, diabetes, hypercholesterolemia, smoking, and atherosclerosis of large and mid-sized intracranial arteries, but there is no increased incidence of these risk factors in patients with lacunar infarcts versus other ischemic strokes. Lacunes are infrequently associated with embolism and extracranial carotid occlusive disease. Lacunes occur in the lenticular nuclei (37%), caudate nucleus (10%), thalamus (14%), internal capsule (10%), and pons (16%). Lacunes are also seen in the corona radiata, external capsule, pyramids, and other brainstem structures.

Clinical presentations of lacunar infarction (see Table 39) are related to size and site of the lesion and range from asymptomatic to classic lacunar syndromes. Onset is often gradual or stepwise. Approximately 30% are preceded by transient ischemic attacks. Defined lacunar syndromes include pure motor hemiparesis, pure sensory syndrome, sensorimotor syndrome, ataxic hemiparesis, dysarthria-clumsy hand, and hemichorea/ballism.

Head CT demonstrates up to 70% of lesions within 7 days. Multiple lacunes are present in 30% of patients. MRI is more sensitive than CT. Thirty percent of lesions on imaging studies are asymptomatic. Treatment consists of antiplatelet agents, control of hypertension, and management of other vascular risk factors. Cerebral angiography is not recommended in pure lacunar syndromes. However, the absence of history or signs of hypertension (such as retinopathy and left ventricular hypertrophy) requires an aggressive workup for sources of embolus, large vessel disease, or unusual causes of stroke. Prognosis is usually favorable, but the probability of recurrence is high.

THALAMIC SYNDROMES

Cerebrovascular disease is the most common cause of discrete thalamic pathology. The thalamic arteries arise from the posterior communicating arteries and from the perimesencephalic segment of the posterior cerebral

TABLE 39

MOST COMMON LACUNAR SYNDROMES

Syndrome	Localization	Clinical Features
Pure sensory stroke	Venticular posterior thalamus	Sensory loss face, arm, leg—same side; no weakness; no visual field deficits; no "cortical" signs
Pure motor hemiparesis	Posterior limb interior capsule, basis pontis, cerebral peduncle	Weakness face, arm, leg—same side; no sensory loss; no visual field deficits; no "cortical" signs
Ataxic hemiparesis	Basis pontis, ventricular anterior thalamus and adjacent interior capsule	Cerebellar ataxia and weakness—same side; often leg > face
Dysarthria—clumsy hand syndrome	Basis pontis, genu interior capsule	Facial weakness, dysarthria, dysphagia, slight weakness and clumsiness of hand—same side

arteries. The following thalamic syndromes result from infarctions and each corresponds to a different arterial territory:

(1) *Inferolateral artery (thalamogeniculate artery)* infarcts with posterolateral thalamic lesions involve mainly the ventral posterior, ventral lateral, and subthalamic nuclear groups. These most commonly include hemisensory loss and pain, hemiataxia, disequilibrium, athetoid posture, and paroxysmal pain.

(2) *Tuberothalamic artery* supplies the anterior regions. Neuropsychologic dysfunction occurs most commonly. Other symptoms include facial paresis for emotional movement, occasional hemiparesis, dysphasia with left-sided lesions, and hemineglect and visuospatial dysfunction with right-sided lesions. Bilateral lesions lead to lethargy, apathy, abulia, and impaired memory.

(3) *Posterior choroidal arteries* supply the lateral geniculate body. With infarction, visual field deficits occur, most commonly quadrantanopia.

(4) *Paramedian arteries* supply the paramedian midbrain and thalamus, including the intralaminar group and most of the dorsomedial nucleus. The triad of common changes is somnolent apathy, memory loss, and abnormalities in vertical gaze. Also occasionally associated with akinetic mutism.

The syndrome of *Dejerine and Roussy (inferolateral thalamic syndrome)* is due to a vascular lesion in the territory of the thalamogeniculate artery. It is characterized by a mild hemiparesis, persistent hemianesthesia for touch, slight hemiataxia and astereognosis, choreoathetotic movements, and pain. *Thalamic pain syndrome* occurs contralateral to the lesion and is described as burning, aching, or boring. It is constant, but often there are paroxysmal increases, spontaneous or observed in patients with lesions in brainstem, internal capsule, basal ganglia, and subcortical parietal lobe. Treatment with tricyclic antidepressants (amitriptyline 10 to 100 mg qhs) or anticonvulsants (carbamazepine or dilantin) is sometimes effective. Conventional analgesics are ineffective.

MOYAMOYA DISEASE

From the Japanese word meaning "puff of smoke," moyamoya refers to the angiographic appearance of small vessels arising from the Circle of Willis in association with gradual occlusion of large vessels. Although the disease is most commonly found in the Japanese, moyamoya occurs in people throughout the world. In previous years, diagnosis of moyamoya was dependent on cerebral angiography. However, with improvement in the quality of MRI and MRA, diagnosis of moyamoya can be made without conventional cerebral angiography. The MRA must demonstrate stenosis or occlusion at the terminal portions of the intracranial internal carotid arteries and at the proximal portions of the anterior communicating arteries and the middle cerebral arteries. Diagnosis with MRA requires visualization of abnormal vascular networks in the basal ganglia on MRA, or demonstration of moyamoya vessels as apparent signal voids in the ipsilateral side of the basal ganglia on MRI. These two findings must be found bilaterally. Diagnosis solely based on MRI and MRA is recommended for children only. With conventional angiography, there must be bilateral stenosis or occlusion at the terminal portions of the intracranial internal carotid arteries and at the proximal portions of the anterior communicating arteries and the middle cerebral arteries. Angiogram must also demonstrate bilateral abnormal vascular networks in the vicinity of the occlusive (or stenotic) lesions in the arterial phase.

Adults and children usually present differently. Children frequently present with hemiparesis, monoparesis, sensory disturbance, involuntary movement, headache, and convulsions. Adults are more likely to have a sudden onset of intraventricular, subarachnoid, or intracerebral hemorrhage. However, symptoms similar to those in children may occur in adults. Conditions associated with moyamoya include Down's syndrome, neurocutaneous syndromes (tuberous sclerosis, neurofibromatosis, Sturge-Weber Syndrome), sickle cell disease, Fanconi's anemia, cyanotic congenital heart disease, pituitary tumor, type I glycogenosis, radiation therapy, vasculitis, and leptospirosis. Moyamoya may be inherited. Although there is no specific treatment, the majority of patients undergo revascularization operations. Patients with mild and transient symptoms tend to undergo conservative treatment. Surgery tends to have a better prognosis. Medical treatment has included vasodilators, antiplatelet agents, antifibrinolytic agents, and fibrinolytic agents.

SICKLE CELL DISEASE

SCD is due to a genetic defect in which valine is substituted for glutamic acid at the sixth position of the beta hemoglobulin chain, which transforms HbA to HbS. Neurologic manifestations are seen in one third of patients with SCD. The frequency of neurologic manifestations is proportional to the propensity for sickling: 6% to 35% in sickle cell disease (SS), 6% to 24% in individuals heterozygous for HbS/HbC and 0% to 6% in sickle cell trait HbA/HbS.

Stroke occurs in as many as 17% of patients with SCD. Cerebral infarction occurs in 25% of all children with SCD, mainly caused by large artery stenosis. The middle cerebral and intracranial internal carotid arteries more commonly develop stenosis. Three intrinsic mechanisms contribute to ischemia in sickle cell disease: (1) large vessel endothelial injury because of sickled cells, resulting in endothelial hyperplasia and vessel occlusion; (2) sludging of sickled cells during a sickle crises, with resultant ischemia in small vessels; (3) the chronic anemia leads to increased cerebral perfusion, vasodilation, and lack of cerebral autoregulatory reserve for regional cerebral metabolic demands. These abnormal, dilated vessels may rupture with resultant hemorrhage. Research suggests evidence for HLA-related susceptibility for stroke in children with SCD; HLA typing may prove useful in identifying patients at higher risk for stroke. There is evidence that elevated homocysteine levels may be a risk factor for stroke development in SCD.

Elevated blood velocities measured by transcranial doppler ultrasonography (TCD) indicate children at risk for stroke. Red blood cell transfusions sufficient to reduce the percentage of HbS by a factor greater than three are associated with a marked reduction in stroke (>90%). Without treatment, the recurrence rate of stroke is approximately 80%. A clinical alert from The National Heart, Lung and Blood Institute recommends TCD baseline testing in children ages 2 to 16 with SCD and follow-up studies every 6 months in children with normal studies. TCDs represent a noninvasive alternative to angiography. Angiography may precipitate sickling unless abnormal hemoglobin is reduced via transfusion.

Other neurologic complications associated with SCD include seizures, behavioral changes (i.e., acute and chronic encephalopathy), alterations in consciousness, CNS infections, visual impairment, and intracranial hemorrhage. Hemorrhages are more commonly subarachnoid in children and intraparenchymal in adults. Seizures occur in 8% to 12% of patients and are typically generalized tonic-clonic. CNS infections in sickle cell patients are commonly due to encapsulated organisms. This is due to the decreased phagocytic ability of the reticuloendothelial system especially in functionally asplenic patients. Visual complications include vitreous, retinal and subretinal hemorrhages, and central retinal artery and other retinal vascular changes. Idiopathic headache is common and may be related to increased cerebral blood flow. Myelopathy can result from vertebral body infarction, extramedullary hematopoiesis, and spinal cord infarction.

VENOUS THROMBOSIS

Thrombosis of the cerebral venous system may involve the cortical veins alone, the dural sinuses alone, or both. Cortical vein thrombosis is rare and characterized by headache, seizures and focal deficits (including cranial nerve VI palsy), somnolence, coma, and death. Papilledema may be present. Subarachnoid hemorrhage resulting from rupture of congested veins or extension of hemorrhagic infarction may occur. Other signs of parasagittal stroke or hemorrhage may be present because of propagation of thrombus into surrounding cortical veins. Thrombosis may also involve the cavernous sinus (usually as a result of facial or orbital infection). Cavernous sinus involvement is characterized by facial pain, proptosis, and involvement of CNs III, IV, and VI. Venous thrombosis may also involve the superior petrosal (prominent facial pain), the inferior petrosal (*Gradenigo's syndrome with retro-orbital pain and CN VI palsy*), the lateral (increased intracranial pressure and ear pain) or internal jugular (use of catheters or pacemakers may involve CN IX, X, and XI) sinuses.

Intracranial venous thrombosis can be aseptic or septic. Intracranial septic venous thrombosis is rare and usually involves the cavernous sinus. Aseptic intracranial venous thrombosis is divided into dural venous sinus thrombosis, deep venous thrombosis, and superficial or cortical vein thrombosis. Superior sagittal sinus thrombosis is the most common type.

Contrast-enhanced CT scan shows a "negative delta" sign, which is characterized by opacification of the sinus wall with noninjection of the clot inside the sinus in only 30% of cases. MRI or magnetic resonance venography may be diagnostic. Venous phase angiography usually shows a filling defect. Results of lumbar puncture, if not contraindicated by mass effect, are nonspecific but may reveal increased pressure and increased levels of protein, polymorphonuclear leukocytes, and red blood cells (if hemorrhage has occurred).

Etiologies of intracranial sinovenous occlusive disease:

1. Trauma: Injury, neck surgery, indwelling IV lines
2. Infection: Facial, orbital, paranasal sinuses, middle ear, meningitis
3. Endocrine: Pregnancy, puerperium, contraceptives
4. Volume depletion: Hyperosmolar coma, inflammatory bowel disease, diarrhea, postpartum, postoperative, dehydration
5. Hematologic: Polycythemia vera, disseminated intravascular coagulation, sickle cell disease, cryofibrinogenemia, paroxysmal nocturnal hemoglobinuria, thrombocytosis, antithrombin III deficiency, transfusion reaction, factor V Leiden
6. Impaired cerebral circulation: Arterial occlusion, congenital heart disease, congestive heart failure, anesthesia in seated position, sagittal sinus webs
7. Carcinoma: Leukemia, lymphoma, meningeal spread, meningioma
8. Drugs/therapies: L-Asparaginase, androgens, cisplatin, etoposide
9. Other: Wegener's granulomatosis, polyarteritis nodosa, systemic lupus erythematosus, Behçet's syndrome, Cogan's syndrome, homocystinuria, cardiac pacemakers

Vein of Galen thrombosis in neonates after trauma or infection may result in extensor posturing, fever, tachycardia, tachypnea, and death. Survivors may have bilateral choreoathetosis.

Previously considered almost universally fatal, cerebral venous thrombosis now has a good long-term prognosis with the use of anticoagulation. In relatively small studies, anticoagulation with heparin, coumadin, or low-molecular-weight heparin has been safely employed even in patients with cerebral hemorrhage. Intracranial hypertension should be controlled during treatment. Management also includes treatment of the underlying cause and supportive care.

REFERENCES

Glucose in ischemia:
Auer R: *Neurology* 51(Suppl 3):S39–S43, 1998.

Anticoagulation:
Harrison L et al: *Ann Int Med* 126:133–136, 1997.
Korczyn AD: *Neurol Clin* 10:209–217, 1992.
Swanson RA: *Neurology* 52:1746–1750, 1999.

ISCHEMIA

Cardioembolic stroke:
Fatkin D et al: *Am J Cardiol* 73:672–676, 1994.
Hart RG, Halperin JL: *Ann Int Med* 131:688–695, 1999.

Antiplatelet therapy:
Bennett CL et al: *Ann Int Med* 128:541–544, 1998.
CAPRIE Steering Committee: *Lancet* 348:1329–1339, 1996.
Diener HC et al: *J Neurol Sci* 143:1–13, 1996.

Thrombolytic therapy:
Adams et al: *Stroke* 27:1711–1718, 1996.
Hacke W et al: *Lancet* 352:1245–1251, 1988.
Hakim AM: *Neurology* 51(Suppl 3):S44–S46, 1998.
Hill et al: *Can Med Assoc J* 162:1281–1284, 2000.

Surgical Therapy:
Chaturvedi S, Halliday A: *Curr Atheroscler Rep* 2(2):115–119, 2000.
Executive Committee for the Asymptomatic Carotid Atherosclerosis Study: *JAMA* 273(18):1421–1428, 1995.
Gomez CR: *Semin Neurol* 18(4):501–511, 1998.
Kondziolka D, Wechsler L et al: *Neurology* 55(4):565–569, 2000.
North American Symptomatic Carotid Endarterectomy Trial Collaborators: *N Engl J Med* 325(7):445–453, 1991.

Stroke risk factors:
Gilon D et al: *N Engl J Med* 341:8–13, 1999.
Hart RG, Halperin JL: *Ann Int Med* 131:688–695, 1991.
Sacco R: *Neurology* 51(Suppl 3):S27–S30, 1998.
Wilterdink JL, et al: *Neurology* 51(Suppl 3):S23–S26, 1998.

Lacunar syndromes:
Gan R et al: *Neurology* 48:1204–1211, 1997.
Horowitz D, et al: *Neurology* 48:325–327, 1997.

Moya Moya:
Barnett HM et al: Stroke: pathophysiology, *diagnosis and management*, ed 3, New York, Churchill, Livingstone, 1998.

Sickle Cell Disease:
Adams RJ: *J Child Neurol* 15:344–349, 2000.
Styles LA et al: *Blood* 95:3562–3567, 2000.

Venous thrombosis:
De Bruijn et al: *Stroke* 30:484–488, 1999.
Perkin GD: *J Neurol Neurosurg Psychiatry* 59:1–3, 1995.
Preter et al: *Stroke* 27:243–246, 1996.

LAMBERT-EATON MYASTHENIC SYNDROME

Lambert-Eaton myasthenic syndrome (LEMS) is an autoimmune disorder of neuromuscular transmission. Antibodies directed at the voltage-gated calcium channels (VGCCs) on presynaptic cholinergic nerve terminals are responsible for the disease. Calcium entry via voltage-gated calcium channels is required to facilitate docking and release of presynaptic acetylcholine vesicles. Antibodies to VGCCs lead to a decrement in the release of presynaptic acetylcholine (ACh) vesicles. Presynaptic ACh stores and the postsynaptic response to individual quanta are normal.

LEMS is a rare disease and usually occurs in older adults with mean age of onset of 50 and ratio of men to women of 1.8:1. LEMS is associated with small cell lung carcinoma (SCLC) in approximately two thirds of cases. The remaining third of cases are mainly idiopathic. Other neoplasms associated with LEMS include carcinomas of the rectum, kidney, stomach and breast, and leukemia. Autoimmune diseases such as systemic lupus erythematosus, rheumatoid arthritis, and Sjögren's syndrome may be related to LEMS. LEMS may precede the diagnosis of cancer by an average of 10 months.

Clinical features: Proximal leg or arm weakness; muscle aching and stiffness worsened by prolonged exercise; difficulty combing hair or rising from a chair. Unlike myasthenia gravis, initial symptoms due to cranial nerve dysfunction are rare. However, transient diplopia, ptosis, dysphagia, dysarthria, and neck flexion weakness can develop in later stages. Eighty percent of patients will experience autonomic involvement, usually dry mouth and impotence, occasionally constipation, blurred vision, and impaired sweating. Sensory complaints are rare.

On examination, proximal weakness of the lower limbs greater than the upper limbs is the most consistent finding. A progressive increase in strength after a few seconds of sustained contraction is usual, with fatigue after continued contraction. Muscle wasting is rare. Limb reflexes are decreased or absent in >90% of cases. However, a potentiation of reflexes after maximal contraction of the involved muscle for 10 to 15 seconds is usually present.

Laboratory findings: On nerve conduction studies, the amplitude of the compound muscle action potentials (CMAP) is reduced. The sensory responses are normal. Nerve conduction velocities and latencies are normal. Slow repetitive stimulation (2 Hz) produces a decremental response of the CMAP amplitude similar to myasthenia gravis. In contrast, the repetitive stimulation performed at high frequencies (>10 Hz) creates a profound incremental response (100% to 200% increase in amplitude of CMAP) due to calcium accumulation in the presynaptic terminal with subsequent enhancement of the release of ACh vesicles. A similar phenomena is present after a brief (10 sec) sustained voluntary exercise (post-exercise facilitation). Antibodies to VGCCs can be tested in blood. LEMS patients sometimes respond to edrophonium but not consistently, and it usually is not useful for the diagnosis.

Treatment is directed at the responsible tumor or underlying autoimmune disorder. Response to cholinesterase inhibitors is variable. Plasmapheresis, immunosuppressive agents (azathioprine), and prednisone (100 mg/day for 1 week followed by a gradual taper to 60 mg every other day) may help, particularly if the LEMS is due to autoimmunity. A drug that facilitates synaptic transmission, *3,4-diaminopyridine (DAP)*, which prolongs the duration of presynaptic action potentials by blocking delayed rectifier potassium channels and leads to increased calcium entry to the presynaptic terminal, may improve strength in LEMS patients in doses of 15 mg four times a day (1 mg/kg/day). Anticholinesterases may facilitate the effect of DAP. Guanidine 10 mg/kg/day may improve strength but is not well tolerated due to severe side effects including bone marrow suppression and renal failure.

The survival of tumor-associated LEMS is poor due to progression of the underlying malignancy, although patients with SCLC and LEMS generally have longer survival time in comparison to patients with SCLC alone. In LEMS without underlying disease the prognosis is good and clinical remission can be achieved in 40% of patients with immunosuppressive agents.

REFERENCES

Lennon VA et al: *N Engl J Med* 332:1467–1474, 1995.
Saunders DB: *Ann Neurol* 37:S63–S73, 1995.

LEARNING DISABILITIES

Learning disability (LD) is defined as difficulty in the acquisition and use of language, reasoning, mathematical abilities, or social skills. Approximately 50% of children with LD have associated attention deficit-hyperactivity disorder (ADHD), conduct disorder, anxiety disorders, and to a lesser extent, mood disorders.

In preschoolers, LD usually becomes evident as language delay. A child who has no meaningful words by age 18 months, no meaningful phrases by age 24 months, or speech unintelligible to strangers by age 3 years should be evaluated for hearing loss and referred for speech therapy.

In school-aged children, LD usually becomes evident as unexpected school failure. Selective reading disability is a common form of LD that can lead to general failure in school if not recognized early. There is often a family history of learning problems. Standard intelligence and achievement tests should be administered to verify normal intelligence and failure to achieve the expected level of performance.

In the U.S. the clinician should ensure that parents are under the Individuals with Disabilities Education Act, which defines the level of disability necessary for a child or adolescent to be eligible for special education services in public schools. The parents, or the clinician on the parent's behalf, should inform the school in writing of the child's needs for special education services. Counseling for associated social, behavioral, and psychiatric symptoms should be tailored to take into account the child's specific language and cognitive deficits. Parent support and consultation and management may be needed to help the family develop a supportive home environment and a consistent home-school behavioral reinforcement program.

REFERENCE

Beitchman JH: *J Am Acad Child Adolesc Psychiatry* 37:1117–1119, 1998.

LIMBIC SYSTEM

The limbic system is brain network subsystem consisting of the cingulate, parahippocampal, and subcallosal gyri, hippocampal formation, dentate gyrus, hypothalamus, mammillary bodies, amygdaloid complex, epithalamus, medial tegmental region of the midbrain, septal nuclei, anterior and dorsomedial thalamic nuclei, and fibrous pathway (fornix, mammillothalamic tract, medial forebrain bundle, and stria terminalis). *Papez circuit* constitutes the principal structure of the limbic system. Lesions and disease in the limbic system lead to abnormalities of memory, emotion, motivation, behavior, and autonomic and endocrine control.

REFERENCES

Carpenter MB: *Core text of neuroanatomy*, ed 4, Baltimore, Williams & Wilkins, 1991.
Strub RL, Black FW: *The mental status examination in neurology*, ed 4, Philadelphia, FA Davis, 2000.

LUMBOSACRAL PLEXUS

The lumbosacral plexus is comprised of the anastomoses derived from the ventral primary rami of T12-S4 (see Figure 23). Etiologies for lumbosacral dysfunction include neoplasms (cervix, prostate, bladder, colorectal, kidney, breast, ovary, and lymphoma), retroperitoneal hemorrhage, psoas abscess (from osteomyelitis), diabetes, inadvertent injections into the gluteal artery or umbilical artery, intravenous heroin, idiopathic retroperitoneal fibrosis, herpes zoster infections, pyelonephritis, appendicitis, retroperitoneal masses, aortic aneurysms, and trauma. Pain, weakness, loss of deep tendon reflexes, and sensory changes may occur in the appropriate distribution (see also Dermatomes, Myotomes).

Lumbosacral plexus neuropathy (less common than idiopathic brachial plexopathy) occurs during labor and delivery, when the descending fetal head may compress the lumbosacral trunk and S1 root at the point where they join and pass over the pelvic rim. It is characterized by a sudden onset of severe pain in the thigh or buttock (followed 5 to 10 days later by weakness in the distribution of the involved plexus and elevated erythrocyte sedimentation rate.

Radiation plexopathy usually occurs one to many years after radiation. Findings include unilateral or bilateral distal leg weakness, mild pain, and EMG showing myokymic discharges (50%). In contrast, plexopathy due to tumor is associated with severe pain at onset and weakness involving proximal and unilateral leg muscles.

CT scan is the imaging procedure of choice for visualizing the retroperitoneal space and lumbosacral plexus, but MRI is advancing rapidly and may have a vital role in nerve imaging in the near future.

Management consists of identifying and treating the underlying etiology. Steroids and intravenous immunoglobulin have been successfully used in cases of idiopathic lumbosacral plexopathy.

L

LUMBOSACRAL PLEXUS

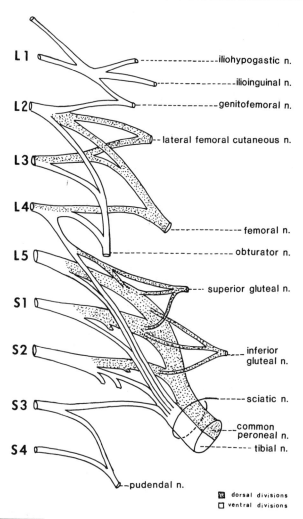

FIGURE 23

Lumbosacral plexus.

REFERENCES

Ismael SS et al: *J Neurol Neurosurg Psychiatry* 68:771–773, 2000.
Triggs WJ et al: *Muscle Nerve* 20:244–246, 1997.

LYME DISEASE

Lyme disease, also called Lyme borreliosis, is a multisystem disease (dermatologic, neurologic, rheumatologic, and cardiac manifestations) caused by a tick-transmitted spirochete, *Borrelia burgdorferi*. Clinically, lyme disease may be divided into three stages.

Stage I: Localized infection (3 days to 1 month) usually begins shortly after a tick bite with flulike syndrome. Skin lesion manifests as a red macule or papule and expands centrifugally to form an annular red lesion with central clearing (*erythema chronicum migrans*). Regional adenopathy and mild systemic symptoms of headache, neck stiffness, lethargy, or mild encephalopathy may occur. The CSF is usually normal.

Stage II: Disseminated infection (up to 9 months) occurs within days or weeks. The spirochete may spread hematogenously. This stage manifests clinically as meningoradiculitis, migratory musculoskeletal pain, acute arteritis, generalized adenopathy, splenomegaly, carditis, severe malaise, and fatigue. Weeks to months after illness the most common neurologic abnormality is lymphocytic meningitis with or without accompanying CNS parenchymal involvement. Radiculoneuritis, when present, may be asymmetrical, painful, and with dermatomal sensory and myotomal motor abnormalities. Variations include mononeuritis, mononeuritis multiplex, brachial or lumbosacral plexopathy, and Guillain-Barré-like syndrome. Electrophysiologic testing usually points to axonal degeneration in distal nerves and roots. Cranial neuropathies develop in about 60% of patients. Facial palsy is most common: 70% to 80% in stage II and 10% of all patients. Cranial nerves III, IV, VI (13%), V (6%), VIII (5%), and II (3%) may also be involved. CSF findings in stage II include increased cell count (100 to 200 WBC/mm^3 with >90% lymphocytes), decreased glucose (<2/3 serum glucose), and increased protein (35% of patients, usually 100 to 300 mg/dl).

Stage III: Late or persistent infection occurs months to years after initial infection. It manifests as attacks of arthritis in large joints, persistent skin infection, and persistent, often progressive, neurologic abnormalities sometimes with a long latency. Neurologic manifestations include chronic progressive encephalomyelitis (meningitis, encephalitis, myelitis, cranial neuritis, radiculoneuritis), focal encephalitis, mild encephalopathy, dementia, seizures, distal axonopathy, and asymmetric polyneuropathy. CSF findings are similar to stage II.

Diagnosis: History of erythema migrans, tick bite or exposure to travel in an endemic area, extraneural involvement, and/or suggestive neurologic syndromes (i.e., unilateral or bilateral Bell's palsy, aseptic meningitis, atypical Guillain-Barré syndrome, and mild polyneuropathy). Not all patients recall the tick bite or the rash. Serologic evidence of IgM and IgG antibodies are measured by ELISA as an initial screen and confirmed by Western blot. CSF Lyme antibody index confirms neurologic Lyme disease but is not invariably elevated. *B. burgdorferi* is virtually impossible to culture and routine biopsy is not helpful. Polymerase chain reaction may be used in the future.

Treatment: Stage I and II with facial palsy: doxycycline 100 mg PO bid for 21 to 30 days or amoxicillin (with probenecid) 500 mg PO qid 21 to 30 days or cefuroxime 500 mg PO bid for 21-30 days. Stage II with neurologic involvement other than facial palsy requires penicillin G 24 MU/day IV for 14 to 21 days or ceftriaxone 2 g/day IV for 30 days or cefotaxime 2 g IV q 8 hr for 30 days or doxycycline 100 to 200 mg PO bid for 21 to 28 days. Stage III treatment is the same as in stage II, except doxycycline is given for 30 days. Parenteral antibiotics are preferred for neurologic Lyme disease associated with CSF abnormalities or CNS Lyme syndromes. Nonspecific problems (fatigue, joint pain, muscle ache) may persist for many months after treatment.

REFERENCE

Halperin JJ et al: *Neurology* 46:619–627, 1996.

MACROCEPHALY

Macrocephaly is head circumference greater than 2 standard deviations above the normal distribution for age. Differential diagnoses of macrocephaly include hydrocephalus (communicating or noncommunicating), megalencephaly, thickening of the skull, and hemorrhage into the subdural or epidural spaces. The causes of megalencephaly are anatomic and metabolic. Anatomic megalencephaly includes conditions in which the brain is enlarged because the number or size of cells increases. These include genetic megalencephaly or megalencephaly with gigantism (Sotos syndrome), neurocutaneous disorders, or other neurologic disorders. These children are macrocephalic at birth but have normal intracranial pressure. Children with metabolic megalencephaly are normocephalic at birth and develop megalencephaly during the neonatal period due to storage of abnormal substances or by producing cerebral edema.

Evaluation includes review of prior head circumference measurements to assess rate of head growth (a rapidly growing head that is crossing percentile lines suggests hydrocephalus), assessment of head shape (frontal bossing is associated with hydrocephalus, lateral bulging with infantile subdural hematoma), measurement of head circumference of parents and siblings (benign familial megalencephaly), and CT, MRI, or ultrasound. If the infant is neurologically and developmentally normal, close observation may be all that is necessary.

A useful rule of thumb for normal rate of head growth follows:

| Premature infants | 1 cm/week |
| 1 to 3 months | 2 cm/month |

| 3 to 6 months | 1 cm/month |
| 6 to 12 months | $\frac{1}{2}$ cm/month |

REFERENCE

Fenichel GM: *Clinical pediatric neurology: a signs and symptoms approach*, Philadelphia, WB Saunders, 1997.

MAGNETIC RESONANCE IMAGING (MRI)

MRI is a form of computed tomography that creates images based on the behavior of various tissues exposed to strong magnetic fields, controlled magnetic field gradients, and radiofrequency (RF) pulses. Image intensity and contrast depends upon the concentration of unpaired protons, typically from hydrogen nuclei; the motion of these nuclei; nuclear magnetic relaxation parameters; and the type of sequence or acquisition that the MRI device is performing.

When tissue protons are placed in a magnetic field, they tend to align themselves either longitudinally (parallel) in a low-energy state or transversely (antiparallel) in a high-energy state to the vector of the imposed magnetic field, although they flip periodically between the two states. Since low-energy states are preferred, more protons align longitudinally than transversely at any given moment. The net magnetization vector, therefore, is longitudinal to the imposed magnetic field (the equilibrium state). A 90-degree RF pulse can be applied, exciting the protons, changing them from longitudinal to transverse alignment. As these protons return to equilibrium within the magnetic field (i.e., longitudinal alignment), they emit energy (as RF signal), which can be detected and converted into meaningful data—the image—by means of certain manipulations discussed below.

TECHNICAL PARAMETERS IN MRI

1. *Repetition time* (TR) defines a duration of a cycle, i.e., the time between successive 90-degree RF pulses. It also sets the "starting intensity" from which the signal decay (T2) is measured.
2. *Echo time* (TE) defines a sampling interval during the cycle, i.e., the time between giving the RF pulse and measuring the amount of RF signal being emitted by the tissue, i.e., "the echo." There may be single or multiple echoes sampled during a given cycle.
3. *Relaxation time* is the time it takes the protons to return to equilibrium within the magnetic field after an RF pulse has been given. MRI signal is based mainly on the relaxation times of the protons within lipids and water. Protons within protein, DNA, and solid structures such as bone, have relaxation properties that are undetectable by typical MRI imaging. Relaxation time is determined by two processes called T1 and T2.

T1 relaxation is based upon how fast the protons return to equilibrium (longitudinal alignment) after being energized. At any given time after the

TABLE 40

T1-WEIGHTED IMAGE

Dark (Low Signal, Long T1)	Bright (High Signal, Short T1)
CSF	Lipid
Deoxyhemoglobin (in intact red blood cells)	Gadolinium
Calcium	Methemoglobin (free or in red blood cells)
Air	Proteinaceous substances
Edema	Hepatic failure (globus pallidus)
Most pathologic lesions	Hypoxia (caudate, putamen)
	Melanotic tumors

RF pulse is given (TE), those elements whose protons re-equilibrate fastest (lipids, for example, with the highest percentage of protons in the longitudinal position), appear brightest on images where the T1 characteristics are selected for (T1-weighted images; T1WI). Those elements whose protons re-equilibrate slower, water for example, will appear darker (see Table 40). The shorter the TE, the greater the difference between the elements. At short TE, a large percentage of the lipid protons have reattained their longitudinal position, whereas few water protons have done so. At longer TE, a large percentage of both lipid and water protons are realigned. The greater the difference between the two elements (the shorter the TE), the greater the contrast on T1WI (T1-weighted images have short TR and short TE).

T2 relaxation is determined by how fast an element "decays" from the transverse alignment to the longitudinal alignment. In this situation, the longer an element maintains its transverse alignment (slower decay), the stronger a signal it will emit (i.e., its brightness, on T2-weighted images; T2WI) (see Table 41). At shorter TE, a high percentage of both lipid and water protons are made in transverse alignment. At a longer TE, most of the lipid protons have returned to longitudinal alignment (fast decay), whereas most of the water protons remain in transverse alignment (slow decay). Therefore, for greatest contrast of T2WI images, choose longer TE (T2WI have long TE and long TR).

TABLE 41

T2-WEIGHTED IMAGE

Dark (Low Signal, Long T2)	Bright (High Signal, Short T2)
Solids	CSF
Cortical bone	Liquids
Calcium	Edema
Hemosiderin	Most pathologic lesions
Deoxyhemoglobin (in intact red blood cells)	
Methemoglobin (in intact red blood cells)	
Ferritin	
Mucinous metastatic lesions	
Air	

TABLE 42

GRADIENT ECHO T2-WEIGHTED IMAGE

Dark (Low Signal)	Bright (High Signal)
Hemosiderin	Flow-related enhancement
Deoxyhemoglobin	
Calcium	
Ferritin	

The degree of brightness or darkness on T1WI and T2WI can thus be determined by tissue fat and water content (see Tables 40–43). In general, pathological conditions are dark on T1WI, bright on T2WI, and bright on spin density images (see below).

The acquisition of data may be performed in a variety of patterns or sequences, which emphasizes these differences in tissue properties. A typical example is the spin echo (SE) sequence in which an initial 90-degree pulse is given, and the echo is recalled at a predetermined point with an additional 180-degree pulse. The 180-degree pulse is necessary because of "dephasing" or spreading of the magnetic vectors of individual protons as they decay; they would eventually cancel each other out until the net vector becomes so weak that the signal emitted would be undetectable. The 180-degree pulse "rephases" or brings back together the individual proton vectors so the echo emitted can be detected. T1WI images, T2WI images, and "intermediate" spin density images (long TR, short TE) may be obtained with this sequence. SD images utilize tissue characteristics between T1WI and T2WI (long TR, short TE).

Another frequently used acquisition sequence is the gradient echo (GE), a "fast scanning" technique that replaces the protons for sampling by means of reversing the magnetic field gradient. The sequence takes less scanning time and is useful for imaging flowing blood (flow-related enhancement), for detecting calcification or hemorrhage, and for mild myelogram effect (white CSF) in the spinal canal. GE images, like SE may be T1- or T2-weighted; usually only T2WI or SD images are employed.

TABLE 43

HEMATOMA

	T1WI	T2WI
Acute	—	Bright rim (intact red blood cells)
	—	Dark core (deoxyhemoglobin)
	—	Edema
Subacute	Bright rim (methemoglobin)	—
	Dark to bright core (methemoglobin)	—
	Less edema	—
Chronic	—	Dark rim (hemosiderin)
	—	No edema

Perfusion-weighted images (PWI) are a recent application for the MRI in evaluating cerebral blood flow using a bolus-tracking method in acquiring repeated images during the first passage of the intravenous paramagnetic contrast (gadolinium). Areas of diminished blood flow are bright on PWI.

Diffusion weighted images (DWI) are another function of the MRI method that study the water motion in brain tissue. Areas with low diffusion appear as high or bright signals. For example, DWI shows the cerebral infarcts as bright signals within 30 minutes of onset and lasts 7 to 21 days. Quantitative measurement using apparent diffusion coefficient (ADC) maps can be generated. ADC may be helpful in the artifact called T2 shine-through, where a bright signal on T2 appears bright on DWI.

DWI and PWI images are vital in taking care of acute stroke patients. Combining both images enables the treating physician to identify the penumbra area, potentially salvageable tissue.

CLINICAL USES OF MRI

1. Vascular: Strokes appear earlier and in better detail on MRI (particularly DWI and PWI) than on CT. This may become standard in acute stroke intervention. For vascular malformations MRI/MRA is the noninvasive test of choice. For aneurysms, MRI/MRA is excellent for screening, but conventional angiography can exclude smaller aneurysms.

   MRI with MRI venography is superior for venous sinus thrombosis. MRI can visualize (early) all types of hemorrhage, i.e., hypertensive, tumoral, and other intraparenchymal, subdural, and epidural bleeds. CT, however, can image blood at least as well and less expensively. MRI is very poor for detecting subarachnoid blood. MRI should be chosen if a subtle hemorrhage (e.g., small contusion) is suspected.
2. Tumors: MRI is the exam of choice to rule out small tumors or for tumor delineation. The ability to map the extent of a tumor (especially with the use of gadolinium) and the multiplanar capability of MRI make it very useful in surgical planning.
3. Infections: Cerebritis is well visualized with MR. Abscess is well delineated with MRI.
4. Meningeal processes: MRI is more sensitive than CT for visualizing both infected and neoplasm-infiltrated meninges.
5. Trauma: Acutely, MRI is not the exam of choice because of the lack of bony detail and the length of time needed to obtain images. CT should be used.
6. Demyelinating disease: MRI is the exam of choice due to the excellent delineation of white matter pathology. Active lesions of multiple sclerosis will enhance with gadolinium.
7. Congenital/structural abnormalities: MRI is excellent for showing heterotopias and other anatomical abnormalities.

8. Spine imaging: Because the spinal cord is a thin, inherently low contrast structure, MRI is the noninvasive exam of choice for all spine pathology. Vertebral bone is well imaged on spinal MRI because it contains fatty marrow. However, small spinal column fractures are better seen on CT. MRI also allows good visualization of the soft tissue and ligaments.
9. Pregnancy: The safety of MRI in pregnancy has yet to be determined, therefore, risk versus benefit must be considered.

ADVANTAGES OF MRI

1. Multiple planar capability: The magnetic field can be adjusted to image in any plane without moving the patient.
2. No ionizing radiation.
3. Superficial soft tissue contrast: Subtle differences in soft tissue proton relaxation characteristics enable visual distinction between soft tissues. This is considered an "inherent" contrast of the soft tissue that can be significantly better appreciated with MRI than any other modality.
4. Vascular anatomy: Flowing blood has different characteristics than stationary soft tissue. Vessels can be imaged in more detail with MRI than other noninvasive modalities; magnetic resonance angiograms and magnetic resonance venograms can be reconstructed by subtracting out the background stationary tissue signal (via longer relaxation times) from the signal from moving protons.
5. MRI can easily image areas that are poorly visualized by CT, e.g., areas encased in thick bones, such as the orbit and optic nerve, posterior fossa, and temporal lobes.
6. Gadolinium is a paramagnetic IV contrast agent analogous to iodinated contrast of x-ray CT, which enhances tissues that are highly vascular or have a damaged blood-brain barrier. Unlike traditional contrast agents, gadolinium has very few contraindications and adverse reactions are rare. Contrast-enhanced MRI is generally obtained with T1WI, where gadolinium enhancement appears bright.

DISADVANTAGES AND LIMITATIONS OF MRI

1. Longer imaging time: It can take between one and a half to three hours, depending on the anatomic area being studied and the complexity of the image acquisition. This has improved markedly with newer generation machines.
2. Sensitivity to motion is very high, resulting in degraded image quality with patient movement. Chloral hydrate, benzodiazepines, barbiturates, or other medications can be used as a sedative, but timing and dosage and possible respiratory depression are important parameters to monitor.
3. Claustrophobia is often due to tighter confinement and longer imaging times than CT. Sedation may be necessary or consider using an open MRI.

4. Metal and electronic devices, e.g., pacemakers, cochlear implants, and foreign bodies often contraindicate MRI. A list may be obtained from the manufacturer, but it is becoming less problematic since the newest metal devices are being made MRI compatible.
5. Calcium is not well visualized. Therefore, bone signal is restricted to that given off by marrow fat and is usually black on MR.
6. Artifacts are common on MRI due to the complex interactions of several types of information, any of which can distort the final image.

INTRAOPERATIVE MRI

The use of open MRI units in the operating room has contributed to an increased extent of tumor removal and a parallel improvement in survival times.

REFERENCES

Atlas SW, ed: *Magnetic resonance imaging of the brain and spine*, New York, Raven Press, 1991.
Black PM et al: *Neurosurgery* 41(4):831–842, 1997.
Wirtz CR et al: *Neurosurgery* 46(5):1112–1120, 2000.

MEMORY

Memory comprises the mental processes of registration, encoding, and storage of experiences and information. It is divided into short-term or working memory (active holding and manipulation of information) and long-term memory (information stored for periods of minutes to decades). Other classifications include declarative (explicit) and nondeclarative (implicit) memory. The anatomy of memory involves many widely distributed neural structures. The medial temporal lobe memory system (hippocampus, amygdala, and adjacent related entorhinal, perirhinal, and parahippocampal cortices and their connections to neocortex) is involved in the processing and storage of long-term memory. Papez circuit plays a critical role in the transfer of information into long-term memory and its emotional components. Damage to basal forebrain structures (septum, nucleus basalis of Meynert, and orbitofrontal regions), as occurs in Alzheimer's disease, is associated with memory disorder often accompanied by other frontal lobe abnormalities.

Damage to diencephalic structures, particularly dorsomedial and other thalamic nuclei, as in Korsakoff's syndrome, leads to amnesia, possibly by disconnection of cortical areas involved in memory processing. Bilateral damage of the limbic system causes severe memory disturbance. Bilateral damage to the amygdaloid region and anterior temporal lobes may produce the *Klüver-Bucy syndrome*, which is characterized by behavioral and cognitive deficits, placidity, apathy, hypersexuality, hyperorality, and visual and auditory agnosia.

Amnestic syndromes include retrograde or antegrade amnesia. Retrograde amnesia commonly follows head injury and involves loss of memory for a variable time before the event. Antegrade amnesia, the inability to incorporate ongoing experience into memory stores, is seen in head trauma, Wernicke-Korsakoff's psychosis or bilateral limbic lesions to the hippocampal-amygdala complex. The latter is usually due to occlusive vascular disease, hypoxic encephalopathy, or encephalitis. Total global retrograde amnesia, in which an individual loses all prior memory, is never due to organic dysfunction.

REFERENCE

Mesulam MM: *Principals of behavioral and cognitive neurology*, New York, Oxford University Press, 2000.

MENINGITIS

Meningitis is an infectious or inflammatory process involving the subarachnoid space. Bacterial meningitis (invariably associated with a cortical encephalitis and often with a ventriculitis) is a medical emergency and should be suspected in any patient with an acute onset of nuchal rigidity, headache, altered mental status, fever, emesis, and photophobia. Meningeal signs are often absent in infants younger than 6 months of age and in elderly individuals. If the diagnosis of acute bacterial meningitis is suspected, blood cultures and head CT are obtained immediately. Antibiotic therapy should be begun before the patient leaves the emergency room for the CT. Antibiotics are chosen based on patient age, severity of clinical situation, and possible organisms (see Table 44). If the CT result is normal, a CSF examination must be performed and sent for blood cell and differential cell counts, glucose and protein levels, and cultures (bacterial, viral, fungal,

TABLE 44

WIDE-COVERAGE ANTIBIOTICS USED IN INITIAL TREATMENT OF ACUTE MENINGITIS BEFORE RETURN OF CULTURES

Patients	Antibiotic Therapy
Neonates	Ampicillin or penicillin G IV IM; aminoglycoside or ampicillin and cefotaxime; appropriate dosages depend on age and weight
Children 1–3 mo	Ampicillin 200 mg/kg per day IV divided q 6 hr and cefotaxime 200 mg/kg per day IV divided q 6 hr
Children >3 mo	Cefotaxime 200 mg/kg per day IV divided q 6 hr or ceftriaxone 100 mg/kg per day divided q 12 hr
Adults	Cefotaxime 1 g IV q 8 hr to 2 g IV q 4 hr or ceftriaxone 1 to 2 g IV q 12 hr

For severe penicillin allergy consider giving chloramphenicol and trimethoprim-sulfamethoxazole. If methicillin-resistant *Staphylococcus* organisms are a consideration, vancomycin 1 g IV q 12 hr is recommended.

and mycobacterial, as appropriate). Organism-specific studies, including cryptococcal antigen studies and counterimmunoelectrophoresis specific for some strains of *Haemophilus influenzae, Neisseria meningitides, Streptococcus pneumoniae*, β-hemolytic streptococci, and *Escherichia coli* are often useful, especially if results of initial CSF cultures are negative (see Table 45).

TABLE 45

CAUSATIVE ORGANISMS IN MENINGITIS ACCORDING TO PATIENT AGE AND CLINICAL SETTING*

Infants < 6 wk old: Group B streptococci, *E. coli, S. pneumoniae, L. monocytogenes, Salmonella* organisms, *P. aeruginosa, S. aureus, H. influenzae, Citrobacter* organisms, herpes simplex 2

Children 6 wk to 15 yr old: *H. influenzae, S. pneumoniae, N. meningitidis, S. aureus*, viruses

Older children and young adults: *N. meningitidis, S. pneumoniae, H. influenzae, S. aureus*, viruses

Adults > 40 yr old: *S. pneumoniae, N. meningitidis, S. aureus, L. monocytogenes*, gram-negative bacilli

Diabetes mellitus: *S. pneumoniae*, gram-negative bacilli, staphylococci, *Cryptococcus* organisms, Mucormycosis

Alcoholism: *S. pneumoniae*

Sickle cell anemia: *S. pneumoniae*

Pneumonia or upper respiratory infection: *S. pneumoniae, N. meningitidis*, viruses, *H. influenzae*

AIDS or other abnormal cellular immunity: *Toxoplasma, Cryptococcus, Coccidiodes*, and *Candida* organisms; *L. monocytogenes, M. tuberculosis* and *avium-intracellulare, T. pallidum, Histoplasma* organisms, *Nocardia, S. pneumoniae*, gram-negative bacilli

Abnormal neutrophils: *P. aeruginosa, S. aureus*, Candida and Aspergillus organisms, Mucormycosis

Immunoglobulin deficiency: *S. pneumoniae, N. meningitidis, H. influenzae*

Ventricular shunt infections: *S. epidermidis, S. aureus*, gram-negative bacilli

Penetrating head trauma, skin lesions, bacterial endocarditis or other heart disease, severe burns, IV drug abuse: *S. aureus*, streptococci, gram-negative bacilli

Closed head trauma, CSF leak, pericranial infections: *S. pneumoniae*, gram-negative bacilli

Following neurosurgical procedures: *S. aureus, S. epidermidis*, gram-negative bacilli

Tick bites: *B. burgdorferi*

Swimming in fresh water ponds: *Naegleria* organisms

Contact with water frequented by rodents or domestic animals: *Leptospira* organisms

Contact with hamsters or mice: Lymphocytic choriomeningitis virus

Exposure to pigeons: *Cryptococcus* organisms

Travel in southwestern United States: *Coccidioides* organisms

---

* Adapted from Mandell GL et al: *Principles and practice of infectious diseases*, ed 2, New York, John Wiley & Sons, 1985.

Laboratory evaluation of CSF includes a Gram stain and india ink examination of centrifuged CSF sediment. Cell counts >1000/mm^3, protein levels >50 mg/dl, and glucose levels <30 mg/dl suggest bacterial infection. There is overlap with ranges more typical of fungal, tuberculous, and viral meningitis (see Cerebrospinal Fluid). A polymorphonuclear (PMN) predominance is more common with bacterial meningitis, and a

TABLE 46

CAUSES OF ASEPTIC, CHRONIC (C), AND RECURRENT (R) MENINGITIS

Infectious
Actinomyces sp. (C)*
Amebas
Blastomyces sp. (C)*
Brucella sp. (C)
Borrelia sp. (C, R)
Candida sp. (C)
Coccidioides sp. (C)
Cryptococcus sp. (C)
Cysticercosis (C)*
Fungi (C, R)
Herpes simplex 1 and 2
Histoplasma sp. (C)
Human immunodeficiency virus (C)
Leptospira sp. (C, R)
Listeria sp.
M. tuberculosis (C, R)
Mycoplasma sp.
Nocardia sp.*
Parameningeal suppurative foci (R)
Partially treated meningitis (R)
Rickettsia sp.
T. pallidum (C)
Toxoplasma sp. (C)*

Noninfectious
Behçet's syndrome (C, R)
Chemical
Drugs (ibuprofen, isoniazide, sulindac, sulfamethoxazole)
Granulomatous angitis (C)
Lupus erythematosus (R)
Meningitis-migraine syndrome (R)
Mollaret's meningitis (R)
Neoplasm (C, R)
Rupture of cyst (R)
Sarcoidosis (C, R)
Uremia
Uveomeningoecephalitis (C, R)
Viruses (R)

* More commonly cause brain abscess or focal lesion.

lymphocytosis with aseptic meningitis. Approximately 10% of bacterial meningitides show a lymphocytosis. Early viral meningitis, especially as a result of mumps, may show a PMN predominance. Hypoglycorrachia (low CSF glucose level) occurs in bacterial, tuberculous, fungal, carcinomatous, or chemical meningitis.

In the subacute presentation (more than 24 hours of symptoms), unless mental status is impaired, a more detailed workup may be done before starting antibiotic therapy. Signs and symptoms of meningoencephalitis lasting for at least 4 weeks with persistently abnormal results of CSF study are consistent with chronic meningitis. Recurrent meningitis is defined as repetitive episodes of meningitis associated with an abnormal result of CSF study followed by symptom-free periods during which the CSF is normal (see Table 46). *Mollaret's meningitis*, also called benign recurrent aseptic meningitis, is associated with herpes simplex virus, type 2, and may improve on administration of prophylactic acyclovir.

Mortality rates for the different forms of meningitis are variable. The three most common bacterial meningitides (pneumococcal, meningococcal, and *H. influenzae*) have an average mortality rate of 10%; neurologic deficits occur in about 20% of survivors. The less common bacterial meningitides can have much higher mortality rates. The frequency of complications correlates with increased duration of symptoms before treatment. Mental status changes, in particular agitation and confusion, are poor prognostic signs, as is an underlying malignancy, alcoholism, diabetes, or pneumonia. Common sequelae include hearing loss, vestibular dysfunction, cognitive and behavioral changes, and seizures.

Glucocorticoid administration suppresses the inflammatory response, with resultant decreased brain edema and lowered intracranial pressure. Children with meningitis who receive treatment with dexamethasone 0.6 mg/kg per day in four divided doses for the initial 4 days of antibiotic therapy have lower rates of sensorineural hearing loss and neurologic sequelae. The advantages of corticosteroids in the treatment of adults with meningitis are unclear, although such treatment may benefit those with increased intracranial pressure.

REFERENCES

Durand ML et al: *N Engl J Med* 328:21–28, 1993.
Quagliarello V, Scheld WM: *N Engl J Med* 327:864–872, 1992.

MENTAL STATUS TESTING

Routine clinical mental status examination should allow for quick screening of focal and global abnormalities. Elements of the mental status examination include state of awareness, attention, mood and affect, speech and language, memory, visual spatial function, praxis, and other aspects of cognition such as calculations, thought content, and judgment. Patients who appear to have difficulties on screening examinations should have a more detailed survey of their cognitive abilities, ranging from short, standardized tests such as the Mini-Mental Status Examination or the short Blessed Test to more detailed neuropsychologic evaluation (see Figure 24).

Interpretation of mental status testing cannot be performed in isolation. An inattentive patient may not perform well on memory tasks or language comprehension, but this is not indicative of primary language or memory disturbance. Visual impairment may complicate constructional testing and naming. General information and proverb testing, although useful as a

M

MENTAL STATUS TESTING

Actual	Possible	
		Orientation
_____	5	What is the date, year, month, day, season?
_____	5	Where are we: state, county, town, hospital, floor?
		Registration
_____	3	Name three objects: 1 second to say each. Then ask the patient to name all three after you have said them. Give one point for each correct answer. Then repeat them until patient learns all three. Count trials and record. Trials _____
		Attention and calculation
_____	5	Serial 7's. One point for each correct. Stop after five answers. As an alternative, spell "world" backwards.
		Recall
_____	3	Ask for the names of the three objects repeated above. Give 1 point for each correct name.
		Language
_____	2	Name a pencil and a watch.
_____	1	Repeat the phrase "No ifs, ands, or buts."
_____	3	Follow a three-stage command: "Take the paper in your right hand, fold it in half, and put it on the floor."
_____	1	Read and obey the following: "Close your eyes."
_____	1	Write a sentence.
_____	1	Copy the design shown here.
_____		**Total** (maximum score, 30)

Assess level of consciousness along the following continuum:

Alert   Drowsy   Stupor   Coma

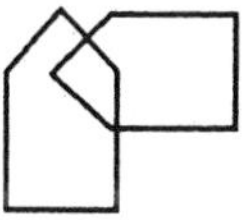

FIGURE 24

Mini mental state examination. (From Folstein MF, Folstein SE, McHugh PR: *Psychiatr Res* 12:189–98, 1975.)

screening test, is highly dependent on educational level, socioeconomic status, and cultural background.

REFERENCES

Crum R et al: *JAMA* 269(18):2386–2391, 1993.
Katzman R et al: *Am J, Psychiatry* 140:734–739, 2000.
Strub RL, Black FW: *The mental status examination in neurology*, ed 4, Philadelphia, FA Davis, 2000.)

METABOLIC DISEASES OF CHILDHOOD

A metabolic disorder should be suspected under the following conditions: (1) neurologic disorder is replicated in sibling or close relative, (2) recurrent episodes of altered consciousness or unexplained vomiting in an infant, (3) recurrent unexplained ataxia or spasticity, (4) progressive CNS degeneration, (5) mental deterioration in sibling or close relative, and (6) mental retardation in the absence of major congenital anomalies.

The following procedures may be performed (1) urine screen, (2) serum ammonia, fasting blood glucose, pH, pCO_2, and lactic and pyruvic acid, (3) serum amino and organic acids, (4) x-ray, (5) serum lysosomal enzyme screen, (6) tissue biopsy for structural and biochemical alterations, and (7) CT or MRI.

CLASSIFICATION BY CLINICAL PRESENTATION

I. *Acute encephalopathy* presents shortly after birth or during early infancy with recurrent vomiting, lethargy, poor feeding, and dehydration. It initially affects the gray matter, and, hence, presents with cognitive impairment, seizures, or vision impairment. Course is rapidly progressive. This presentation is usually caused by "small-molecule diseases" (amino acids, organic acids, and simple sugars) and represents an "intoxication" or toxic encephalopathy. Intoxications result from accumulation of toxic compounds proximal to the metabolic block. Serum lactate and ammonia, blood gas, and urine ketones permit classification of the metabolic disorders into those with: (1) ketosis (maple syrup urine disease [MSUD]), (2) ketoacidosis and acidosis (organic acidurias), (3) lactic acidosis, (4) hyperammonemia with ketoacidosis (urea cycle disorders), and (5) no ketoacidosis or hyperammonemia (nonketotic hyperglycinemia [NKH], sulfite oxidase deficiency, and peroxisomal/lysosomal) (see Table 47).

II. *Chronic or progressive encephalopathy* manifests during late infancy, childhood, or adolescence. It initially affects white matter and presents with gradual onset of long-tract signs such as spasticity, ataxia, or hyperreflexia. Dementia may develop later. Liver, heart, muscle, or kidneys are frequently involved. This clinical presentation is caused by large-molecule (glycogen, glycoprotein, lipids, and mucopolysaccharides) or storage diseases and represents intoxication, energy deficiency, or both. Glycogen storage diseases, congenital lactic acidosis, fatty acid oxidation defects, mitochondrial

TABLE 47

DETECTION OF NEUROMETABOLIC DISORDERS: A PRACTICAL CLINICAL APPROACH

History (early infancy)	Routine Laboratory Studies				Special Laboratory Studies			Enzyme Studies			Disorder
	Blood gases	Ketone	Lactic acid	Ammonia	Organic acids	Amino acids	Sulfites	WBC	Fibroblasts	Tissue	
Acute encephalopathy	–	+	–	–	+	+	–	+	+	+	MSUD
	+	+	–	–	+	–	–	+	+	–	Organic aciduria
	+	+	+	–	+	–	–	+	+	+	Lactic acidosis
	–	–	+	+	–	+	–	–	–	+	Urea cycle disorder
	–	–	–	–	–	+	–	+	+	–	NKH
	–	–	–	–	–	–	+	+	+	–	Sulfite oxidase deficiency

History (older child)	Routine Laboratory Studies		Special Laboratory Studies			Enzyme Studies			Disorder
	Urine MPS	Urine oligosaccharides	Lysosomal enzymes	VLCFA	Inclusion bodies	WBC	Fibroblasts	Tissue	
Chronic encephalopathy	–	–	+	–	–	+	+	+	Sphingolipidosis
	+	–	+	–	–	+	+	+	Mucopolysaccharidoses
	–	+	+	–	–	+	+	+	Glycoprotein degradation disorder
	–	–	–	+	–	–	+	+	Peroxisomal disorder
	–	–	–	–	–	+	+	+	Fatty acid oxidation disorder
	–	–	–	–	+	–	–	–	Neuronal ceroid lipofuscinosis

M

METABOLIC DISEASES OF CHILDHOOD

respiratory disorders, and peroxisomal disorders belong to this group. Routine metabolic screening tests are seldom helpful. Neuroimaging and EEG, evoked potentials, electromyography and nerve conduction studies (EMG-NCV) and specialized genetic/metabolic testing are often necessary to elucidate the diagnosis.

The following metabolic disorders require early recognition and prompt treatment:

1. Phenylketonuria (PKU): Autosomal recessive (AR); defect of phenylalanine hydroxylase; 2 months, vomiting and irritable; 4 to 9 months, mental retardation; later seizures, eczema, reduced hair pigmentation; early treatment with phenylalanine-restricted diet can lead to normal IQ.
2. MSUD: AR; defect in branched chain amino acids (valine, leucine, isoleucine); first week, opisthotonos, intermittent hypertonia, and irregular breathing; 50% with hypoglycemia; sweet smelling urine; if a diet restricted in branched-chain amino acids is started within first 2 weeks of life, normal or near-normal IQ may be achieved.
3. Homocystinuria: (AR); cystathionine synthase defect; presents between 5 and 9 months; strokes or seizures; ectopia lentis; sparse, blond and brittle hair; treatment is methionine-restricted diet with or without pyridoxine 250 to 1200 mg/day.
4. Bassen-Kornzweig disease (abetalipoproteinemia): AR; first year, steatorrhea; second year, ataxia, retardation, retinitis pigmentosa; hypocholesterolemia, acanthocytosis; treat with vitamin E, A, and K.
5. Galactosemia: AR; defect in galactose-1-uridyl transferase; normal at birth; first week, listless, jaundice, vomiting, diarrhea, and no weight gain; second week, cataracts, hepatosplenomegaly; may be hypotonic and have pseudotumor cerebri; treat with lactose-free diet; visuoperceptual deficits persist despite early treatment; susceptible to *Escherichia coli* sepsis.
6. Hypothyroidism: Post-term, macrosomia, jaundice, large posterior fontanelle, mottled skin, big belly; second month, hypotonia, grunting cry, macrocephaly, coarse hair; later, developmental delay, deafmutism, and spasticity; if thyroid replacement not started within first 3 months of life, cerebellar and speech defects may persist.
7. Pyridoxine deficiency: Neonatal seizures and EEG abnormalities respond only to pyridoxine; requiring lifelong treatment.

REFERENCE

Menkes JH: *Texbook of child neurology*, Baltimore, Lippincott Williams & Wilkins, 2000.

MICROCEPHALY

Microcephaly refers to head circumference smaller than 2 standard deviations (SD) below the normal distribution for age, sex, and race. Head circumference smaller than 3 SD of age norms usually indicates later mental retardation.

A small head circumference at birth establishes the antepartum timing of brain damage but does not distinguish primary from secondary microcephaly. Primary microcephaly encompasses conditions in which the brain is small and never formed properly because of genetic (microcephaly vera) or chromosomal abnormalities. Defective neurulation (anencephaly, encephalocele), defective prosencephalization (callosal agenesis, holoprosencephaly), and defective cellular migration also give rise to primary microcephaly. Secondary microcephaly implies that the brain was forming normally but a disease process impaired further growth. These include intrauterine disorders (infection, toxins, vascular), perinatal brain injuries (hypoxic ischemic encephalopathy [HIE], intracranial hemorrhage, meningitis, and encephalitis, stroke) and postnatal systemic diseases (chronic cardiopulmonary or renal disease, malnutrition).

Cranial MRI may be helpful in distinguishing between primary and secondary microcephaly. In primary microcephaly, MRI is either normal or may show a cerebral malformation. MRI is usually abnormal in secondary microcephaly and may reveal ventriculomegaly, cerebral atrophy, or porencephaly.

REFERENCE

Fenichel GM: *Clinical pediatric neurology: a signs and symptoms approach*, Philadelphia, WB Saunders, 1997.

MOTOR NEURON DISEASE

AMYOTROPHIC LATERAL SCLEROSIS (ALS)

ALS is a progressive neurodegenerative disorder that primarily affects motor neurons. Annual incidence of ALS varies from 0.2 to 2.4 per 100,000 population. The majority of the cases are sporadic. Five percent to 10% of cases are familial, with 20% of the familial cases related to the mutation in the Cu/Zn superoxide dismutase (SOD) gene located on chromosome 21. A combination of ALS, parkinsonism, and dementia occurs in several regions of western pacific islands, which may originate from a different pathogenesis.

The disorder often starts at age 55 to 75 years, with a younger age in the familial cases. Male to female ratio is 1.4:1 to 2.5:1.

Clinical presentation is characterized by the presence of both upper motor neuron and lower motor neuron signs. Painless weakness and atrophy of distal muscles in the limbs are common symptoms. The distribution of weakness may be asymmetric and over time progress to adjacent myotomes in the same limb and the opposite limb. Upper motor neuron complaints such as loss of fine movement and spasticity are also present. Lower and upper motor neuron bulbar involvement resulting in dysarthria, dysphagia, and sialorrhea occurs as an initial presentation in 19% to 28% of all cases (*bulbar onset ALS*). On clinical examination, patients have upper motor neuron signs (spasticity, increased tone, hyperreflexia) and/or lower motor neuron signs (muscle atrophy, weakness, and fasciculation) in bulbar or spinal innervated muscles or both (see Table 48). A typical picture of ALS

TABLE 48

CLASSIFICATION OF MOTOR NEURON DISEASE BY INITIAL PRESENTATION

	Spinal Cord	Brain Stem
Lower motor neuron (atrophic)	Spinal muscular atrophy	Progressive bulbar palsy
Upper motor neuron (spastic)	Primary lateral sclerosis	Progressive pseudobulbar palsy

with generalized upper and lower motor neuron findings is the rule. Death is usually caused by respiratory insufficiency or aspiration pneumonia.

Rarely, the true "progressive bulbar palsy" clinical picture occurs, and the disease does not progress beyond weakness involving the bulbar region. Two percent to 3.7% of all ALS cases present as a pure spinal cord upper motor neuron syndrome (*primary lateral sclerosis*), which presents with spastic paraparesis and progresses at a much slower rate. *Progressive muscular atrophy* or the pure lower motor neuron type of ALS is rare and has a more favorable outcome.

Diagnosis is based on clinical examination and electromyography, which reveals low-amplitude compound muscle action potentials on nerve conduction studies with normal sensory studies. Needle EMG shows widespread fibrillation potentials and fasciculations in multiple segments of limb muscles and bulbar muscles, with a reduced number of increased duration and amplitude motor unit action potentials firing rapidly. Imaging studies of the spine may be needed to rule out cervical spondylosis or radiculopathies in certain cases. Laboratory evaluation to look for other causes of motor neuron disorder such as hyperparathyroidism or paraneoplastic motor neuron syndrome may be useful if indicated by clinical history.

Differential diagnosis: (1) Neurodegenerative diseases that can present with pyramidal tract or lower motor neuron involvement (such as multiple systemic atrophy, certain types of spinocerebellar ataxia); (2) Disorders affecting brain stem and spinal cord (such as cervical spondylosis, cervical polyradiculopathies, syringomyelia, multiple sclerosis, adrenomyeloneuropathy, vitamin B_{12} deficiency, familial spastic paraparesis, and tropical spastic paraparesis); (3) Muscle diseases (such as inclusion body myositis, myotonic dystrophy, oculopharyngeal muscular atrophy); and (4) Disorders affecting anterior horn cells (such as spinal muscular atrophy, adult-onset hexosaminidase deficiency).

Management of ALS: (1) Symptomatic: Daytime sialorrhea can be treated with anticholinergic medications such as trihexyphenidyl, atropine, or glycopyrrolate. Depression may be treated with antidepressants. Nutritional support is beneficial, particularly in the patient with dysphagia. Percutaneous endoscopic gastrostomy (PEG) may be performed, but before the forced vital capacity (FVC) falls below 50% of normal. Pain from cramps and spasticity should be managed. Serial pulmonary function tests (PFT) can help in appropriately planning ahead. Dyspnea and progressive decline in PFT both predict poor prognosis, and the issue of resuscitation and whether the patient wishes to be placed on a mechanical ventilator should be discussed beforehand. (2) Antiglutamate agent: Riluzole 50 mg bid, when used early, slows ALS progression, and in the bulbar onset group, prolongs survival by a few months. However, riluzole provides little benefit with more advanced disease and does not show any positive impact on the patient's quality of life or muscle strength. Monthly follow-up of liver function tests and complete blood count is necessary at the beginning and then every 3 months afterward.

Prognosis: Mean duration from onset of symptoms to death is approximately 3 years. Patients with bulbar onset ALS often have a shorter survival, whereas patients with primary lateral sclerosis and progressive muscular atrophy have a longer survival time.

ATYPICAL MOTOR NEURON DISEASES

Several disorders primarily affect the motor system and mimic ALS. These disorders are often referred to as atypical motor neuron diseases (see Table 49). Most of these conditions present with atypical clinical manifestations for ALS and may be distinguished based on clinical, laboratory,

TABLE 49

ATYPICAL MOTOR NEURON DISEASES

1. Immune-mediated motor neuropathies
   Multifocal motor neuropathy with conduction block
2. Nonimmune-mediated lower motor neuron syndromes
   Spinal muscular atrophy
   X-linked bulbospinal muscular atrophy (Kennedy's disease)
   Distal spinal muscular atrophy
   Monomelic amyotrophy (benign focal amyotrophy)
   Fazio-Londe disease
3. Multiple system disorders with motor signs
   Adult hexosaminidase A deficiency
   Spinocerebellar degenerations
       Machado-Joseph disease
       Autosomal dominant cerebellar ataxia
4. Other multiple system disorders
   Shy-Drager syndrome
   Guamanian Parkinson-Amyotrophic lateral sclerosis-dementia complex
   Hallervorden-Spatz disease
   Creutzfeldt-Jakob disease
   Huntington's disease
   Pick's disease
5. Hyperparathyroidism
6. Electrical injury associated with motor neuron disease
7. Infectious/postinfectious
8. Retroviral-associated syndrome
9. Post-radiation motor neuron disease
10. Paraneoplastic disorders with motor neuron dysfunction
11. Toxins/drugs
12. Postpolio syndrome

electrophysiologic, and pathologic characteristics. There are some clinical clues that may help differentiate these patients from patients with ALS, which include long duration of illness, lack of bulbar involvement after 1 year, onset before age 35 years, presence of family history, and absence of concurrent upper and lower motor neuron signs in the same spinal segment. Absence of muscle wasting in chronically weak limbs may suggest that the weakness is a consequence of focal conduction block with preservation of motor axon, as seen in multifocal motor neuropathy. The presence of sensory involvement, bowel or bladder dysfunction, cerebellar or extrapyramidal dysfunction, and extraocular muscle weakness on neurologic examinations should also lead the search toward other multisystemic disorders that do not exclusively affect the motor system. The recognition of these other disorders is important because several disorders are potentially treatable or may not carry the same grave prognosis as ALS.

REFERENCES

Motor neuron disease: ALS I, ALS II, and familial ALS. *Continuum* 3:48–74, 1997.
Quality Standards Subcommittee of the AAN: *Neurology* 49:657–659, 1997.

MULTIPLE SCLEROSIS

Multiple sclerosis (MS) is the most common demyelinating disease affecting 250,000 to 350,000 people in the United States and over 1 million people worldwide. Onset of the disease is usually between the ages of 10 and 60 years, with peak age between 20 and 30. The cause remains unknown but are suspected to be autoimmune. The incidence of MS increases with latitude in temperate climates. Risk for development of the disease correlates with the latitude at which one lived before the age of 15 years. There is a familial predisposition for its development; women are more affected than men, and whites more so than blacks or Asians. Approximately 80% of patients will have relapsing-remitting MS, while 20% follow a primary progressive course. Of the patients with relapsing-remitting disease, 50% will develop secondary progressive MS.

Clinical features are fatigue, limb weakness, spasticity, hyperreflexia, paresthesias, Lhermitte's sign (sensation of "electricity" down the back associated with neck flexion), ataxia, tremor, nystagmus, optic neuritis, internuclear ophthalmoplegia, diplopia, vertigo, bowel or bladder dysfunction, impotence, depression, emotional lability, and cognitive abnormalities. The *Uhthoff* phenomenon is the worsening of a sign or symptom with exercise or increased temperature.

The *diagnosis* of MS is made on clinical grounds and can be classified as clinically definite, laboratory-supported definite, clinically probable, or laboratory-supported probable by using established criteria. For diagnostic purposes, symptomatic attacks should have objective dysfunction lasting a minimum of 24 hours that occur in different locations in the CNS involving primarily white matter and be separated by a period of at least 1 month (separated by space and time).

Radiologic and laboratory studies may support the clinical diagnosis. CT results are usually normal but can show areas of decreased attenuation in the white matter, areas of contrast enhancement, or both. MRI is far more sensitive than CT for detecting MS plaques and is the imaging procedure of choice. Focal enhancement with gadolinium is considered evidence of an "active" plaque. T2 imaging frequently demonstrates finger-like extensions along the small or medium blood vessels called "Dawson's fingers," while T1 imaging reveals areas of decreased signal called "black holes." CSF may have normal to mildly elevated protein, normal glucose, moderate lymphocytic pleocytosis (usually 5 to 20 cells/mm^3), elevated IgG, and oligoclonal IgG bands in 90% of cases. Free kappa light chains and/or myelin basic protein are elevated during flares. Visual, auditory, and somatosensory-evoked potentials may reveal abnormalities in their respective pathways. Cystometrics may show an uninhibited, spastic, or flaccid bladder or detrusor-sphincter dyssynergia.

General management includes avoidance of heat and excessive fatigue. Fever and hot weather can decrease conduction and exacerbate symptoms. A small, spastic bladder can be treated with oxybutynin, propantheline, imipramine, or tolterodine (long acting). Sphincter dyssynergia and a spastic bladder often coexist and are treated with phenoxybenzamine, or diazepam, or both. A large, flaccid bladder is treated with Valsalva or Crede maneuvers, catheterization (intermittent or permanent), or pharmacologic agents such as bethanechol and phenoxybenzamine.

Spasticity is treated most commonly with baclofen at doses of 40 to 80 mg/day or tizanidine in doses up to 24 mg/day with diazepam or dantrolene as needed to control spasms. Chronic pain or neuralgia is treated with carbamazepine, gabapentin, phenytoin, or amitriptyline. Selective serotonin reuptake inhibitiors (SSRIs) can be used for depression.

Treatment options for relapsing-remitting MS include interferon beta-1b (Betaseron) 8 million units SC every other day, interferon beta-1a (Avonex) 30 μg IM weekly, or glatiramer acetate (Copaxone) 20 μg SC daily. These reduce relapses and the formation of new lesions on MRI. Side effects of beta-interferon include flulike symptoms, erythema or tenderness of injection site, elevated liver function tests, depressed lymphocyte counts, and depression. Glatiramer acetate injections also may cause irritation at the injection site or brief episodes of chest tightness, palpitations, or shortness of breath. Interferon beta-1b is also being used in the treatment of secondary progressive MS. Mitoxantrone (Novantrone), an antineoplastic agent with immune-modulating effect, has been approved for treating patients with secondary progressive MS.

The cumulative maximum dose is $120\,mg/m^2$ over a 3-year period to limit its cardiac toxicity. Many variables must be weighed, including individual lifestyle, cost, side effects, and disease course before initiating therapy.

Methylprednisolone is used for acute relapses. The usual dose of 1000 mg daily for 3 to 5 days with oral prednisone taper (1mg/kg/day) shortens the time to recovery. Plasma exchange has been used in patients not responding to steroids. A variety of other immunosuppressive therapies including azathioprine, methotrexate, cyclophosphamide, and cyclosporine have been tested, but none have been shown to alter the course of the disease.

REFERENCES

Noseworthy JH et al: *N Engl J Med* 343:938–952, 2000.
Rudick RA et al: *N Engl J Med* 337:1604–1611, 1997.

MUSCLE DISEASES AND TESTING

Bedside examination of the muscles involves assessment of *bulk*, *tone*, and *strength*. In certain neurologic diseases, *fatigue* of muscular response may be important. Subtle weakness may not be demonstrated by action against resistance but may be revealed with provocative postures or movement, such as pronator drift or arm-rolling. Quantitative measures of force generation by specific muscle groups may be helpful in the context of rehabilitation and physical/occupational therapy (see Table 50). In addition to clinical muscle testing, histopathological classification to different types of muscle fibers (Table 51) is vital for sorting out the various muscle diseases (Table 52).

TABLE 50

GRADING OF MUSCLE STRENGTH

Grade	Strength
0	No perceptible contraction.
1	Trace contraction is observed, but no movement is achieved.
2	Movement is achieved in horizontal plane but not against gravity.
3	Movement is achieved against gravity but not against additional resistance.
4–	Movement is achieved against slight resistance.
4	Movement is achieved against moderate resistance.
4+	Movement is achieved against large resistance but is less than expected, given patient age and fitness.
5	Intact strength.

Aids to the examination of the peripheral nerves, ed 3, East Sussex, Balliere Tindall, 1986.

TABLE 51

CHARACTERISTICS OF MUSCLE FIBER TYPES

Characteristic	Type 1	Type 2a	Type 2b
Speed	Slow	Fast	Fast
Metabolism	Oxidative	Oxidative-glycolytic	Glycolytic
Fatigue resistance	+	+	−

TABLE 52

SYNDROMIC CLASSIFICATION OF MUSCLE DISEASES

I. Acute (evolving in days) or subacute (weeks) paretic or paralytic disorders of muscle.
  A. Rarely fulminant myasthenia gravis or myasthenic syndrome from a "mycin" antibiotic or hypokalemia.
  B. Idiopathic polymyositis and dermatomyositis.
  C. Viral polymyositis.
  D. Acute paroxysmal myoglobinuria.
  E. "Alcoholic" polymyopathy.
  F. Familial (malignant) hyperpyrexia precipitated by anesthetic agents.
  G. Neuroleptic malignant syndrome.
  H. First attack of episodic weakness may enter into differential diagnosis (see below).
  I. Botulism.
  J. Organophosphate poisoning.
II. Chronic (i.e., months to years) weakness or paralysis of muscle, usually with severe atrophy.
  A. Progressive muscular dystrophy.
    1. Sex-linked recessive.
      a. Duchenne.
      b. Becker.
      c. Benign with early contractures (Dreifuss-Emery).
      d. Scapuloperoneal.
    2. Autosomal recessive.
      a. Scapulohumeral (limb-girdle).
      b. Autosomal recessive dystrophy of childhood (Erb).
      c. Congenital.
    3. Autosomal dominant.
      a. Facioscapulohumeral (Landouzy-Dejerine).
      b. Scapuloperoneal.
      c. Late-onset recessive (Erb).
      d. Distal—adult onset.
      e. Distal—childhood onset.
      f. Ocular (Hutchinson-Fachs).
      g. Oculopharyngeal (Victor-Hayes-Adams).
      h. Myotonic dystrophy.
  B. Chronic polymyositis or dermatomyositis (may be subacute).
    1. Idiopathic.
    2. With connective tissue disease.
    3. With occult neoplasm.
    4. Inclusion body myositis.
  C. Chronic thyrotoxic and other endocrine myopathies.
  D. Chronic, slowly progressive, or relatively stationary polymyopathies.
    1. Central core and multicore diseases.
    2. Rod-body and related polymyopathies.
    3. Mitochondrial and centronuclear polymyopathies.
    4. Other congenital myopathies (reducing-body, fingerprint, zebra-body, fiber-type atrophies, and disproportions).
    5. Glycogen storage disease.
    6. Lipid myopathies (carnitine deficiency myopathy and undefined lipid myopathies).
III. Episodic weakness of muscle.
  A. Familial (hypokalemic) periodic paralysis.

Table continued on next page

TABLE 52 —cont'd

SYNDROMIC CLASSIFICATION OF MUSCLE DISEASES

B. Normokalemic or hyperkalemic familial periodic paralysis.

C. Paramyotonia congenita (von Eulenberg).

D. Nonfamilial hyperkalemic and hypokalemic periodic paralysis (including primary hyperaldosteronism).

E. Acute thyrotoxic myopathy (also thyrotoxic periodic paralysis).

F. Conditions in which weakness fluctuates.
  1. Myasthenia gravis, immunologic type.
  2. Myasthenia associated with:
    a. Lupus erythematosus.
    b. Polymyositis.
    c. Rheumatoid arthritis.
    d. Nonthymic carcinoma.
  3. Familial and sporadic nonimmunologic types of myasthenia.
  4. Myasthenia resulting from antibiotics and other drugs.
  5. Lambert-Eaton syndrome.

G. Exercise intolerance.
  1. Myoadenylate deaminase deficiency.
  2. Ca-adenosine triphosphate deficiency.
  3. Hypothyroidism.
  4. "Fibromyositis" syndrome.
  5. Hypoparathyroidism.
  6. Glycogenosis (debranching enzyme deficiency).

IV. Disorders of muscle presenting with myotonia, stiffness, spasm, and cramp.

A. Myotonic dystrophy, congenital myotonia (Thomsen's disease), paramyotonia congenita, and Schwartz-Jampel syndrome.

B. Hypothyroidism with pseudomyotonia (Debré-Sémélaigne and Hoffman (syndromes).

C. Tetany.

D. Tetanus.

E. Black window spider bite.

F. Myopathy resulting from myophosphorylase deficiency (McArdle's disease), phosphofructokinase deficiency, and other forms of contracture.

G. Contracture with Addison's disease.

H. Idiopathic cramp syndromes.

I. Myokymia and syndromes of continuous muscle activity.

V. Myalgic states.

A. Connective tissue diseases (rheumatoid arthritis, mixed connective tissue disease, Sjögren's syndrome, lupus erythematosus, polyarteritis nodosa, scleroderma, polymyositis).

B. Localized multifocal fibrositis (myogelosis).

C. Trichinosis.

D. Myopathy of myoglobinuria and McArdle's disease.

E. Myopathy with hypoglycemia.

F. Bornholm disease and other forms of viral polymyositis.

G. Anterior tibial syndrome.

H. Other.
  1. Hypophosphatemia.
  2. Hypothyroidism.
  3. Psychiatric illness (hysteria, depression).

VI. Localized muscle mass(es).

A. Rupture of a muscle.

B. Muscle hemorrhage.

C. Muscle tumor.
  1. Rhabdomyosarcoma.
  2. Desmoid.
  3. Angioma.
  4. Metastatic nodules.

D. Monomyositis multiplex.
  1. Eosinophilic type.
  2. Other.

E. Localized and generalized myositis ossificans.

F. Fibrositis (Fibromyalgia).

G. Granulomatous infections.
  1. Sarcoidosis.
  2. Tuberculosis.
  3. Wegener's granulomatosis.

H. Pyogenic abscess.

I. Infarction of muscle in the diabetic.

From Adams RA, Victor M: *Principles of neurology,* ed 5, New York, McGraw-Hill, 1993.

REFERENCES

The guarantors of brain: Aids to the examination of the peripheral nervous system, ed 4, Philadelphia, WB Saunders, 2000.
Wolf JK: *Segmental neurology*, Baltimore, University Park Press, 1981.

MUSCULAR DYSTROPHY (MD)

Muscular dystrophy refers to a group of hereditary diseases that cause progressive muscle weakness.

1. *Duchenne muscular dystrophy (DMD)* is a severe X-linked recessive inherited MD. The defective gene is located in the p21 region of chromosome X, encoding for the protein "dystrophin," which is absent or present in less than 3% of normal quantity in 95% of males with DMD. Dystrophin is a part of the dystrophin glycoprotein complex, which is a group of membrane-associated proteins that span the muscle sarcolemma and provide linkage between the intracellular cytoskeleton and the extracellular matrix, providing membrane stability.

The incidence of DMD is approximately 30 per 100,000 live male births. Delayed motor milestone may be seen in some but not all cases. Weakness is more clearly manifested later on, between 3 and 6 years of age, with difficulty walking. Affected boys then often develop a waddling gait with lumbar lordosis and often stand on their toes due to shortening of calf muscles. By approximately 10 years of age, patients no longer climb stairs or stand from the floor independently. By 12 years, most are confined to a wheelchair. Once in a wheelchair, contractures and kyphoscoliosis develop. Death usually occurs in the third decade due to respiratory insufficiency and infection. Involvement of other organ systems includes cardiac conduction defects, intestinal pseudo-obstruction, and lower than average IQ.

Initially, weakness is proximal, with hips more involved than shoulders. Due to proximal lower extremity weakness, to get up from the floor, the boys turn their faces to the floor, spread their legs, elevate their hips, and climb up from the floor using their hands to assist (Gower's sign). Muscles are hard and rubbery, and certain groups of muscles such as the calves, gluteals, and deltoids may be enlarged (pseudohypertrophy). Deep tendon reflexes are normal initially but disappear early in the disease.

Laboratory investigations reveal elevated creatine kinase (CK) (as high as 15,000 to 20,000 U/L), which is seen in early disease and falls as the disease progresses. Myoglobin may be present. Serum CK levels are also elevated in 50% to 70% of female carriers and may be falsely low during pregnancy. ECG abnormalities are present in 80%. True cardiomyopathy is rare. Nerve conduction studies are normal. Needle EMG examination shows polyphasic motor unit action potentials with normal or early recruitment. Muscle biopsy reveals marked variability of fiber size, scattered hypercontracted muscle fibers, and proliferation of endomysial connective tissue. The absence of dystrophin-positive fibers or the presence of only a few scattered positive fibers, when staining muscle with dystrophin anti-bodies, provides the confirmation for diagnosis. DNA analysis for deletions or duplications within the dystrophin gene is available and beneficial in identifying patients or carriers.

Treatment involves physical therapy including appropriate stretching exercises to help prevent contracture. Night splints and bracing may delay contracture and prolong the ability to stand. Surgical measures such as Achilles tendon releases and spinal stabilization may be necessary to correct the contracture and scoliosis. Pulmonary care is important. Prednisone (0.75 mg/kg/day) is demonstrated to significantly improve strength by increasing muscle mass and decreasing muscle degradation, with major benefit in prolonging the independent ambulation time only early in the course. Other techniques, such as gene therapy or myoblast transfer, are still experimental.

2. *Becker muscular dystrophy (BMD)* is an X-linked dystrophinopathy closely resembling DMD, with the gene defect at the same location as DMD. In BMD the deletion is different and dystrophin still can be produced, although the protein structure may be abnormal or the amount produced is small.

Patients develop the same proximal hip and shoulder weakness, calf hypertrophy, and tendency to walk on their toes. However, onset is later, the disease is less severe, and survival is prolonged. Most patients walk until 16 years. Mental retardation is less common in BMD, there is less tendency for contractures, and skeletal deformities are less marked than in DMD.

Serum CK is elevated. ECG is abnormal in 30% to 40% and is less specific than in DMD. Muscle biopsy reveals findings similar to, but less severe than, DMD. Sixty percent of carriers have elevated CK. As in Duchenne's, the same gene product, dystrophin, of region Xp21, is defective. While dystrophin is absent in DMD, it is often present in Becker's cases, but is often of abnormal size and in normal or decreased amount.

3. *Facioscapulohumeral (Landouzy-Dejerine) dystrophy (FSHD)* is autosomal dominant, with strong penetrance but variable expression. Ten percent to 30% of cases arise from de novo mutation. Recent studies have demonstrated genetic linkage to a locus on the long arm of chromosome 4 (4q35).

The disease presents with a characteristic pattern of weakness of the face and scapular stabilizer muscles. Onset is variable, usually beginning during the first or second decades; 90% of the patients have some weakness on examination by the age 20. The course is slowly progressive and patients usually live a full, productive life. Initially there is facial weakness, inability to purse the lips, and incomplete eye closure. Muscles of the upper extremities may be involved simultaneously with facial muscles. Scapular fixation is lost and biceps/triceps are involved early, with relative sparing of the forearm giving a "Popeye" arm. Weakness of the hips and dorsiflexors may develop, making differentiation from scapuloperoneal dystrophy difficult. Intellect is normal. The cardiovascular system is rarely involved.

Serum CK is mildly elevated in 75% of patients. EMG examination is important in establishing that the disease is myopathic in origin. EMG findings often reveal findings associated with chronic myopathy. Muscle biopsy shows no pathognomonic findings but can help provides assurance that the underlying process is myopathic. Detection of the deletion site on chromosome 4 has high sensitivity and specificity (85% to 95%) for FSHD, even in the sporadic cases from new mutation.

There is no specific treatment for FSHD. Conservative treatment with nonsteroid anti-inflammatory drugs, range of motion exercises, and gentle stretching exercises may help with discomfort and pain in the shoulder and back. Custom fit lumbosacral corsets or abdominal binders may help support the weak abdominal musculature. In carefully selected patients with relatively good deltoid function, surgical fixation of the scapula to the rib cage can improve arm function and enable the patient to carry or lift objects. The procedure is usually done unilaterally.

4. Scapuloperoneal dystrophy presents with clinical presentation and overlaps with FSHD. Inheritance is autosomal dominant. The age of onset varies from childhood to mid-life. Weakness may begin in the anterior tibial and peroneal muscles, causing foot drop, or in the shoulder girdle and scapular muscles. Some of the patients also have mild facial weakness. The weakness is slowly progressive and usually will not result in severe disability. Serum CK is mildly elevated. EMG examination and muscle biopsy show nonspecific myopathic changes. Genetic testing for the deletion site on chromosome 4 seen with FHSD will be negative. The disorder needs to be differentiated from FSHD, which causes weakness in the shoulder girdle and scapular muscles and Emery-Dreifuss muscular dystrophy, which can present with weakness in the humeroperoneal distribution but spare scapular muscles.

5. Emery-Dreifuss muscular dystrophy (EDMD) is an X-linked disorder with onset usually in the first or second decade. The gene responsible for the disease is located at the long arm of the X chromosome. Mutation of the gene leads to diminished synthesis of the protein emerin, which is located at the nuclear membrane of skeletal, cardiac, and smooth muscles.

The clinical presentation is characterized by wasting and weakness of muscles in a scapulohumeroperoneal distribution, with prominent early contractures of elbows, posterior neck, and Achilles tendon. The weakness is slowly progressive. Cardiac conduction abnormalities are constant findings, and the patients and carriers are at risk for sudden death. Skeletal muscle weakness and contractures are rare in female carriers.

Diagnosis is based on clinical presentation, distribution of weakness, and presence of contracture and cardiac conduction defects. Serum CK is usually elevated (less than 10 times). Mild elevation of CK can be seen in female carriers. The earliest ECG abnormalities seen are low-amplitude or absent P waves and first-degree heart block. The cardiac conduction defects will eventually progress to second-degree or complete heart block. Other cardiac arrhythmias such as atrial fibrillation, bradycardia, and ventricular arrhythmia can develop as the disease progresses. EMG findings are influenced by the stage of disease and the muscles chosen to study. The needle EMG examination shows predominantly myopathic findings but may reveal neurogenic features as well. No pathognomonic features are seen in the muscle biopsy. Definite diagnosis of EDMD requires detection of the defect in the emerin gene on the X chromosome.

The disease has no specific treatment. Early contractures can be managed by physical therapy and surgical release. All of the patients should be followed up with a cardiologist, and annual cardiac evaluation (ECG, Holter monitor) is required. A cardiac pacemaker should be considered when indicated because the patient is at risk of early sudden death. The female carriers are also at risk of cardiac arrhythmia and sudden death, and annual ECG should be performed.

6. *Limb-girdle muscular dystrophy (LGMD)* was originally a general term describing disorders with a variety of causes, with a common presentation of progressive shoulder and hip weakness, and without dystrophinopathies. The diseases are inherited through autosomal dominant or recessive mode. The new approach is to classify LGMD into the autosomal dominant type (LGMD1) and the autosomal recessive type (LGMD2). Most cases of LGMD2 are the result of a mutation of the gene encoding for protein in the dystrophin sarcoglycan complexes, and the specific gene defects are known.

There is variation in age of onset, progression of disease, and inheritance between the types of LGMD. Most commonly, onset is during the second or third decade, with hip weakness followed by shoulder weakness shortly thereafter. There may be marked atrophy of the biceps. The course is slowly progressive over decades. Certain types of LGMD may also have prominent weakness in distal muscles (LGMD2B). Patients may eventually be confined to a wheelchair, but skeletal abnormalities are rare. Cardiomyopathy and cardiac conduction defects are less predictable in comparison to those in dystrophinopathies.

Serum CK is elevated up to 10 times normal and tends to be higher in the recessive LGMD than the dominant. EMG and muscle biopsy show nonspecific myopathic changes. The disorders need to be differentiated from dystrophinopathies, spinal muscular atrophy, polymyositis, and metabolic myopathies. There are commercially available antibodies for identifying components of the sarcoglycan complex by tissue staining. However, the specific diagnosis with muscle tissue staining without genetic testing is still difficult, because a disorder of one protein in the sarcoglycan complex will also affect other proteins, leading to confusing results on tissue staining. Commercial genetic testing is still not available.

As with dystrophinopathies, there is no current specific treatment for LMGD. Patients can benefit from physical therapy, stretching exercises, and bracing to reduce contracture and maintain functional capabilities. In patients with cardiac abnormalities, follow-up with a cardiologist is required.

7. *Oculopharyngeal dystrophy (OPMD)* is an autosomal-dominant adult-onset disorder that is prevalent in French Canadians and Spanish Americans. An autosomal recessive type of OPMD has been described. The disorders are both caused by a short trinucleotide repeat expansion in the PABP2 gene on the long arm of chromosome 14 (14q). Onset is in the fourth to sixth decade with ptosis, which may be asymmetrical early in the course. Dysphagia follows, and some degree of facial weakness develops. Extraocular muscle impairment varies in degree, but usually does not progress to complete ophthalmoplegia. Weakness of hips and shoulders is common, but mild. Dysphagia becomes incapacitating with weight loss and inability to clear secretions.

Muscle enzymes are usually normal or elevated three to four times normal. There may be conduction defects on ECG. EMG examination shows myopathic changes. Muscle biopsy shows characteristic small subsarcolemmal, rimmed vacuoles lined with granular material. Electron microscopy shows intranuclear tubular filaments (8.5 nm in diameter, which are different in size with the filament seen in inclusion body myositis) in muscle nuclei. Genetic testing is available for the patient and carriers.

There is still no specific treatment for the disease. Surgical treatments are available to correct the ptosis and improve dysphagia in moderately to severely affected patients.

8. *Distal myopathies* refer to a group of myopathies that have unusual clinical presentation of weakness of the distal lower extremities. Most of the disorders are certain types of muscular dystrophies, although some metabolic and inflammatory myopathies can also present with distal weakness. Table 53 provides the classifications, genetic localization, and clinical presentation of different types of distal myopathies. The first and most reported type of distal myopathy is Welander distal myopathy (late adult-onset type 1), which is an autosomal dominant disorder and occurs mostly in Scandinavian countries.

9. *Congenital muscular dystrophies(CMD)* are a rare heterogenous group of autosomal recessive disorders that begin during the infancy period. The group can be roughly divided based on clinical grounds into those with minimal or prominent involvement of the central nervous system. Laminin alpha chain-deficient CMD and A7-deficient CMD are examples of disorders that present with minimal central nervous system involvement. *Fukuyama congenital muscular dystrophies*, *Walker-Warberg syndrome*, and *muscle eye brain disease* present with prominent central nervous system involvement.

Patients with CMD present with generalized weakness sparing the eye muscles, normal or absent reflexes, variably increased serum CK, and normal EMG. Muscle biopsy shows variation in fiber size, necrosis, swollen hyalinized fibers with extensive fibrosis, and fatty infiltration. The disorders with prominent central nervous system involvement are often accompanied

TABLE 53

TYPES OF DISTAL MYOPATHIES

Type	Inheritance	Gene (gene protein)	Initial Weakness	Creatine Kinase	Biopsy
Late adult onset type I (Welander)	AR	2p13 (dynactin)	Hands, finger and wrist extensors	Normal, or slightly increased	Myopathic vacuolar occasionally
Late adult onset type II (Markesbery-Udd)	AD	2q31	Legs, anterior compartment	Normal, or slightly increased	Vacuolar myopathy
Early adult onset type I (familial IBM, Nonaka)	AR or sporadic	9p1-q1	Legs, anterior compartment	Slightly to moderately increased (<5x normal)	Vacuolar myopathy
Early adult onset type II (LGMD 2B, Miyoshi)	AR or sporadic	2p13 (Dysferin) 10	Legs, posterior compartment	Increased 10-150x normal	Myopathic without vacuoles.
Early adult onset type III (Laing)	AD	14	Legs, anterior compartment	Slightly increased (<3x normal)	Moderately myopathic, no vacuoles.
Myofibrillar: Onset in childhood to 7th decade	AD or sporadic ? AR, or X-linked	11q21-23 (αB-crystallin) 2q35 (Desmin)	Hands or legs	Moderately increased (<5x normal)	Myopathic vacuolar occasionally, myofibrillar destruction, cytoplasmic inclusions, desmin accumulation

by severe brain malformations including lissencephaly, agyria, pachygyria, and hydrocephalus. Children with disorders that minimally affect the central nervous system carry a better prognosis, and a majority of the patients have normal intelligence and a long, stable clinical course.

   10. *Myotonic dystrophy* (see Myotonia).

REFERENCES

Barohn RJ, Amato AA: *Semin Neurol* 9:45–58, 1999.
Brais B, Rouleau GA, Bouchard JP, et al: *Semin Neurol* 19:59–66, 1999.
Griggs RC, Mendell JR, Miller RG: In Reinhardt RW, ed: *Evaluation and treatment of myopathies*, Philadelphia, FA Davis, 1995, 93–153.
Tawil R, Figlewicz DA, Griggs RC, et al: *Ann Neurol* 43:279–282, 1998.
Tsao CY, Mendell JR: *Semin Neurol* 19:9–24, 1999.
Zacharias AS, Wagener ME, Warren ST, et al: *Semin Neurol* 19:67–79, 1999.

MYASTHENIA GRAVIS

Myasthenia gravis (MG) is a disease affecting the neuromuscular junction (NMJ), characterized by muscle fatigue and fluctuating weakness. There are both congenital and acquired forms of MG.

   Congenital myasthenic syndromes are classified by the pattern of inheritance or the site of defect, which can be presynaptic or postsynaptic. Patients with congenital myasthenia present in infancy or early childhood with fatigable weakness involving ocular, bulbar, and limb muscles and positive family history.

   The acquired form of myasthenia gravis is more common and results from autoantibodies directed against the post-synaptic acetylcholine receptor. MG may begin at any age. Neonatal myasthenia affects newborns of mothers with MG. Females are more commonly affected than males and tend to develop the disease at an earlier age, with peak incidence between ages of 10 to 40 years; in males, the peak age is from 50 to 70 years. Acquired MG has an incidence of 2 to 10 per 100,000 and a prevalence of 4 per 100,000.

   Clinical features: MG classically presents with muscle fatigue and weakness. Degree of weakness varies from day to day. Weakness tends to improve after rest or in the morning and worsen as the day proceeds. Ocular muscles and bulbar muscles are predisposed to weakness in MG. Weakness of ocular muscle is the initial manifestation of the disease in about half of the cases and is eventually involved in 90% of the cases. Ocular myasthenia with isolated ocular muscle weakness occurs in approximately 15% of the patients, although later on the patient can progress to have generalized myasthenia. Weakness of bulbar muscles, including muscles of facial expression, mastication, swallowing, and speech, is also common. Examination reveals weakness of the involved muscles, which worsens after sustained or repeated activity and improves after a brief rest. There is no muscle atrophy, and deep tendon reflexes are intact. Fatigability can be demonstrated by having patients look up for several minutes to determine the presence of ptosis or repetitively testing the proximal limb or neck muscles. Cooling of the frontalis muscles and eyelids (ice-pack test) can result in improvement in the ptosis.

Diagnosis is made on clinical grounds, with confirmation by the following diagnostic investigations:

1. *Tensilon test:* Edrophonium (Tensilon) is an ultra short-acting cholinesterase inhibitor. IV injection of Tensilon causes immediate improvement of the weak muscle. The usual dose of Tensilon given in the test is 10 mg. Initially a 2-mg dose is given IV to observe for side effects such as bradycardia, hypotension, or other arrhythmias. If tolerated, the other 8 mg is given in 2- to 3-mg increments over the next 2 to 3 minutes. Atropine sulfate 1 mg should be immediately available as an antidote for cardiac side effects. To maximize sensitivity and specificity, an objectively weak muscle should be selected for testing. Ptosis and major ocular muscle limitation are easily evaluated, but diplopia is subjective and not easily evaluated; limb weakness changes are harder to evaluate. False-positives can occur.
2. *EMG examination:* Routine nerve conduction studies and needle EMG examination are normal in MG, which will help to differentiate MG from other conditions such as myopathy. Ten percent or more decrement in compound muscle action potential (CMAP) amplitude is observed in response to slow repetitive stimulation in 50% to 70% of the patients with generalized myasthenia but may be normal in ocular myasthenia. The diagnostic yield is increased by stimulation of the proximal nerves (e.g., spinal accessory or facial nerve).
3. *Serum anti-acetylcholine receptor antibody titers:* sensitivity as high as 90%.
4. *Single-fiber EMG:* demonstrates abnormal *jitter* (variation in time interval between the firing of adjacent single muscle fibers from the same motor unit, which primarily reflects variation in NMJ transmission time) in 95% to 99% of the patients with generalized MG. However, although single-fiber EMG is very sensitive, it is not specific. Single-fiber EMG can also be abnormal in several other neuropathic and myopathic diseases. Interpretation of single-fiber EMG needs to be used in combination with clinical presentation and routine EMG examination.

Other useful laboratory investigations are chest x-ray and CT of the chest to evaluate for thymoma. Tests of thyroid function, erythrocyte sedimentation rate, antinuclear antibodies (ANA) titers, and vitamin B_{12} level can be helpful in looking for evidence of other autoimmune diseases. Baseline pulmonary function testing is also helpful.

Treatment:

1. Anticholinesterase agents increase the amount of acetylcholine available at the neuromuscular junction, resulting in higher possibility for

acetylcholine to bind to the acetylcholine receptor at the postsynaptic neuromuscular junction. Pyridostigmine (Mestinon) is started at 30 to 60 mg every 3 to 4 hours. Dosage ranges from 60 to 240 mg every 3 to 6 hours. It is available as a 60-mg tablet, a 12 mg/ml syrup, and an 180-mg sustained release preparation for bedtime use. Side effects are due to the muscarinic acetylcholine receptor binding and include excess salivation, abdominal cramping, and secretory diarrhea. Diarrhea can be controlled with anticholinergic medications. Cholinergic crises due to medication excess should be suspected in patients with respiratory failure who have been on high dosage of Mestinon with miosis, sialorrhea, diarrhea, bronchorrhea, cramps, and fasciculations. Treatment consists of withdrawal of anticholinesterases.

2. Thymectomy is mandatory if thymoma is present and usually indicated in young patients with severe MG. Thymectomy has been shown in some studies to induce remission when done early on in younger patients. The patient's status should be optimized by plasma exchange before thymectomy.

3. Immune-modulating agents such as corticosteroids may be used before thymectomy, although some authorities recommend reserving steroids for when thymectomy fails. They are not recommended for ocular myasthenia except in extreme circumstances. Weakness may occur early on before improvement when starting prednisone. Steroids can be started at lower doses and slowly increased up to 1 to 1.5 mg/kg/day. This dose should be maintained until remission is induced, then switched to alternate-day dosing. Anticholinesterases should be tapered first to verify remission. Steroids are then tapered over 6 to 12 months. If the patient relapses, tapering is stopped and the dose-response optimized.

Azathioprine and cyclosporine have been used in conjunction with steroids for their steroid-sparing effect and they have been used alone. There may be a 6-month lag before they becomes effective.

Plasmapheresis and intravenous immunoglobulin are used in myasthenic crisis. Patients with severe weakness and symptoms and signs of respiratory compromise need to be hospitalized, and their respiratory status should be closely monitored. In the patients who are on high-dose anticholinesterase, the possibility of cholinergic crisis, which sometimes is difficult to differentiate clinically from myasthenic crisis, needs to be considered. Precipitating causes of myasthenic crisis such as infection and medications that interfere with neuromuscular transmission should be searched for and treated. These include muscle relaxants such as quinine and curare; antiarrhythmic drugs such as quinidine, procainamide, and propranolol; certain antibiotics; trimethadione; penicillamine; and fever.

Ocular MG might best be treated by merely patching an eye if the patient has double vision (provided the other eye has good motility), but it is reasonable to try a small dose of pyridostigmine. If the therapeutic effect is still suboptimal, further increases are not indicated when the weakness is limited to the eyes. Often, pyridostigmine will relieve a unilateral ptosis, only to unmask diplopia. In addition, it might make a large-angle diplopia into a more disconcerting small degree of diplopia. If diplopia is the problem and a low dose is ineffectual, the patient should be patched. If bilateral ptosis is the problem, ptosis crutches attached to spectacles by an optician may be helpful. Steroids are beneficial in treating ocular myasthenia, but, because of risk-versus-benefit considerations, steroids should be reserved for extreme severe cases such as bilateral ophthalmoplegia with frozen eyes, severe bilateral ptosis that renders the patient functionally blind, and strong insistence by the patient despite being warned of the risk of long-term steroid therapy. Thymectomy, immunosuppression, and plasmapheresis usually are not necessary in pure ocular myasthenia gravis, considering the risk-benefit ratio.

REFERENCES

Drachman DB: *N Engl J Med* 330:1797–1810, 1994.
Engel A, Franzini Armstrong C, eds: *Myology*, New York, McGraw Hill, 1994, 1798–1835.
Lindstrom JM: *Muscle Nerve* 23:453–477, 2000.

MYELOGRAPHY

Myelography is an imaging technique that combines conventional x-ray of the spine with injection of radiopaque dyes into the subarachnoid space; it is indicated for evaluation of spinal cord and root compression. It is useful for detecting intradural and extradural defects resulting from tumors, as well as herniated disks. Myelography does not provide information about the cord itself other than its size and shape. Side effects of metrizamide myelography include nausea, vomiting, headache, meningitis, seizures, and transient encephalopathy.

Myelography is rapidly being replaced by MRI as the diagnostic imaging procedure of choice for evaluation of the spinal cord because MRI is noninvasive and allows visualization of cord pathology, such as intramedullary tumors and syrinx. CT myelography can complement MRI in the preoperative evaluation of abnormalities of the vertebrae or disks. In comparisons with MRI in the evaluation of cervical spondylotic myelopathy/radiculopathy, CT myelography tends to upgrade the degree of spinal stenosis, neural foraminal stenosis, and cord compression. Magnetic resonance myelography (MRM) is noninvasive, has comparable sensitivity to conventional myelography in visualizing lumbar nerve roots, and allows overall assessment of the spinal canal even in the presence of cerebrospinal fluid block.

REFERENCE

Shafaie F et al: *Spine* 24:1781–1785, 1999.

MYOCLONUS

Brief arrhythmic or repetitive muscular contractions of cortical, reticular, or spinal origin; the contractions are irregular in amplitude and frequency, asynchronous, and asymmetric in distribution. Clonus refers to monophasic rhythmic contractions and relaxations of a group of muscles (compare with Tremors). Precipitants of myoclonus include sensory stimuli, physical contact, and anxiety, which may modulate the intensity of the myoclonus.

Segmental and focal myoclonus can be rhythmic or arrhythmic, involving somatotopic areas such as head and neck (without palatal myoclonus) or limbs and torso (spinal myoclonus). It is associated with myelopathies resulting from infection, degenerative disease, osteoarthritis, neoplasm (especially colon carcinoma), and demyelination.

Palatal myoclonus: Rhythmic, synchronous contractions of the palate at an average rate of 120 to 130 per minute can be either bilateral or unilateral and may be associated with contractions of extraocular muscles, larynx, neck, diaphragm, trunk, or limb. Palatal myoclonus persists during sleep. There is hypertrophic degeneration of the contralateral inferior olivary nucleus if the myoclonus is unilateral. The lesion can be anywhere within the Guillain-Mollaret triangle—red nucleus, inferior olivary nucleus, and contralateral dentate nucleus—and the connecting pathways (central tegmental tract and crossing dentatoolivary pathway). The movements disappear after damage to the pathways of corticobulbar or corticospinal motor neurons. Palatal myoclonus is seen in cerebrovascular disease, multiple sclerosis, encephalitis and occasionally is idiopathic.

CLASSIFICATION

I. Physiologic (in persons with normal health).
   A. Sleep jerks (hypnic jerks).
   B. Anxiety induced.
   C. Exercise induced.
   D. Hiccough (singultus).
   E. Benign infantile myoclonus with feeding.
II. Essential myoclonus (no known cause and no other gross neurologic deficit).
   A. Hereditary (autosomal dominant).
   B. Sporadic.
III. Epileptic myoclonus (seizures predominate, and encephalopathy is absent, at least initially).
   A. Fragments of epilepsy.
      1. Isolated epileptic myoclonic jerks.
      2. Epilepsia partialis continua.
      3. Idiopathic stimulus-sensitive myoclonus.
      4. Photosensitive myoclonus.
      5. Myoclonic absences in petit mal.
   B. Childhood myoclonic epilepsies.
      1. Infantile spasms (West syndrome).

      2. Myoclonic astatic epilepsy (Lennox-Gastaut syndrome).

      3. Juvenile myoclonic epilepsy (Janz).

  C. Benign familial myoclonic epilepsy.

  D. Progressive myoclonus epilepsy: Baltic myoclonus (Unverricht-Lundborg).

IV. Symptomatic myoclonus (progressive or static encephalopathy dominates).

  A. Storage diseases.

      1. Lafora body disease.

      2. Lipidoses (such as GM_2 gangliosidosis, Tay-Sachs disease, and Krabbe's disease).

      3. Ceroid lipofuscinosis (Batten disease and Kuf disease).

      4. Sialidosis.

  B. Spinocerebellar degenerations.

      1. Ramsay Hunt syndrome.

      2. Friedreich's ataxia.

      3. Ataxia-telangiectasia.

  C. Basal ganglia degenerations.

      1. Wilson's disease.

      2. Torsion dystonia.

      3. Hallervorden-Spatz disease.

      4. Progressive supranuclear palsy.

      5. Huntington's disease.

      6. Parkinson's disease.

  D. Dementias.

      1. Creutzfeldt-Jakob disease.

      2. Alzheimer's disease.

  E. Viral encephalitides.

      1. Subacute sclerosing panencephalitis.

      2. Encephalitis lethargica.

      3. Arboviral encephalitis.

      4. Herpes simplex encephalitis.

      5. Postinfectious encephalomyelitis.

  F. Metabolic.

      1. Hepatic failure.

      2. Renal failure.

      3. Dialysis syndrome.

      4. Hypoglycemia.

      5. Infantile myoclonic encephalopathy (polymyoclonus) (with or without neuroblastoma).

      6. Nonketotic hyperglycemia.

      7. Multiple carboxylase deficiency.

      8. Biotin deficiency.

      9. Mitochondrial encephalomyopathy with ragged red fibers.

  G. Toxic encephalopathies.

      1. Bismuth.

    2. Heavy metal poisonings.
    3. Methyl bromide and DDT.
    4. Drugs (levodopa, penicillin, amitriptyline, imipramine, morphine, meperidine, L-tryptophan plus monoamine oxidase inhibitor, lithium, and phenytoin).
  H. Physical encephalopathies.
    1. After hypoxia (Lance-Adams syndrome).
    2. Posttraumatic.
    3. Heat stroke.
    4. Electric shock.
    5. Decompression injury.
  I. Focal CNS damage.
    1. After stroke.
    2. After thalamotomy.
    3. Tumor.
    4. Trauma.
    5. Palatal myoclonus.

TREATMENT

Treatment of myoclonus depends on the underlying pathology; however, the degree of disability determines whether treatment is warranted. The following drugs have been helpful, especially in segmental or focal myoclonus:

1. Treat/remove underlying cause (drug, etc.).
2. Clonazepam: 1 to 1.5 mg/day in divided doses with a gradual increase if necessary.
3. Valproic acid: The drug of choice for many of the myoclonic epilepsies but also used in essential myoclonus, posthypoxic myoclonus, and other secondary myoclonic conditions such as Huntington's disease with myoclonus. Initial dosage is 250 mg per day, increasing up to a usual therapeutic dosage of 1200 to 1400 mg per day.
4. 5-OH tryptophan: 100 mg per day in divided doses, increasing by 200 mg every 2 to 3 days up to a total of 1000 to 4000 mg per day; carbidopa, 75 to 150 mg per day, may be given to prevent extracerebral decarboxylation of 5-OH tryptophan to serotonin. This regimen is reported to help many patients with posthypoxic myoclonus and some with progressive myoclonic epilepsy.
5. Many other medications have been used, mostly anecdotally, including alcohol, estrogens, botulinum toxin (palatal myoclonus), tetrabenazine, trihexyphenidyl, and benztropine.

REFERENCE

Fahn S, Marsden CD, Van Woert MH: In Fahn S, Marsden CD, Van Woert MH, eds: *Advances in neurology*, vol 43, New York, Raven, 1986.

MYOGLOBINURIA

Myoglobin in the urine is due to rhabdomyolysis that occurs within several hours of acute muscle necrosis.

CLASSIFICATION

I. Hereditary myoglobinuria.
   - A. Enzyme deficiency known.
     1. Phosphorylase deficiency (McArdle's disease).
     2. Phosphofructokinase deficiency (Tarui disease).
     3. Carnitine palmityltransferase deficiency (DiMauro).
   - B. Incompletely characterized syndromes.
     1. Excess lactate production (Larsson syndrome).
   - C. Uncharacterized.
     1. Familial, no clear biochemical abnormality.
     2. Familial susceptibility to succinylcholine or general anesthesia ("malignant hyperthermia").
     3. Repeated attacks in an individual; no known biochemical abnormality.
II. Sporadic myoglobinuria.
   - A. Exertional myoglobinuria in untrained individuals.
     1. Squat-jump and related syndromes, including "march myoglobinuria."
     2. Anterior tibial syndrome.
     3. Convulsions, high-voltage electric shock.
   - B. Crush syndrome.
     1. Compression by fallen weights.
     2. Compression in prolonged coma.
   - C. Ischemic myoglobinuria.
     1. Arterial occlusion.
     2. Ischemic element in compression and anterior tibial syndrome.
   - D. Metabolic abnormalities.
     1. Metabolic depression.
        a. Barbiturate, carbon monoxide, narcotic coma.
        b. Diabetic acidosis.
        c. General anesthesia.
        d. Hypothermia.
     2. Exogenous toxins and drugs.
        a. Haff disease.
        b. Heroin, cocaine.
        c. Alcoholism.
        d. Toluene.
        e. Malayan sea-snake bite poison.
        f. Malignant neuroleptic syndrome.
        g. Plasmocid.
        h. Fluphenazine.

          i. Succinylcholine, halothane.
          j. Glycyrrhizate, carbenoxolone, amphotericin B.
      3. Other disorders.
          a. Chronic hypokalemia.
          b. Heat stroke.
          c. Toxic shock syndrome.
   E. Myoglobinuria with progressive muscle disease.
   F. Myoglobinuria resulting from unknown cause.

Diagnosis depends on further characterization of pigmenturia (myoglobin, hemoglobin, porphyrins) by spectrophotometry, electrophoresis, or immunoprecipitation. Myalgia or fever and malaise, or both, may be present. Serum muscle enzyme levels are elevated.

Complications include acute tubular necrosis with oliguria and azotemia, hyperkalemia, hypercalcemia, hyperuricemia, and uncommonly, respiratory failure.

Myoglobinuria is life threatening only if there is renal injury, which should be treated with mannitol or alkalinizing agents or both.

REFERENCE

Rowland LP: *Can J Neurol Sci* 11:1–13, 1984.

MYOPATHY

CLASSIFICATION

I. Inflammatory.
II. Endocrine.
III. Metabolic.
IV. Toxic.
V. Congenital.
VI. Muscular dystrophies (see Muscular Dystrophy).
VII. Myotonic disorders (see Myotonia).
VIII. Periodic paralysis (see Periodic Paralysis).

I. *Inflammatory myopathies* (see Table 54).
Polymyositis (PM) and *dermatomyositis* (DM) are inflammatory, usually sporadic, myopathies. Age distribution is bimodal, with peaks at 5 to 15 years of age and 50 to 60 years. Clinical presentation includes symmetric, painless, proximal greater than distal limb weakness that progresses over weeks to months. Dysphagia or respiratory muscle weakness can occur, more commonly with DM. There may be spontaneous exacerbations and remissions. On examination muscle wasting is absent until late in the course, and reflexes are normal. The typical "heliotrope" rash of DM consists of a lavender discoloration of the eyelids and malar areas. A scaly red rash appears over the metacarpophalangeal and proximal interphalangeal joints (Gottron's sign). In group IV there is a generalized

TABLE 54	
CLASSIFICATION OF POLYMYOSITIS/DERMATOMYOSITIS	
Group I	Primary, idiopathic polymyositis (PM)
Group II	Primary, idiopathic dermatomyositis (DM)
Group III	DM or PM associated with carcinoma
Group IV	Childhood DM or PM associated with a vasculitis
Group V	DM or PM with another associated collagen vascular disease (overlap syndrome)

Adapted from Bohan A, Peter JB: *N Engl J Med* 292:344, 1975.

necrotizing vasculitis that may produce multiple infarctions of the GI tract, lungs, skin, nerves, and brain. In group V the associated collagen vascular disorders include scleroderma, systemic lupus erythematosus, rheumatoid arthritis, polyarteritis nodosa, and Sjögren's syndrome. The level of creatine kinase (CK) is usually elevated. Electrocardiography (ECG) results may be abnormal, usually with a conduction block. Electromyography (EMG) results show increased insertional activity, fibrillations, and short, low-amplitude polyphasic motor unit potentials. Muscle biopsy specimens demonstrate interstitial and perivascular inflammation, muscular fiber atrophy, necrosis, regeneration, and characteristic "ghost fibers." Occult malignancy should be excluded in older patients with PM or DM. Treatment begins with the administration of prednisone, 60 to 100 mg per day until weakness resolves (1 to 4 months), followed by a slow taper. Fifty percent of patients respond to corticosteroid therapy. Cyclosporine, azathioprine, methotrexate, IV immunoglobulin, and plasmapheresis have benefited some patients.

Inclusion body myositis consists of slowly progressive, painless, distal greater than proximal muscle weakness and wasting. Onset is after the age of 50 years. Men are affected twice as often as women. The level of CK is normal or mildly elevated; EMG findings resemble those in PM and DM. In addition to the inflammatory changes seen in PM and DM, muscle biopsy specimens show characteristic basophilic rimmed vacuoles and nuclear and cytoplasmic eosinophilic inclusions. No treatment is available. This condition may mimic spinal muscular atrophy on clinical examination.

Sarcoid myopathy is characterized by noncaseating granulomata in muscle as well as other organs. About 50% of sarcoid patients have muscle involvement on biopsy, and most of those are asymptomatic. Chronic, proximal myopathy is the most common clinical muscle presentation. Women are affected four times as often as men. Corticosteroid therapy is the treatment of choice.

Polymyalgia rheumatica is characterized by muscle pain and stiffness that worsen with rest and abate with continued exercise. There is no muscle weakness. Onset is after the age of 55 years, and twice as many women as men are affected. Shoulder muscles are most commonly involved. Temporal arteritis may develop in 55% to 75% of patients.

Erythrocyte sedimentation rate (ESR) is elevated, and anemia is often present. The level of CK, EMG results, and muscle biopsy specimens are usually normal. Treat with prednisone 30 to 50 mg per day for 2 months, then taper. Clinical response and ESR must be followed up during the taper.

REFERENCES

Dalakos MC: *N Engl J Med* 325:1487, 1991.
Walton J: *J Neurol Neurosurg Psychiatry* 54:285, 1991.

II. *Endocrine myopathies.*
Fifty percent to 80% of patients with *Cushing's disease* and 2% to 21% of patients with chronic corticosteroid use have weakness. The distribution is proximal greater than distal, and legs are more involved than arms. Biopsy specimens show type 2 atrophy. To treat, decrease the steroid dose, change to alternate-day dosing, or change to a nonfluorinated steroid.

Adrenal insufficiency (Addison's disease). Twenty-five percent to 50% of patients have general weakness, muscle cramps, and fatigue that resolve with corticosteroid replacement. The results of EMG are usually normal, and the biopsy specimen is unremarkable. Hyperkalemic periodic paralysis (see Periodic Paralysis) can develop in patients with adrenal insufficiency.

Thyrotoxic myopathy develops in approximately 60% of thyrotoxic patients. There are weakness and wasting proximally or myalgias, or both; bulbar muscles are usually spared. Serum muscle enzyme levels are normal to low. Treat by restoring the euthyroid state. Thyrotoxic periodic paralysis resembles familial hypokalemic periodic paralysis (see Periodic Paralysis, Thyroid).

Hypothyroidism causes proximal weakness, fatigue, exertional pain, myalgias and stiffness, cramps, and occasionally, myoedema and muscle enlargement. Deep tendon reflex relaxation time is prolonged. Women are affected 10 times as often as men. The level of CK may be elevated. Treat by restoring the euthyroid state (see Thyroid).

Acromegaly (increased growth hormone): Fifty percent have paroxysmal muscle weakness, decreased exercise tolerance, and slight enlargement of muscles.

Hypopituitarism in adults causes severe weakness and fatigability with disproportionate preservation of muscle mass.

Hyperparathyroidism: Of these patients 25% have fatigue, proximal muscle weakness and atrophy, myalgias, and stiffness. Bulbar muscles are spared. Deep tendon reflexes are brisk. Levels of CK and aldolase are normal. Alkaline phosphatase and calcium levels are elevated, and the phosphorus level is low.

Hypoparathyroidism is usually not associated with significant weakness, but muscle cramping and tetany are common. Tapping the facial nerve causes muscular contraction (Chvostek's sign), and occluding venous return of the arm causes carpopedal spasm (Trousseau's sign).

MYOPATHY

Osteomalacia: In 50% of patients proximal muscle weakness, wasting, myalgias, and characteristic bony changes develop.

REFERENCE

Ruff R, Weissman J: *Neurol Clin* 6(3):575–592, 1988.

III. *Metabolic myopathy.*

Metabolic myopathy refers to muscle disease caused by abnormalities of glycogen or lipid metabolism or a defect of the respiratory chain. Intramuscular glycogen provides energy for short-term, strenuous exercise, whereas fatty acids provide energy for endurance exercise. Thus glycogenoses usually become evident as weakness or cramps, or both, on heavy or intense short-term exercise, whereas lipidoses become evident as poor endurance (Figures 25 and 26).

A. *Glycogenoses.*

Glycogenoses are most often autosomal recessive. Muscle biopsy specimen shows abnormal accumulation of glycogen. The specific enzyme abnormality is diagnosed by biochemical analysis of the affected tissue (muscle, leukocytes, skin, and the like). Glycogenoses in general show blunted or no rise in venous lactate levels with ischemic forearm exercise testing. Acid maltase deficiency is the exception.

Myophosphorylase deficiency (McArdle's disease) and *phosphofructo-kinase deficiency (PFK)* cause early exercise intolerance. Strenuous exercise results in muscle pain, contractures, and myoglobinuria.

Phosphoglycerate kinase deficiency resembles McArdle's disease and PFK deficiency on clinical study but is distinguished by lack of increased glycogen on biopsy and x-linked transmission.

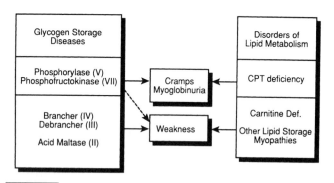

FIGURE 25

The two clinical syndromes associated with disorders of muscle glycogen and lipid metabolism. *Dotted line* represents less common clinical variant of phosphorylase and phosphofructokinase deficiencies. (Courtesy of the Continuing Professional Education Center, Princeton, NJ.)

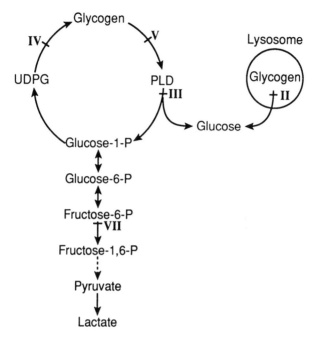

FIGURE 26

Scheme of glycogen metabolism and glycolysis, indicating the metabolic blocks in the five glycogenoses affecting muscle: *II*, acid maltase deficiency; *III*, debrancher deficiency; *IV*, brancher deficiency; *V*, phosphorylase deficiency; *VII*, phosphofructokinase deficiency. *PLD*, phosphorylase-limit dextrin; *UDPG*, uridine-diphosphate-glucose. (Courtesy of the Continuing Professional Education Center, Princeton, NJ.)

Lactate dehydrogenase (LDH) deficiency and *phosphoglycerate mutase deficiency*, both autosomal recessive, also resemble McArdle's disease and PFK deficiency on clinical study. In distinction, both give a rise (although blunted) of lactate level with forearm exercise testing, during which LDH deficiency also has a rise in pyruvate level.

Acid maltase deficiency (Pompe's disease) results in generalized deposition of glycogen in all tissues. Quadriparesis in these patients is due to muscle, peripheral nerve, and CNS involvement. In the infantile type, death occurs by 1 year of age. In the adult type, there is proximal limb-girdle weakness with prominent respiratory involvement. Results of EMG may show myotonia. Life expectancy is normal or slightly decreased. Inheritance is autosomal recessive.

Debranching enzyme deficiency (Forbes-Cori disease), also autosomal recessive, is characterized by abnormal glycogen accumulation in the heart, liver, spleen, and muscle. There is muscle wasting and weakness. Onset may be in infancy or adulthood.

Brancher enzyme deficiency is probably autosomal recessive. Amylopectin accumulates in the liver, spleen, and nervous system. The deficiency is associated with cirrhosis, hypotonia, areflexia, and muscle wasting and is fatal by age 5 years.

B. *Lipid metabolism myopathies.*

Primary carnitine deficiency occurs in two forms, myopathic and systemic. Both begin with progressive weakness during childhood or later. In the systemic form, in addition to weakness, there are recurrent episodes of hepatic encephalopathy. Muscle biopsy specimens and studies of histochemistry in both forms show abnormal lipid accumulation; biochemical analysis of muscle shows decreased carnitine content. Serum concentration of carnitine is normal in the myopathic form and decreased in the systemic form. Results of EMG show myopathic features. Prognosis in the systemic form is poor: death occurs in the late teens or early twenties. Most of the cases are sporadic, but there is evidence of autosomal recessive inheritance in some cases. Treatment with high-dose oral carnitine or prednisone may be effective. Secondary carnitine deficiency may occur in cirrhosis, renal dialysis, dystrophies, organic acidemia, mitochondrial myopathies, chronic illness, and parenteral nutrition.

Carnitine palmityltransferase (CPT) deficiency. Symptoms begin in childhood with weakness, myoglobinuria, and painful cramps (contractures) in response to prolonged exercise or fasting, or both. Strength between episodes is normal. Creatine kinase level rises during attacks. Forearm ischemic exercise testing shows normal rise in lactate level. Biochemical analysis of muscle and leukocytes shows markedly decreased CPT activity. Glycogen metabolism is normal; therefore the ability to perform intense exercise of short duration is not impaired. The deficiency is more common in males. Treatment with high-carbohydrate, low-fat diet may reduce the frequency of attacks.

Acyl coenzyme A (acyl-CoA) dehydrogenase deficiencies are lipid myopathies with variable proximal muscle weakness, metabolic acidoses, and episodic hypoglycemia with minimal ketonuria. Biopsy specimen shows lipid myopathy. One variety becomes evident in early childhood with the preceding symptoms, as well as cardiomegaly, hepatomegaly, and hypotonia.

Multisystem triglyceride storage disorder consists of congenital ichthyosis, hepatosplenomegaly, vacuolized granulocytes, and lipid myopathy. There may be nystagmus, retinal dysfunction, cataracts, corneal opacities, and sensorineural hearing loss.

REFERENCES

Carroll JE: *Neurol Clin* 6(3):563–574, 1988.
Servidei S, DiMauro S: *Neurol Clin* 7(1):159–178, 1989.

TABLE 55

MITOCHONDRIAL SYNDROMES

KSS	MELAS	MERRF
Ophthalmoplegia	Vomiting	Myoclonic epilepsy
Retinal degeneration	Strokelike episodes	Ataxia
Heart block	Seizures	Central hypoventilation
CSF protein increase	Positive family history	Positive family history
Ataxia		

KSS, Kearns-Sayre syndrome; MELAS, mitochondrial encephalopathy with lactic acidosis and strokelike episodes; MERRF, myoclonic epilepsy with ragged red fibers.

M

MYOPATHY

C. *Mitochondrial disorders.*

Abnormal mitochondrial function results in disorders of the CNS or muscle, or both. Defects of oxidative metabolism may involve pyruvate metabolism, Krebs cycle, or the respiratory chain. These defects typically result in lactic acidosis in blood and CSF. When the defect involves mitochondrial DNA, the muscle biopsy specimen usually contains abnormal mitochondria that are seen as ragged red fibers on trichrome stains.

Mitochondrial myopathies result in weakness and exercise intolerance. In severe forms patients have profuse sweating and heat intolerance at rest without hyperthyroidism. The mitochondrial encephalomyopathies are primarily CNS disorders. They include the three clinical syndromes described in the next paragraph, whose common features include short stature, weakness, spongy degeneration of brain, dementia, and sensoneural hearing loss (see Table 55).

Kearns-Sayre syndrome (KSS) becomes evident before 20 years of age with ophthalmoplegia, retinal degeneration, heart block, and weakness. The defect is a mitochondrial DNA deletion. Mitochondrial encephalopathy with lactic acidosis and strokelike episodes (MELAS) becomes evident in the first decade of life with episodic vomiting, recurrent hemiparesis or hemianopsia, and seizures. The defect is in complex I of the respiratory chain and is maternally inherited. Myoclonic epilepsy with ragged red fibers (MERRF) becomes evident before 20 years of age with myoclonus, seizures, and ataxia. These patients have a maternally inherited defect in complex IV of the respiratory chain.

Treatment consists of avoiding conditions that increase the body's energy demands (fasting, infection, overexertion, and extreme temperatures) as well as medications that inhibit respiratory chain function (phenytoin and barbiturates) and medications inhibiting mitochondrial protein synthesis (tetracycline and chloramphenicol). The administration of coenzyme Q may benefit some patients with KSS.

D. Adenylate deaminase deficiency affects 1% to 2% of the population. It is probably not a true myopathy but becomes evident with cramps.

REFERENCES

DeVivo DC, DiMauro S: *Int Pediatr* 5:112–120, 1990.
Tritschler HJ, Medori R: *Neurology* 43:280–288, 1993.

TABLE 56

RECOGNIZED TOXINS THAT CAUSE MYOPATHY

Myopathy With Neuropathy	Myopathy With Cardiomyopathy
Aminodarone (Cordarone)	Chloroquine (Aralen)
Chloroquine (Aralen)	Clofibrate (Atromid)
Clofibrate (Atromid)	Colchicine
Colchicine	Doxorubicin (Adriamycin)
Doxorubicin (Adriamycin)	Emetine, Ipecac
Ethanol	Ethanol
Hydroxychloroquine (Plaquenil)	Hydroxychloroquine (Plaquenil)
Organophosphates	Metronidazole (Flagyl)
Vincristine (Oncovin)	

IV. *Toxic myopathies.*

Alcohol myopathy takes two forms. There may be an acute attack of muscle pain, tenderness, swelling, weakness, and myoglobinuria after "binge" drinking. Thigh muscles are most commonly involved. The second form consists of a chronic, slowly progressive, proximal muscle weakness. The level of CK is slightly elevated. Results of biopsy are nonspecific.

Table 56 lists recognized toxins that cause a myopathy classified according to presence or absence of neuropathy or cardiomyopathy.

REFERENCES

Harris JB, Blain PG: In *Baillière's clinical endocrinology and metabolism*, 4:665–686, 1990.
Kuncl RW, Wiggins WW: *Neurol Clin* 6:593–621, 1988.
Urbano-Marquez A et al: *N Engl J Med* 320:409–415, 1989.

V. *Congenital myopathies.*

Symptoms are usually present from birth and include a "floppy infant" with hypotonia, decreased deep tendon reflexes, decreased spontaneous movement, muscular weakness, and often an abnormal consistency of muscle on palpation. Associated anomalies are variable and include scoliosis, high-arched palate, elongated facies, ophthalmoplegia, and pectus excavatum. Symptoms are nonprogressive or slowly progressive. The level of CK is often normal. Results of EMG show small-amplitude, polyphasic motor units. It is usually not possible to discern the specific types of myopathy on clinical basis alone; biopsy of a muscle specimen is necessary for classification.

Central core disease becomes evident as hypotonia, proximal weakness, delayed motor milestones; bulbar musculature is relatively spared. Biopsy specimens show a well-circumscribed circular region in the center of muscle fibers and a predominance of type I fibers.

Nemaline myopathy is usually associated with dysmorphic features and bulbar involvement (poor suck-and-swallow reflexes with a weak cry). The severe congenital type can result in respiratory failure and death.

Biopsy specimens show a predominance of type I fibers and dark-staining rods originating from Z lines.

There are many other, less common congenital myopathies with specific abnormalities on biopsy, including myotubular myopathy, congenital fiber-type disproportion, multicore disease, fingerprint body myopathy, and sarcotubular myopathy.

REFERENCES

Banker BQ: In Engel AG, Banker BQ, eds: *Myology*, New York, McGraw Hill, 1986.
Bodensteiner J: *Neurol Clin* 6:499–518, 1988.

MYOTOMES (*Table 57*)

TABLE 57
MYOTOMES

Muscle	Nerve	Root
Levator scapulae	C3,4 and dorsal scapular	C3,*4*,5
Rhomboids (major and minor)	Dorsal scapular	C4,5
Supraspinatus	Suprascapular	C5,6
Infraspinatus	Suprascapular	C5,6
Deltoid	Axillary	C5,6
Biceps brachii	Musculocutaneous	C5,6
Brachioradialis	Radial	C5,6
Supinator	Radial	C5,6
Flexor carpi radialis	Median	C6,*7*
Pronator teres	Median	C6,*7*
Serratus anterior	Long thoracic	C5,6,*7*
Latissimus dorsi	Thoracodorsal	C6,*7*,8
Pectoralis major		
Clavicular head	Lateral pectoral	C5,*6*,7
Sternal head	Medial pectoral	C6,*7*,8, T1
Triceps brachii	Radial	C6,*7*,8
Extensor carpi radialis longus	Radial	C6,*7*
Anconeus	Radial	C7,8
Extensor digitorum	Radial	C7,8
Extensor carpi ulnaris	Radial	C7,8
Extensor indicis proprius	Radial	C7,8
Palmaris longus	Median	C7,8, T1
Flexor pollicis longus	Median	C7,8, T1
Flexor carpi ulnaris	Ulnar	C7,8, T1
Flexor digitorum sublimis	Median	C7,8
Flexor digitorum profundus	Median	C7,8, T1
	Ulnar	
Pronator quadratus	Median	C8, T1
Abductor pollicis brevis	Median	C8, T1
Opponens pollicis	Median	C8, T*1*
Flexor pollicis brevis	Median	C8, T*1*

Table continued on following page

TABLE 57 —cont'd

MYOTOMES

Muscle	Nerve	Root
Lumbricals I and II	Median	C8, *T1*
First dorsal interosseous	Ulnar	C8, *T1*
Abductor digiti minimi	Ulnar	C8, *T1*
Iliopsoas	Femoral	*L2,3,4*
Adductor longus	Obturator	*L2,3,4*
Gracilis	Obturator	*L2,3,4*
Quadriceps femoris	Femoral	*L2,3,4*
Anterior tibial	Deep peroneal	*L4,5*
Extensor hallucis longus	Deep peroneal	*L4,5*
Extensor digitorum longus	Deep peroneal	*L4,5*
Extensor digitorum brevis	Deep peroneal	*L4,5*, S1
Peroneus longus	Superficial peroneal	*L5*, S1
Internal hamstrings	Sciatic	*L4,5*, S1
External hamstrings	Sciatic	*L5, S1*
Gluteus medius	Superior gluteal	*L4,5*, S1
Gluteus maximus	Inferior gluteal	L5, *S1,2*
Posterior tibial	Tibial	*L5*, S1
Flexor digitorum longus	Tibial	*L5*, S1
Abductor hallucis brevis	Tibial (medial plantar)	L5, *S1,2*
Abductor digiti quinti pedis	Tibial (lateral plantar)	*S1,2*
Gastrocnemius lateral	Tibial	L5, *S1,2*
Gastrocnemius medial	Tibial	*S1,2*
Soleus	Tibial	*S1,2*

Italics in root column denote major root supply.

MYOTONIA

Myotonia refers to a delay in muscle relaxation demonstrated after voluntary action (such as hand grip or forced eye closure) or percussion of a muscle such as the thenar or wrist extensor muscles (*percussion myotonia*). Results of EMG show repetitive discharges with waxing and waning amplitude and frequency, giving a characteristic "dive bomber" sound. Myotonia results from several different abnormalities of muscle membrane and is treated with membrane-stabilizing drugs such as quinine, procainamide, phenytoin, or tocainamide. If potassium sensitivity is demonstrated, acetazolamide may be used. These medications treat myotonia with variable success but are often unable to improve associated weakness.

Myotonic dystrophy is the most common adult-onset muscular dystrophy (1 in 7500 persons). It becomes evident as weakness in excess of myotonia, particularly involving the face and distal limbs. Atrophy of the temporalis and masseter muscles causes the jaw to hang open, producing a characteristic "hatchet-head" and "fish-mouth" appearance. Frontal balding, ptosis, and neck muscle atrophy add to this appearance. Other neurologic features include hypersomnia, dysarthria, dysphagia with nasal

TABLE 58

CHARACTERISTICS OF THE MYOTONIAS

| | Myotonic Dystrophy | Myotonia Congenita | | Paramyotonia Congenita | Hyperkalemic Periodic Paralysis |
		Thomsen's Disease	Becker's Disease		
Inheritance	Autosomal dominant	Autosomal dominant	Autosomal recessive	Autosomal dominant	Autosomal dominant
Defect	Protein kinase	Chloride channel	Chloride channel	Sodium channel	Sodium channel
Gene locus	19q	7q	7q	17q	17q
Age of onset	Teens to twenties	Infancy to childhood	Childhood	Infancy	Childhood
Course	Slowly progressive	Nonprogressive	Rarely progressive	Variable weakness	Variable weakness
Presenting complaint	Distal weakness; Systemic features	Diffuse stiffness	Diffuse stiffness, weakness	Cold-induced stiffness	Episodic weakness
Other features	Typical facies	Absence of type II fibers	± Muscle hypertrophy; Absence of type II fibers	Paradoxic myotonia	May have cardiac arrhythmia

MYOTONIA

N

regurgitation, and cognitive dysfunction. Systemic features include cardiac conduction defects, impaired gastric motility, testicular atrophy, glucose intolerance resulting from decreased insulin sensitivity, early subcapsular cataracts, and increased risk associated with general anesthesia. The course is slowly progressive; death typically occurs in the sixth decade of life as a result of cardiac or respiratory complications. Muscle enzyme levels are often elevated. Muscle biopsy specimens show internal nuclei, type I fiber atrophy, and ring fibers. "Anticipation," or earlier onset of more severe disease in successive generations, has been linked to an increasing number of repetitions of an unstable DNA sequence on chromosome 19 found in offspring of patients. Linkage analysis has been used for genetic counseling.

A congenital form of myotonic dystrophy associated with maternal inheritance becomes evident as generalized hypotonia and bulbar and respiratory weakness. Affected children have "shark mouth" and club feet, and 70% have mental retardation. Treatment is symptomatic for adult and congenital forms of disease.

Patients with myotonia congenita (*Thomsen's disease* is the autosomal dominant form; *Becker's disease* is the autosomal recessive form) typically complain of diffuse muscle stiffness (that is, myotonia) after resting, which relaxes with exercise. In paramyotonia congenita (Eulenberg's disease) the stiffness, often induced by cold, worsens with exercise (paradoxic myotonia). Muscles of the face and distal upper extremities are most often involved. Table 58 delineates the clinical features of the myotonias.

REFERENCE

Ptacek LJ, Johnson KJ, Griggs RC: *N Engl J Med* 323(7):482–489, 1993.

NEGLECT

Neglect is the failure to report, respond to, or orient to novel and meaningful stimuli presented to the side opposite a brain lesion when this failure cannot be attributed to either sensory or motor dysfunction. Components of neglect include inattention or sensory neglect, motor neglect, spatial neglect, personal neglect, allesthesia (hallucination of perception in response to a stimulus), and anosognosia. Bedside tests for neglect include visual confrontation, double simultaneous stimulation, letter or figure cancellation, figure drawing, and line bisection. Lesions associated with neglect correlate with the type of neglect syndrome. Attention system defects with sensory neglect are associated with right parietal lobe lesions. Motor neglect with varying degrees of akinesia and motor impersistence can be seen in frontal lesions. Defects in the representational system are often associated with right hemisphere lesions because the right hemisphere is important as an attention system for left and right hemispace, whereas the left hemisphere is primarily important only for attention to right hemispace. Another explanation posits a bihemispheric network of attention systems, which is overrepresented in the right hemisphere.

REFERENCE

Heilman KH, Watson RT, Valenstein E: In Heilman KH, Valenstein E, eds: *Clinical neuropsychology*, ed 3, New York, Oxford University Press, 1993.

NEUROCUTANEOUS SYNDROMES

Neurocutaneous syndromes, or phakomatoses (Greek *phakos*=lens shaped, mole, freckle), represent disordered development early in embryogenesis, which produces defects in multiple organ systems roughly according to germ cell layers. They may be divided into disorders affecting ectodermal derivatives (neural and cutaneous tissue) or those involving mesodermal tissue (vascular elements, widespread) or classified by mode of inheritance.

AUTOSOMAL DOMINANT INHERITANCE

Neurofibromatosis type 1 (NF-1, Von Recklinghausen's disease) is a neuroectodermal disorder related to genetic abnormality on chromosome 17. It occurs in approximately 1 in 3,000 people. The diagnoses requires at least two of the following:

1. Six or more cafe au lait spots greater than 5 mm in diameter.
2. Axillary or inguinal freckles.
3. Two neurofibromas of any type or one or more plexiform neurofibromas. (Neurofibromas occur along peripheral nerves and are made from Schwann cells, fibroblasts, vascular elements, or pigmented cells. They are pedunculated, nodular, or diffuse but not encapsulated. A neurofibroma that extends into the surrounding tissue is a plexiform neurofibroma; these have a 5% lifetime risk of malignant transformation).
4. Optic nerve or chiasmatic glioma.
5. Two or more Lisch nodules (pigmented hamartomas of the iris, best seen with slit lamp exam of the iris and more common in older patients).
6. First-degree relative with NF-I by foregoing criteria.
7. Bony abnormalities such as thinning of cortical long bone or sphenoid dysplasia. Other associated features of NF-I include tumors (pheochromocytoma, Wilm's tumor, leukemia), pseudoarthroses of radius and tibia, kyphosis, and endocrine dysfunction secondary to hypothalamic and pituitary compression from an optic glioma.

Neurofibromatosis type 2 (NF-2) is due to a genetic abnormality on chromosome 22. It occurs in approximately 1 in 50,000 people.

NEUROCUTANEOUS SYNDROMES

Symptoms usually develop in adolescence and early adulthood; these include headache, dizziness, tinnitus, hearing loss, and facial weakness. The diagnostic criteria include the following:

1. Bilateral eighth nerve tumors (acoustic neuromas).
2. Unilateral eighth nerve tumor and a first-degree relative with NF-2.
3. A first-degree relative with NF-2 and two of the following: glioma, schwannoma, presenile posterior cataract, astrocytoma, neurofibroma of another type, plexiform neurofibroma, or retinal hamartoma.

Tuberous sclerosis (Bourneville's disease) has multiple manifestations, including generalized or partial complex seizures after 3 months of age, occasionally associated with mental retardation or hemiparesis. Neuroradiologic features are multiple subependymal nodular calcification, cortical tubers, and ventricular dilatation. Development of giant astrocytomas is relatively frequent. Cutaneous manifestations include facial angiofibroma (hamartomas of facial skin that usually appear after the age of 5), adenoma sebaceum depigmented nevi, subungual fibromas, or Shagreen patches (hamartomas in the dermis that appear like cobblestone pavement, commonly located in the posterior neck and lumbar back region). Other associated conditions include renal angiolipomas and cysts, cardiac rhabdomyomas, pulmonary cysts, and retinal hamartomas.

Von Hippel-Landau disease (VHD). Diagnostic criteria include hemangioblastoma of the CNS (most commonly found in the cerebellum, medulla, spinal cord, or cerebral hemispheres) or retina and one additional characteristic lesion or a direct relative with the disease. Characteristic lesions include hypernephroma, renal cell carcinoma, pheochromocytoma, renal, pancreatic, or epididymal cysts, and islet cell tumors. Secondary polycythemia may occur due to production of an erythropoietic factor produced by a cerebellar or renal tumor. Retinal hemangioma may be the earliest sign and can appear in the first decade of life. Exudate from the hemangioblastoma may accumulate under the retina, causing detachment and blindness. Therefore, people at risk for VHD should be examined periodically after age 6 to prevent blindness from retinal lesions. Treatment involves surgical removal of the hemangioblastoma or radiotherapy (if inoperable).

AUTOSOMAL RECESSIVE INHERITANCE

Xeroderma pigmentosa is a rare disorder resulting from a defect in cellular repair of damaged DNA. This results in accelerated aging in tissue exposed to solar light and degeneration of neurons. Skin and eye manifestations usually occur within the first months of life. Neurologic findings are not present in all patients but may include microcephaly, ataxia, spasticity, and choreoathetosis. Peripheral nerve involvement results in hyporeflexia occasionally progressing to areflexia. The diagnosis is made by family history and laboratory tests showing deficient DNA repair in fibroblasts.

Chediak-Higashi syndrome is a disorder of lysosomal abnormality resulting in large granulations in leukocytes, neurons, pigment cells, and platelets. Cellular immunity is deficient, and recurrent pyogenic infections include otitis media, bronchitis, pharyngitis, cellulitis, and subcutaneous abscesses. Leukemias are frequent in this syndrome. Neurologic symptoms occur in approximately 50% of patients and include mental retardation, seizures, cerebellar ataxia, increased intracranial pressure, and a chronic polyneuropathy with a stocking-glove type of sensory loss, weakness, and atrophy. The diagnoses is made by finding large granulations in leukocytes in peripheral blood, marrow, or giant lysosomes in the cytoplasm of Schwann cells.

Ataxia-telangiectasia is an autosomal recessive (AR) disease, caused by a defect in the repair mechanism of the damaged DNA. It presents with progressive cerebellar ataxia, oculomotor apraxia, and choreoathetosis beginning in childhood. Telangiectasias of the conjunctiva, ears, and flexor surfaces appear later. Systemic manifestations include decreased IgA and IgE, increased alpha-fetoprotein, recurrent pulmonary infections, and development of reticuloendothelial tumors.

NONHEREDITARY NEUROCUTANEOUS DISEASES

Neurocutaneous melanosis occurs predominantly in white patients and is characterized by large pigmented nevi that are light to dark brown. Melanin-containing cells in the pia may develop into intracranial or intraspinal melanomas. Hydrocephalus may result secondary to obstruction of the arachnoid villi. Patients rarely live beyond 20 years of age.

Sturge-Weber syndrome (meningofacial angiomatosis with cerebral calcifications) is a sporadic congenital malformation of the cephalic venous microvasculature, resulting in neurologic, cutaneous, and optic symptoms. Pathologically, there are venous angiomas with torturous vessels involving the face, leptomeninges, and choroid, in addition to calcification of layers 2 and 3 of the parietal-occipital cortex. Neurologic manifestations include unilateral seizures, cerebral hemiatrophy with hemiparesis, hemisensory deficits, visual field defects, and mental abnormalities. Cutaneous lesions vary in extent from a small "port wine nevus" on the upper eyelid to those involving the entire face and other parts of the body. Ocular manifestations include congenital glaucoma.

OTHER NEUROCUTANEOUS SYNDROMES

1. *Klippel-Trenaunay-Weber syndrome* (limb hypertrophy and hemangiomas).
2. *Osler-Weber-Rendu syndrome* (hemorrhagic telangiectasias).
3. *Wyburn-Mason syndrome* (facial angioma, retinal AVM's, cerebrovascular anomalies, and seizures)
4. *Incontinentia pigmenti* (bullous lesions of skin, micropolygyria, microcephaly, and mental retardation), hypomelanosis of Ito (skin whorls, mental retardation seizures, and ocular deficits).

5. *Fabry's disease* (papular eruption, painful sensory neuropathy, and stroke) and *linear nevus syndrome* (linear yellow papules, mental retardation, and seizures).

REFERENCES

Herron J et al: *Clin Radiol* 55:82–98, 2000.
Kerrison JB et al: *Neurosurg Clin N Am* 10:775–787, 1999.
King A et al: *Neurology* 54:4–5, 2000.

NEUROLEPTICS

Neuroleptics include several classes of compounds whose primary common feature is blockade of dopamine receptors, although all of them have other effects at other receptors, such as anticholinergic activity. An exception is clozapine and other "atypical antipsychotics" (Olanzapine, Quetiapine) which block serotonin receptors and has little dopamine receptor blockade. The primary clinical use of neuroleptics is in the treatment of psychosis and agitation. Neuroleptics are also used for control of hyperkinetic movement disorders (chorea, tics, and dystonia), for suppressing nausea, for control of vertigo, neuralgic pain, and acute and refractory migraines, and for treating the abdominal pain of porphyric crises.

Aliphatic phenothiazines such as chlorpromazine (Thorazine) are strongly sedating. Potent α-adrenergic antagonism results in postural hypotension. Antiemetic and anticholinergic effects are significant. Extrapyramidal and dystonic symptoms occur with medium frequency.

Piperidine phenothiazines such as thioridazine (Mellaril) and mesoridazine (Serentil) have a relative potency similar to that of the aliphatic compounds. Sedative and α-adrenergic antagonism are less than with aliphatic compounds. Antiemetic effects are negligible. This class has a low incidence of extrapyramidal and dystonic side effects.

Piperazine phenothiazines, such as prochlorperazine (Compazine), trifluoperazine (Stelazine), perphenazine (Trilafon), and fluphenazine (Prolixin), have the highest relative potency and the strongest antiemetic effects. They also have the highest incidence of extrapyramidal and dystonic symptoms. Sedation and α-adrenergic antagonism are minimal.

The pharmacologic features of butyrophenones such as haloperidol (Haldol) closely resemble those of the piperazines. They have strong dopaminergic-blocking effects and a high incidence of extrapyramidal and dystonic symptoms. Relatively less orthostatic hypotension and sedation occur than with lower potency neuroleptics.

Pimozide (Orap), a diphenylbutylpiperidine, is similar in effect to haloperidol and is used in the United States primarily for the treatment of Tourette's syndrome.

The thioxanthenes resemble the phenothiazines. Thiothixene (Navane) resembles the piperazines, with greater dystonic and extrapyramidal side effects.

Atypical antipsychotics differ from typical psychotics in their "limbic-specific" dopamine type 2 (D2)-receptor binding and high ratio of serotonin type 2 (5-HT2)-receptor binding to D2 binding. Clozapine, olanzapine, risperidone, quetiapine, and ziprasidone. Clozapine use has fallen due to agranulocytosis in 1% to 2% of patients and significant lowering of seizure threshold. Complete blood counts must be closely monitored if clozapine is used. These medications can be sedating and associated with weight gain and anticholinergic side effects.

EXTRAPYRAMIDAL SIDE EFFECTS

Dystonia may occur early (1 to 3 weeks) in the course of neuroleptic therapy or after a single parenteral injection. It may consist of generalized torsion dystonia, opisthotonos, torticollis, retrocollis, oculogyric crisis, trismus, or focal appendicular dystonia. Dystonia is more common in younger patients, especially children or adolescents, and in black males. It usually resolves spontaneously within 24 hours of stopping use of the drug but may be terminated within minutes with benztropine (Cogentin) 1 mg IM or IV or diphenhydramine (Benadryl) 50 mg IV; oral therapy may be continued for 24 to 48 hours.

Parkinsonian symptoms of stiffness, "cog-wheeling," tremor, and shuffling gait are dose related and may begin as early as a few days to 4 weeks after starting therapy. The neuroleptic dosage should be decreased or an anticholinergic agent may be added. Anticholinergic agents in use include benztropine 0.5 to 4.0 mg bid, biperiden (Akineton) 2.0 mg qd to tid, and trihexyphenidyl (Artane) 2 to 5 mg tid. Anticholinergics carry the risk of precipitating anticholinergic delirium, which may mimic psychotic symptoms; therefore prophylactic use should be limited to patients at high risk for extrapyramidal symptoms.

Akathisia is a subjective sensation of motor restlessness with an urge to move around that generally occurs within several weeks of starting neuroleptic therapy. It improves on decreasing the dose of neuroleptic or adding β blockers or benzodiazepines. Neuroleptic dose should not be increased to treat this form of "agitation," which may mimic the initial psychotic symptoms.

Tardive dyskinesia, consisting of oral-lingual-facial-buccal movements or other choreoathetoid or ballistic movements, may occur after prolonged neuroleptic therapy. Its incidence may be decreased by using neuroleptics only when indicated, keeping doses as low as possible and duration of therapy as short as possible, and early detection through careful monitoring. The more advanced the dyskinesia, the less likely is resolution. Primary treatment consists of tapering and withdrawing the neuroleptic. Treatment with reserpine 0.25 mg per day, increasing by 0.25 mg per day to 1 to 5 mg per day in divided doses, with care to avoid orthostatic hypotension, may help. Neuroleptics themselves have no role in the treatment of tardive dyskinesias.

A *withdrawal syndrome*, seen particularly in children and consisting of choreic movements, may occur when long-term administration of neuroleptics is suddenly stopped. The syndrome usually resolves within 6 to 12 weeks but can be avoided by restarting the drug therapy and tapering more slowly.

The *neuroleptic malignant syndrome* is rare but often (20% to 30%) fatal. Hyperthermia, hypertonia of skeletal muscles, fluctuating consciousness, and autonomic instability are characteristic. Laboratory findings include elevated creatine kinase level, leukocytosis, and liver function abnormalities. The differential diagnosis includes heat stroke (neuroleptics may potentiate by decreasing sweating), malignant hyperthermia associated with anesthesia, idiopathic acute lethal catatonia, drug interactions with monoamine oxidase inhibitors, and central anticholinergic syndromes. Treatment begins with discontinuing the neuroleptic and providing cooling blankets, antipyretics, and IV hydration. Dantrolene sodium 0.8 to 10 mg/kg per day IV has been used. Bromocriptine, 2.5 to 10 mg PO tid, amantadine, and levodopa with carbidopa have also been used effectively.

Neuroleptics lower the seizure threshold and may precipitate seizures. Their use in patients with epilepsy is not contraindicated unless seizure control is a significant problem.

REFERENCES

Kaplan HI, Sadock BJ, eds: *Synopsis of psychiatry*, ed 6, Baltimore, Williams & Wilkins, 1991.

Stip E: *J Psychiatry Neurosci.* 25:137–53, 2000.

NEUROPATHY

CLINICAL CLASSIFICATION OF NEUROPATHY

I. Polyneuropathies.
  A. Acute predominantly motor neuropathy with variable sensory involvement.
    1. Acute inflammatory demyelinating polyradiculoneuropathy (Guillain-Barré syndrome).
    2. Polyneuropathy associated with:
      a. Diphtheria.
      b. Porphyria.
      c. AIDS.
      d. Thallium.
      e. Triorthocresyl phosphate, dapsone.
  B. Acute motor neuropathy.
    1. Diabetic multiple mononeuropathy (asymmetric proximal diabetic neuropathy, diabetic amyotrophy).
  C. Acute asymmetric sensorimotor polyneuropathy (multiple mononeuropathy or mononeuritis multiplex).
    1. Polyarteritis nodosa.
    2. Wegener's granulomatosis.
    3. Diabetes.

    4. AIDS.

    5. Other angiopathies, vasculitides.

D. Subacute symmetric sensorimotor neuropathy.

    1. Toxic.

       a. Heavy metals—arsenic, mercury, thallium.

       b. Drugs.

          (1) Antibiotics—clioquinol, ethambutol, isoniazid, nitro-
furantoin, streptomycin.

          (2) Antineoplastic—vinca alkaloids, cisplatin, chlorambucil,
methotrexate, daunorubicin.

          (3) Cardiovascular—clofibrate, disopyramide, hydralazine.

          (4) Other—gold salts, colchicine, phenylbutazone,
methaqualone, penicillamine, chloroquine, disulfiram,
cyclosporine A.

       c. Industrial chemicals—triorthocresyl phosphate, acrylamide,
methyl bromide, n-hexane, methyl-n-butyl ketone.

    2. Nutritional deficiency—vitamin B_{12}, niacin (pellagra), thiamine
(beriberi), pyridoxine, vitamin E.

    3. Uremia.

    4. Chronic alcoholism (nutritional deficiency).

    5. Early chronic relapsing demyelinating polyneuropathy.

E. Subacute to chronic, predominantly sensory neuropathy.

    1. Diabetes.

    2. Drugs—chlorambucil, metronidazole, ethambutol, pyridoxine,
phenytoin (rare), propylthiouracil.

    3. Sjögren's syndrome.

    4. Leprosy.

    5. Paraneoplastic.

    6. AIDS.

    7. Idiopathic nonmalignant inflammatory sensory
polyganglionopathy.

    8. Vitamin deficiency: B_{12} and E.

F. Subacute to chronic, predominantly motor neuropathy.

    1. Diabetes—proximal diabetic motor neuropathy ("amyotrophy").

    2. Lead.

G. Chronic sensory motor neuropathy.

    1. Diabetes—mixed sensory-motor-autonomic neuropathy.

    2. Associated with multiple myeloma.

    3. Other dysproteinemias—macroglobulinemia, cryoglobulinemia,
ataxia-telangiectasia.

    4. POEMS syndrome—*p*olyneuropathy, *o*rganomegaly (lympha-
denopathy, splenomegaly, or hepatomegaly), *e*ndocrinopathy
(usually hypogonadism or hypothyroidism), *m*onoclonal
gammopathy, and *s*kin changes.

    5. Paraneoplastic.

    6. Uremia.

      7. Leprosy.
      8. Amyloidosis.
      9. Chronic inflammatory demyelinating polyradiculoneuropathy (CIDP).
    10. Sarcoidosis.
  H. Hereditary motor and sensory neuropathies (HMSN), types I to IV.
  I. Hereditary sensory neuropathies (HSAN), types I to IV.
  J. Hereditary neuropathies with known or suspected metabolic defects.
      1. Fabry's disease (alpha galactosidase deficiency, X-linked).
      2. Metachromatic leukodystrophy (aryl sulfatase A deficiency, autosomal recessive).
      3. Refsum's disease (phytanic oxidase deficiency, autosomal recessive).
      4. Adrenomyeloneuropathy (X-linked).
      5. Tangier's disease (hypo-alpha-lipoproteinemia, autosomal recessive).
      6. Krabbe's disease (globoid cell leukodystrophy, galactosyl ceramidase deficiency, autosomal recessive).
  K. Other hereditary neuropathies.
      1. Familial amyloid neuropathy.
      2. Hereditary predisposition to pressure palsies.
      3. Giant axonal neuropathy.
      4. Friedreich's ataxia.
II. Mononeuropathies.
    1. Trauma—fractures and dislocations, penetrating injuries, and pressure palsies.
      a. Brachial plexus—fracture of clavicle or humerus, birth trauma, traction injuries.
      b. Axillary nerve—as for brachial plexus, also IM injections, shoulder subluxation.
      c. Radial nerve—fracture of head of humerus, compression at the radial groove ("Saturday palsy" and "bridegroom's palsy").
      d. Ulnar nerve—fracture of radius or ulna.
      e. Median nerve—carpal tunnel syndrome, anterior interosseous syndrome.
      f. Sciatic nerve—fracture of pelvis (S-I joint), fracture of acetabulum, IM gluteal injections.
      g. Femoral nerve—fracture of femur, lithotomy position, renal transplants.
      h. Lateral femoral cutaneous nerve (meralgia paresthetica).
      i. Tibial nerve—fracture of tibia or fibula.
      j. Common or superficial peroneal nerve—pressure palsy at fibular head from crossed legs or after weight loss.
    2. Entrapment (see Carpal Tunnel Syndrome, Ulnar Neuropathy).
    3. Carcinomatous infiltration.

4. Vasculitis.
5. Leprosy.

CLINICAL FEATURES OF SELECTED NEUROPATHIES
HMSN (Charcot-Marie-Tooth Disease) (CMT), Types I to IV

Hereditary neuropathies are common and may occur in subtle forms. Careful family history taking and examination of family members (including foot examination for pes cavus and EMG) is important in diagnosis. The differential diagnosis of HMSN types includes Friedreich's ataxia, hereditary distal spinal muscular atrophy, and chronic inflammatory demyelinating polyneuropathy (CIDP), which has slight asymmetries in involvement of different peripheral nerves as opposed to the hereditary types, which demonstrate uniform involvement.

CMT I: Hypertrophic form of Charcot-Marie-Tooth (peroneal muscular atrophy, Roussy-Levy syndrome). Inheritance is autosomal dominant with variable penetrance, rarely autosomal recessive. Onset is usually in the second decade but may be later. Many patients have subtle findings and are undiagnosed. There is slowly progressive distal weakness and atrophy with little sensory loss. The lower extremities are more involved than the upper. Palpably thickened nerves occur in 50% of cases. Total areflexia is common. Foot deformity (pes cavus, calluses, hammer toes) results from unopposed flexor action of the posterior compartment muscles and may be the only clinical finding. Life span is usually normal, with only rare wheelchair confinement. Nerve conduction velocities are decreased by 40% to 75%. EMG reveals dispersed compound muscle action potentials with low amplitude due to chronic denervation. EMG abnormalities may precede and be more extensive than clinical involvement. The CSF is usually normal. Pathologically, there are hypertrophic (*"onion bulb"*) changes and myelinated axon loss due to chronic demyelination and remyelination.

Genetic testing for subtypes of CMT 1 showed that CMT1-A subtype is linked to chromosome 17p11.2-12 duplication, and CMT1-B subtype is linked to chromosome 1q22-23 point mutations. The linkage of CMT1-C is still undetermined.

CMT II: Neuronal form of Charcot-Marie-Tooth (peroneal muscular atrophy). Inheritance is as in CMT I, except that onset is slightly later. CMT II is distinguished from CMT I by the absence of hypertrophic changes, later age of onset, slower progression, less involvement of upper extremities, and greater involvement of lower extremities (atrophy of ankle flexors, inverted champagne bottle). Nerve conduction velocities are normal or slightly slowed, but amplitudes are severely diminished. EMG reveals spontaneous activity and denervation changes. CSF is usually normal. Pathologically there are no hypertrophic changes and demyelination is mild; axonal number is decreased in distal myelinated nerves. Linkage studies showed that CMT2-A subtype is linked to chromosome 1p36, CMT2-B subtype is linked to chromosome 3q-22, and CMT2-D subtype is linked to chromosome 7p14. The CMT2-C subtype linkage is undetermined.

CMT III: Dejerine-Sottas disease (hypertrophic neuropathy of child-hood, congenital hypomyelination neuropathy). Inheritance is autosomal recessive. Onset is congenital or in infancy. The congenital form is more severe. Motor milestones are initially delayed and then lost. Walking occurs after 15 months and as late as 3 to 4 years. Best motor perform-ance occurs late in the first or early in the second decade. Patients are confined to a wheelchair by the end of the second decade. Severe progres-sive weakness and atrophy is initially distal, but eventually affects proximal muscles. There is severe sensory loss and sensory ataxia. Skeletal deform-ities (short stature, kyphoscoliosis, hand and foot deformities) are more severe and frequent than in CMT I or II. Motor nerve conduction velocities are extremely slow and sensory nerve action potentials are unrecordable. CSF protein is elevated. Pathologically, in addition to hypertrophic changes, myelin sheaths are thin or absent. Linkage studies show that CMT3-A subtype is linked to chromosome 17p11.2-12 duplication, and CMT3-B subtype is linked to chromosome 1q22-23 point mutation.

CMT IV: Inheritance is autosomal recessive. It is characterized by early onset in childhood and progressive weakness leading to inability to walk in adolescence. NCS are slow and CSF protein is normal. Nerve biopsy shows loss of myelinated fibers, hypomyelination, and onion bulbs. Genetic testing showed that CMT4 is linked to chromosome 8q13-21.1.

X-linked CMT is clinically similar to CMT type I, but shows an X-linked pattern of inheritance. There is no male to male transmission. Symptoms usually start between ages 5 and 15. Genetic studies showed that it is linked to chromosome Xq13.3 point mutation.

There are other complex, poorly characterized forms of CMT, which show pyramidal tract signs, optic atrophy, spinocerebellar degeneration, or deafness, in addition to neuropathy.

Hereditary Sensory and Autonomic Neuropathies (HSAN), Types I to IV

HSAN I: Dominantly inherited sensory neuropathy (Hereditary Sensory Neuropathy of Denny-Brown). Inheritance is autosomal dominant. Onset is in the second to third decade. There is progressive distal lower-extremity dissociated sensory loss; pain and temperature are relatively more involved. There is distal hyporeflexia. Autonomic function is normal, except for impaired distal sweating. Painless ulcerations and foot deformities may be present. Mild distal lower extremity weakness and atrophy are late findings. Upper extremity sensory loss is mild. Life expectancy is normal. NCS of the lower extremity reveal decreased sensory amplitudes and normal or mildly decreased sensory conduction velocities; motor nerve conduction studies are normal. Pathologically, axonal degeneration causes decreased numbers of small myelinated fibers and unmyelinated fibers. Differential diagnosis includes diabetic neuropathy, hereditary amyloidosis (prominent autonomic dysfunction), and syringomyelia.

HSAN II: Infantile and congenital sensory neuropathy (Morvan's disease). Inheritance is autosomal recessive. HSAN II is clinically similar to HSAN I except that onset is in infancy, and involvement of all sensory modalities is equal, severe, and proximal as well as distal. The lips and tongue may be affected. Strength is normal. Painless ulcerations and fractures are common. There is distal areflexia. Sensory nerve action potentials are unrecordable; motor nerve conduction studies are normal. Pathologically, the number of all myelinated axons is severely decreased, with moderately decreased numbers of unmyelinated fibers and some segmental demyelination and remyelination.

HSAN III: Familial dysautonomia (Riley-Day syndrome). Inheritance is autosomal recessive, and it occurs primarily in Ashkenazi Jews. Onset of symptoms is usually shortly after birth, with episodic cyanosis, vomiting, unexplained fever, poor suck, and an increased susceptibility to infection. There is characteristic blotching of the skin and no fungiform papilla on the tongue. Autonomic symptoms include decreased lacrimation, hyperhidrosis, fluctuating body temperature, and episodic hypotension (usually postural). There is a dissociated sensory loss with predominant involvement of pain and temperature, causing corneal ulcerations, painless skin lesions, and deformed joints. Areflexia is generalized. Strength, sweating, and sphincter function are normal. Intelligence is usually normal. Prognosis is generally poor, but occasional individuals survive to middle age. Sensory nerve action potentials are severely diminished; motor nerve conduction studies may be mildly abnormal. Peripheral nerves show marked depletion of unmyelinated fibers.

HSAN IV: Congenital sensory neuropathy. Inheritance is autosomal recessive. This very rare disorder is characterized by congenital anhidrosis, generalized insensitivity to pain and temperature, mental retardation, and episodic pyrexia.

Diabetic Neuropathy

This is a clinical or subclinical disorder of the somatic or autonomic peripheral nervous system that occurs in patients with diabetes mellitus without other causes for peripheral neuropathy. Proposed etiologic factors include localized endoneurial hypoxia, chronic hyperglycemia, episodic hypoglycemia, polyol accumulation, myoinositol deficiency, and impaired axonal transport. Microangiopathy and infarction have been proposed as the mechanism for diabetic multiple mononeuropathies. The following diabetic neuropathy syndromes are recognized:

Symmetrical polyneuropathies include the following:

a. *Distal sensory polyneuropathy* is the most common. Onset is usually insidious, but may occur acutely following an episode of diabetic coma or hypoglycemia. Usually, clinical manifestations reflect involvement of all fiber types. However, occasionally a large or small fiber pattern is more prominent. The large fiber pattern presents with paresthesias in the feet and loss of distal reflexes, position sensation, and vibratory sensation. The small fiber pattern is loss of thermal and pinprick sensation associated with burning pain. Autonomic neuropathy often accompanies the small fiber pattern. Pathologically, there is distal axonal loss with variable degrees of segmental demyelination. NCS show reduced sensory action potential amplitude and variable slowing of motor nerve conduction velocity (related to degree of demyelination). EMG shows denervation, despite little or no weakness.

b. *Autonomic neuropathy* presents with symptoms including abnormal pupillary reaction, postural hypotension, abnormalities of heart rate, peripheral edema, anhidrosis, abnormalities of reflex vasoconstriction, abnormal gastrointestinal motility, diarrhea, atonic bladder, and impotence. Sudden death may occur from lack of reaction to hypoglycemia or cardiorespiratory arrest.

c. *Symmetric proximal lower extremity motor neuropathy ("amyotrophy")* presents with slowly progressive, symmetrical weakness, which is distinct from asymmetric "amyotrophy," which is discussed under the focal diabetic neuropathies. Initial manifestations include lower back and proximal lower extremity pain, which is followed by progressive proximal weakness, loss of patellar reflexes, and atrophy. Sensation is spared, but a distal sensory polyneuropathy may coexist. Initial EMG shows reduced motor-unit recruitment, while evidence of denervation appears later. Prognosis for recovery varies, but is generally worse with insidious onset of symptoms. Control of hyperglycemia may promote recovery.

Focal and multifocal diabetic neuropathies include the following:

a. *Trunk and limb mononeuropathy* (including mononeuropathy multiplex) occur acutely, most often in the ulnar, median, radial, femoral, lateral cutaneous, thoracic, and peroneal nerves. These lesions often occur at the same sites as entrapment neuropathies. It is important to exclude other etiologies, such as radiculopathy. It may not be possible to distinguish between a diabetic mononeuropathy and an entrapment syndrome. Prognosis for recovery is good.

b. *Cranial neuropathies* most commonly affect the extraocular muscles (see Ophthalmoplegia) and may be associated with facial pain or headache. Third nerve lesions show rapid onset and pupillary sparing, whereas aneurysmal compression typically has an unresponsive pupil.

c. *Asymmetric proximal lower limb motor neuropathy* is the unilateral form of "amyotrophy." Onset of unilateral pain and proximal weakness is sudden, progressing over 1 to 2 weeks. The patellar reflex is lost, and proximal atrophy eventually develops. Although the etiology remains uncertain, prognosis is good. There have been reports of successful treatment with steroids, plasma exchange and intravenous gamma globulins.

Inflammatory Demyelinating Polyneuropathies

Guillain-Barré syndrome ([GBS], Guillain-Barré-Strohl syndrome, acute inflammatory demyelinating polyradiculoneuropathy [AIDP]) is probably immunologically mediated, involving both cellular and humoral responses, but no single autoantigen has been identified.

The typical clinical presentation is paresthesias in the distal extremities, followed by lower extremity weakness. The weakness then ascends to involve the arms and face. Bilateral sciatica is common. Initial examination shows symmetrical limb weakness, absent or greatly diminished deep tendon reflexes, and minimal sensory loss. Progression to involve respiration, eye movements, swallowing, and autonomic function occurs in severe cases. Weakness progresses form 1 to 3 weeks before stabilizing and then recovering. Severity of symptoms varies among individual cases. In severe cases, complications of pneumonia, sepsis, adult respiratory distress syndrome, pulmonary embolus, and cardiac arrest are responsible for most severe morbidity and mortality.

GBS is often preceded by an infection, usually viral. Important associated infections include human immunodeficiency virus (HIV), Epstein-Barr virus, cytomegalovirus, influenza virus, and *Campylobacter jejuni* enteritis. Underlying systemic diseases such as systemic lupus erythematosus (SLE), Hodgkin's disease, and sarcoidosis are very occasionally associated with GBS. Surgery and vaccinations may also precede GBS.

Confirmatory test findings include CSF protein greater than 55 mg/dL with little or no pleocytosis (*"albuminocytologic dissociation"*) starting about 1 week after onset of symptoms. CSF protein is often normal during the first few days of the illness. NCS show signs of demyelination early, before CSF protein changes. Differential diagnosis includes spinal cord disease, myasthenia gravis, neoplastic meningitis, vasculitic neuropathy, paraneoplastic neuropathy, botulism, diphtheria, heavy-metal intoxication, poliomyelitis, and porphyria.

There are several GBS variants. These share signs of diminished reflexes, demyelination pattern on nerve conduction studies, and elevated CSF protein. Variant syndromes include *Fisher syndrome* (ophthalmoplegia, ataxia, and areflexia with little associated weakness), weakness without paresthesias and sensory loss, pharyngeal-cervical-brachial weakness, paraparesis, pure sensory and pure ataxia.

Plasma exchange significantly alters the progression and severity of GBS, decreasing the need for mechanical ventilation by approximately 50%. The efficacy of intravenous immunoglobulin treatment (IVIg) is probably comparable with plasmapheresis. IVIg given daily at 0.4 g/kg for 1 week is the preferred treatment in unstable patients; recent literature suggests a better response for IVIg in anti-GM1b-positive GBS (axonal variant). Corticosteroids are inefficacious in GBS but may be used for pain control. Dysautonomia is a major cause of morbidity and should be treated aggressively with hydration, vasoactive drugs, and pacemakers if needed.

Chronic inflammatory demyelinating polyradiculoneuropathy (CIDP or chronic relapsing dysimmune polyneuropathy) is similar to GBS but shows a protracted, often relapsing course, pronounced sensory involvement, response to corticosteroid treatment, and greater association with systemic disease. Worsening of symptoms for longer than 2 months, with subacute onset and fluctuation of symptoms over years, is characteristic of CIDP. Sensory involvement often accompanies proximal extremity and neck flexor weakness and diminished reflexes. Corticosteroids, plasmapheresis, immunosuppressive drugs, and IVIg can treat CIDP. Treatment regimens include prednisone 100 mg/day for 4 weeks, tapering gradually over 1 year to a dose of 10 to 20 mg qod. Plasma exchange is usually given in three to five exchanges over 1 to 2 weeks. Plasmapheresis with lower dose prednisone may be tried as initial therapy. IVIg given at 0.4 g/kg/day for 5 days is efficacious according to some but not all studies. Immunosuppressive drugs are used only in refractory cases.

Underlying systemic diseases causing a syndrome indistinguishable from CIDP include monoclonal gammopathies, lymphoma, connective tissue disease (polyarteritis nodosa, cryoglobulinemia, SLE), anti-MAG-associated polyneuropathies, Lyme disease, HIV infection, and sarcoidosis.

GENERAL PRINCIPLES OF TREATMENT OF NEUROPATHIES
A. Patient education and counseling.
B. Genetic counseling.
C. Withdrawal of medications suspected of causing neuropathy.
D. Withdrawal from toxic exposure.
E. Correction of nutritional and vitamin deficiencies.
F. Treatment of alcoholism.
G. Blood glucose control in diabetic neuropathies.
H. Specific drug therapies.
   1. Chelating agents in lead neuropathy.
   2. Hematin infusions in acute intermittent porphyria.
   3. Long-term prednisone or other immune modifying regimens in CIDP.
   4. Phytanic acid (reduced) diet in Refsum's disease.
I. Plasmapheresis in AIDP and other autoimmune disorders.
J. Pain control.
   1. Improve blood glucose control in diabetic neuropathies.
   2. Simple analgesics—aspirin and acetaminophen.
   3. Gabapentin, phenytoin, and carbamazepine—achieve anticonvulsant levels.
   4. Tricyclic drugs—amitriptyline and imipramine.
   5. Transcutaneous electrical nerve stimulation.
K. Meticulous foot care.
L. Orthotic devices and splints.
M. Surgical correction of entrapment neuropathies.
N. Physical and occupational therapy.

REFERENCES

Dalakas MC: *Muscle Nerve* 22:1479–1497, 1999.
Dyck PJ et al: *Neurology* 47:10–17, 1996.
Yuki N et al: *Ann Neurol* 47:314–321, 2000.

NUTRITIONAL DEFICIENCY SYNDROMES

Vitamin A deficiency may complicate disorders of fat malabsorption like sprue, biliary atresia, and cystic fibrosis and produces night blindness (nyctalopia). Vitamin A excess can cause pseudotumor cerebri.

Thiamine (B₁) deficiency occurs most commonly in chronic alcoholism but may complicate other conditions associated with poor nutritional status, such as hyperemesis of pregnancy, malignancy, dialysis, prolonged intravenous feeding, or refeeding after starvation. Neurologic manifestations include *Wernicke-Korsakoff syndrome, sensorimotor polyneuropathy*, and *optic neuropathy* (usually retrobulbar) (see Alcoholism). Treatment consists of thiamine therapy, 50 to 100 mg daily, administered parenterally if GI absorption is unreliable. Thiamine should be given before IV glucose or refeeding to avoid exacerbating the effects of thiamine deficiency in patients with unknown nutritional histories.

Pyridoxine (B₆) deficiency in children causes recurrent *seizures* refractory to conventional anticonvulsants. It is due to inadequate dietary intake or an autosomal recessive disorder known as pyridoxine dependency. It usually becomes evident within a few days of birth with severe seizures, which cease after administering 50 to 100 mg of IV pyridoxine, and requires lifelong supplementation of 2 to 30 mg/kg per day of pyridoxine.

Pyridoxine deficiency in adults is rarely caused by deficient diets but is caused by medications such as isoniazid, hydralazine, or penicillamine, which interfere with pyridoxine activity. The deficiency causes a *sensorimotor polyneuropathy* prevented by concomitant supplementation of 50 mg pyridoxine qd PO.

Pyridoxine overdose causes a *sensory neuropathy* characterized by diminished reflexes, impaired position and vibration sense, and sensory ataxia; strength and pain and temperature sensation are relatively spared.

B₁₂ (cyanocobalamin) deficiency is almost always due to malabsorption; causes include pernicious anemia, gastrectomy, ileal diseases such as tropical sprue, regional enteritis and bacterial overgrowth, and rarely, inherited metabolic conditions. Neurologic manifestations include *subacute combined degeneration*, that is, *myelopathy* involving the posterior columns and lateral corticospinal tracts; *dementia; sensorimotor polyneuropathy*; and *optic neuropathy* (usually retrobulbar). Laboratory evaluation includes complete blood cell count; serum levels of cyanocobalamin, and folate; homocystine and methylmalonic acid levels; and the Schilling test. Treatment consists of IM injections of 100 μg daily or 1000 μg twice weekly for 2 weeks, followed by weekly injections of 1000 μg for another 2 to 3 months. If the B₁₂ deficiency results from malabsorption, the patient should be placed on lifelong maintenance therapy of monthly 1000 μg injections. Oral repletion (500 mg per day) may also be effective if GI absorption is normal.

Folate deficiency is due to poor intake (alcoholism or pregnancy), malabsorption (small-intestine–like inflammatory bowel disease), or drug antagonism (for example, phenytoin). Whether postnatal folate deficiency causes neurologic disease remains controversial; syndromes attributed to folate deficiency include *subacute combined degeneration* of the spinal cord, *sensorimotor polyneuropathy*, and *dementia*. Treatment consists of 1 mg of folate orally per day. Low-folate diets have been associated with CNS dysraphic states (spina bifida and anencephaly), and supplementation with 0.4 mg per day early in the first trimester of gestation may be preventative. Supplementation of grains with folate has reduced neural tube defect incidence in the U.S. and several other countries.

Niacin (nicotinic acid) deficiency causes *pellagra*, which is characterized by the triad of *dermatitis, diarrhea*, and *dementia*. Pellagra is endemic to areas where corn, a poor source of niacin, is the staple food and the intake of meat, which contains the niacin precursor tryptophan, is low. The major neurologic manifestation is an *encephalopathy* or *dementia*. *Polyneuropathy, optic neuropathy*, or *myelopathy* may also occur. Treatment consists of 50 mg of oral niacin several times per day.

Vitamin D deficiency causes rickets and osteomalacia and may be associated with hypocalcemia. Long-term therapy with phenytoin, phenobarbital, or primidone may result in vitamin D deficiency and osteomalacia. Treatment is vitamin replacement.

Vitamin E deficiency occurs (1) in patients with severe fat malabsorption resulting from chronic cholestatic diseases, especially biliary atresia, intestinal resection, cystic fibrosis, and Crohn's disease, and (2) as part of inherited metabolic diseases like abetalipoproteinemia (Bassen-Kornzweig syndrome) and familial isolated vitamin E deficiency. The hallmark of vitamin E deficiency is *spinocerebellar degeneration* variably associated with a *peripheral neuropathy*, resulting in areflexia, ataxia, and impaired position and vibration sense. In this regard it appears similar to Friedreich's ataxia on clinical study. *Pigmentary retinitis* (with night blindness), *nystagmus, ophthalmoplegia*, and *proximal muscle weakness* may also occur. Treatment is with very high-dose oral vitamin E.

Vitamin E has anti-oxidant properties and doses of 2000 IU per day may slow funtional decline in Alzheimer's disease.

REFERENCES

Kayden JH: *Neurology* 43:2167–2169, 1993.
So YT et al: In Bradley WG et al, eds: *Neurology in clinical practice*, Boston, Butterworth-Heinemann, 2000.

NYSTAGMUS

A biphasic ocular oscillation in which at least one phase is slow. The nystagmus direction is defined as the direction of the fast component. The direction may be horizontal, vertical, diagonal, or rotational. There are two general types, jerk and pendular. In jerk nystagmus the slow phase is always centripetal and the fast (saccadic) phase returns the eye to the target. In pendular nystagmus the oscillations are of equal velocity in both directions. When examining a patient with nystagmus, observe changes in amplitude and frequency with change in gaze direction. Nystagmus is of value in indicating dysfunction somewhere in the posterior fossa, that is, vestibular system (including the end organ), brainstem, or cerebellum.

Congenital nystagmus is present at birth or noted in early infancy at the time of development of visual fixation, and it persists throughout life. Some cases are familial. It may accompany primary visual defects and is a cardinal feature of albinism. It is almost always binocular, of similar amplitude in both eyes, and uniplanar (usually horizontal). It increases with attempts to fixate, decreases with convergence, disappears in sleep, often has a "null" position, and may have "inversion" of the optokinetic reflex. There may be associated head oscillations that are not compensatory or head tilt or turn that helps bring the eyes to the null position. Being present from infancy, it is not associated with oscillopsia.

Latent nystagmus is a form of congenital nystagmus. There is no nystagmus with binocular vision, but when one eye is occluded, jerk nystagmus develops in both eyes, with the fast phase toward the viewing eye. Latent nystagmus can be elicited by the intention of viewing with one eye. *Manifest latent nystagmus* occurs in patients with amblyopia, strabismus, or other eye disease who fixate monocularly. The fast phase is in the direction of the fixating eye.

Acquired nystagmus in infants may be due to progressive bilateral visual loss in early childhood, CNS disease, or spasmus nutans. Spasmus nutans is a syndrome of nystagmus, head nodding, and anomalous head positions. The nystagmus is pendular, rapid, of small amplitude, and usually bilateral but can differ in each eye; it may be monocular in a horizontal, rotary, or vertical direction. The nystagmus may vary with the direction of gaze. It begins in infancy (4 to 18 months of age) and spontaneously remits within 1 to 2 years after onset. There are usually no associated neurologic abnormalities. Some cases are familial.

Acquired pendular nystagmus is usually horizontal but may be vertical, diagonal, elliptic, or circular and may be associated with head tremor. There may be marked dissociation between the two eyes. It is associated with vascular or demyelinating lesions of the brainstem or cerebellum. In demyelinating disease it usually indicates a cerebellar lesion. Rarely, it is associated with visual dysfunction.

Vestibular nystagmus (see also Calorics, Vertigo) results from dysfunction of the vestibular end-organ, nerve, or brainstem connections and from acute lesions of the cerebellar flocculus. It is usually present in primary position, increases with gaze toward fast phase, and decreases with gaze toward the slow phase (with central lesions it may reverse direction). Vertigo usually coexists. The hallmarks of peripheral lesions are that the nystagmus can be suppressed by fixation and is accentuated when fixation is removed. For further differentiation of peripheral from central vestibular nystagmus, see Vertigo.

Gaze-evoked nystagmus, the most common form of nystagmus, is elicited by attempting to maintain an eccentric eye position. If this cannot be maintained, the eyes drift back toward primary position. Quick corrective phases then bring the eyes back to the eccentric position. The fast phase is in the direction of gaze. Gaze-evoked vertical nystagmus almost always occurs with the horizontal type. There may be a torsional component to the nystagmus. With severe intoxications nystagmus may be horizontal pendular in primary position. Drugs are the most common cause of bidirectional gaze-evoked nystagmus. Offending agents include anticonvulsants, barbiturates, tranquilizers, ethanol, and phenothiazines. If the patient is not receiving any medications, gaze-evoked nystagmus indicates vestibulocerebellar, brainstem, or cerebral hemispheric dysfunction; neuromuscular fatigue; or muscular weakness. More precise localization requires assessment of the associated signs and symptoms.

Downbeat nystagmus occurs in primary position, increases in down gaze and lateral gaze, and may be accentuated by convergence. It is highly suggestive of a dysfunction at the craniocervical junction affecting posterior midline cerebellum and underlying medulla. When downbeat nystagmus is seen in cerebellar disease, other cerebellar eye signs are usually present, most commonly impaired vertical smooth pursuit and vertical vestibulo-ocular reflex. For differential diagnosis see Table 59.

Upbeat nystagmus occurs in primary position and is usually secondary to lesions at the pontomesencephalic and pontomedullary junctions. Drug intoxication is an uncommon cause. Other causes are listed in Table 59.

Physiologic (end-point) nystagmus occurs in normal individuals in the extremes of horizontal or upward gaze. It is a small-amplitude, variably sustained jerk nystagmus that is often dissociated (more marked in the abducting eye).

See-saw nystagmus consists of one eye intorting and rising while the opposite eye extorts and falls. Repetition in alternating directions produces a see-saw effect. It can occur in all fields of gaze but may be limited to primary position or downward gaze. It is seen with diencephalic dysfunction, frequently caused by parasellar tumors expanding within the third ventricle. The pathogenesis is unknown but believed to involve the interstitial nucleus of Cajal.

Periodic alternating nystagmus is a horizontal jerk nystagmus that periodically changes directions. Typically it beats for 90 seconds in one direction, then is in a neutral phase for about 10 seconds, and then beats 90 seconds in the opposite direction. It may persist during sleep. It may be congenital or may be due to craniocervical junction abnormalities or brainstem and cerebellar disease; it frequently becomes evident after visual loss.

Rotary (torsional) nystagmus occurs around the globe's anteroposterior axis and is seen in medullary disease. In vestibular disease a rotational component is usually combined with a prominent horizontal or vertical nystagmus.

Dissociated nystagmus refers to a significant asymmetry in either amplitude or direction between the two eyes. It occurs in internuclear ophthalmo-

TABLE 59

CAUSES OF VERTICAL NYSTAGMUS

Upbeat Nystagmus

Cerebellar degenerations and atrophies

Multiple sclerosis

Infarction of medulla or cerebellum

Tumors of the medulla, cerebellum, or midbrain

Wernicke's encephalopathy

Brainstem encephalitis

Behçet's syndrome

Meningitis

Leber's congenital amaurosis or other congenital disorder of the anterior visual pathways

Thalamic arteriovenous malformation

Congenital

Organophosphate poisoning

Tobacco

Associated with middle ear disease

Transient finding in otherwise normal infants

Downbeat Nystagmus

Cerebellar degeneration, including familial periodic ataxia and paraneoplastic degeneration

Craniocervical anomalies, including Arnold-Chiari malformation, Paget's disease, and basilar invagination

Infarction of brainstem or cerebellum

Dolichoectasia of the vertebrobasilar artery

Multiple sclerosis

Cerebellar tumor

Syringobulbia

Encephalitis

Head trauma

Anticonvulsant medication

Lithium intoxication

Alcohol, including cerebellar degeneration

Wernicke's encephalopathy

Magnesium depletion

Vitamin B_{12} deficiency

Toluene abuse

Congenital

Midbrain infarction

Increased intracranial pressure and hydrocephalus

Transient finding in otherwise normal infants

From Leigh RJ, Zee DS: *The neurology of eye movements*, ed 3, Philadelphia, FA Davis, 1999.

N

NYSTAGMUS

plegia, in pendular nystagmus in patients with multiple sclerosis, and in a variety of posterior fossa lesions.

Rebound nystagmus is a transient nystagmus that develops on return to primary gaze after maintaining an eccentric gaze. The fast phase is in the opposite direction of prior gaze. It occurs most frequently in cerebellar disease.

Circular or elliptic nystagmus is a form of pendular nystagmus (horizontal and vertical pendular oscillations 90 degrees out of phase) with a continuous oscillation in a fine, rapid, circular, or elliptic pattern.

Diagonal (oblique) nystagmus occurs when simultaneous, pendular, horizontal, and vertical components are in phase or 180 degrees out of phase.

Nystagmus in myasthenia gravis may manifest as a gaze-evoked nystagmus in any direction with asymmetry between the two eyes. Muscle fatigue is seen as an increase in the nystagmus. Such nystagmus of the abducting eye occurring with impaired adduction of the contralateral eye constitutes the "pseudointernuclear ophthalmoplegia" of myasthenia gravis.

Voluntary "nystagmus" consists of bursts of rapid, conjugate, horizontal oscillations that are actually voluntarily produced back-to-back saccades. They can rarely be sustained for more than 10 to 30 seconds at a time.

Lid nystagmus is of three types. Upward jerking of the eyelids synchronous with vertical ocular nystagmus is nonlocalizing. Rapid twitching of the eyelids synchronous with the fast phase of horizontal ocular nystagmus induced by lateral gaze may occur with the lateral medullary syndrome. Lid nystagmus induced by convergence (Pick's sign) is associated with medullary lesions.

Convergence-retraction nystagmus is caused by lesions of the mesencephalon that involve the posterior commissure, classically, pineal tumors as part of Parinaud's syndrome.

Treatment of symptomatic nystagmus relies on physical and pharmacologic methods. Congenital nystagmus can be treated with prisms, surgery, and contact lenses. Baclofen may benefit acquired periodic alternating nystagmus. Trihexyphenidyl may be useful for pendular nystagmus in multiple sclerosis. Gabapentin may also help acquired nystagmus in multiple sclerosis. Botulinum toxin A is under investigation.

REFERENCE

Dell'Osso LF et al: In Duane TD, Jaeger EA, eds: *Clinical ophthalmology*, Philadelphia, Lippincott, 1988.

OCCIPITAL LOBE

The occipital lobe extends from the parieto-occipital fissure on the medial surface of the brain to the lateral surface, where it merges with the parietal and temporal lobes. The calcarine sulcus marks the boundary of the primary visual area (Brodmann's area 17), and the rest of the occipital lobe constitutes the visual association cortex. Its function is mainly concerned with visual perception and interpretation. *Clinical syndromes* associated with occipital lesions include visual field defects, cortical blindness, visual agnosias, achromatopsia, metamorphopsias, illusions, and hallucinations.

Visual anosognosia (*Anton's syndrome*) or cortical blindness includes lack of awareness of the defect and is associated with bilateral lesions. *Balint's syndrome*, seen with bilateral occipital and parieto-occipital infarctions, consists of optic ataxia, paralysis of gaze and disturbance of visual attention, and simultanagnosia. Visual symptoms referable to the occipital lobe occur commonly in migraine. Occipital lobe epilepsy may present with visual phenomena, and postictal blindness may also occur.

OCULAR OSCILLATIONS

The following abnormal oscillatory eye movements are distinct from nystagmus because of waveform differences. (e.g., no distinct slow and fast phases).

Ocular bobbing consists of intermittent downward jerks of both eyes, followed by a slow drift to primary position. It is seen with extensive destructive lesions of the pons but also occurs with pontine compression, obstructive hydrocephalus, or metabolic encephalopathy. *Ocular dipping* is an inverse movement (slow downward, fast upward) with less reliable localization.

Ping-pong gaze denotes slow, horizontal, conjugate drift of the eyes that alternates every few seconds and is associated with bilateral hemispheric dysfunction.

Ocular myoclonus refers to pendular vertical oscillations seen with brainstem lesions and often accompanied by rhythmic movements of the palate and other midline structures.

The term *saccadic oscillations* includes several specific entities. *Saccadic dysmetria* can produce oscillation when overshooting saccades are followed by one or more corrective saccades. *Square-wave jerks*, seen most prominently in cerebellar disorders and progressive supranuclear palsy, and *macro square-wave jerks*, seen in multiple sclerosis and olivopontocerebellar atrophy, are saccades that interrupt fixation with normal intersaccadic intervals.

Flurries of rapid eye movements without an intersaccadic interval are termed *ocular flutter* if purely horizontal and *opsoclonus,* if multidirectional. Both can be secondary to viral infection, drug effects, tumor, or can occur in paraneoplastic syndromes such as neuroblastoma in children or with anti-Purkinje's cell antibodies in adults (mostly women with gynecologic tumors).

Superior oblique myokymia is a monocular torsional oscillation of small-amplitude, high-frequency contractions of a monocular superior oblique muscle. It causes oscillopsia, diplopia, or visual blurring. Although sometimes seen with brainstem disease, it is usually idiopathic and may respond to carbamazepine therapy.

Spasmus nutans is an ocular oscillation accompanied by head nodding and torticollis. It appears before 18 months of age and remits spontaneously, usually by age 3 years. The abnormal eye movements are usually dysconjugate and vary in direction. Although usually benign, this entity must not be confused with signs of intracranial tumor; the presence of poor feeding, optic atrophy, or raised intracranial pressure should be investigated by neuroimaging studies.

REFERENCES

Abel LA: In Daroff R, Neetens A, eds: *Neurological organization of ocular movement*, Berkeley, Kugler, 1990.

Leigh RJ, Zee DS: *The neurology of eye movements*, ed 3, Philadelphia, FA Davis, 1999.

OLFACTION

The sense of smell is mediated by the first cranial nerve. *It is the only sensory modality without a thalamic relay*. Complaints may include anosmia, hyposmia, parosmia, or loss of appreciation of flavors in food. Smell is tested clinically using nonirritating aromatic compounds such as oil of wintergreen, cloves, coffee, almond oil, or lemon oil. The stimulus is presented to one nostril with the other occluded. The ability to appreciate the presence of a substance, even if not properly identified, is evidence that anosmia is not present.

More detailed olfactory testing using the UPSIT (University of Pennsylvania Smell Identification Test) can distinguish hyposmia, anosmia or malingering. Unilateral anosmia is more often due to a structural lesion rather than a diffuse process. Causes of anosmia or hyposmia include the following:

1. Infection: Rhinitis, sinusitis, basilar meningitis, frontal abscess, osteomyelitis (frontal, ethmoidal), viral hepatitis, syphilis, influenza.
2. Toxic or metabolic disorders: Pernicious anemia, zinc deficiency, lead and calcium intoxication, diabetes mellitus, hypothyroidism, medication effects.
3. Neoplasms: Frontal tumor, olfactory groove or sphenoid meningioma, radiation therapy.
4. Trauma to cribriform plate.
5. Congenital: olfactory agenesis (Kallmann's syndrome) and septo-optic dysplasia (De Morsier's syndrome).
6. Others: hydrocephalus, amphetamine and cocaine abuse, aging, smoking, trigeminal lesions (causing mucosal atrophy), anterior cerebral artery disease, nasal polyps, multiple sclerosis, Alzheimer's disease, and Parkinson's disease.

Hyperosmia is seen in hysteria, migraine, hyperemesis gravidarum, cystic fibrosis, Addison's disease, and strychnine poisoning.

Olfactory hallucinations can occur with neoplasms or vascular disease involving the inferomedial temporal lobe, near the hippocampus or uncus.

They may also be seen in psychiatric disease (olfactory reference syndrome). *"Uncinate fits"* are so called because of the presence of olfactory or gustatory hallucinations as part of complex partial or simple partial seizures; these may be triggered or even be arrested by olfactory stimulation. Anosmia is not present in such cases. Multiple chemical sensitivities syndrome (MCS) is associated with unexplained odor sensitivity and excitability to multiple chemical and environmental stimuli. Sensitization by low levels of chemicals, fragrances, and perfumes are frequently associated with the reporting of MCS symptoms

REFERENCES

Dawes PJ: *Clin Otolaryngol* 23:484–490, 1998.
Ross PM: *Prev Med* 28:467–480, 1999.

OPALSKI'S SYNDROME

Refers to ipsilateral hemiplegia and lateral medullary syndrome. Infarction is usually located lower than that found in Wallenberg's syndrome (submedullary syndrome of Opalski). The syndrome is usually caused by vertebral artery occlusion. A related syndrome is Babinski-Nageotte syndrome, with contralateral hemiparesis due to hemimedullary infarct before the pyramidal tract decussation.

REFERENCES

Monataner J, Alvarez-Sabin J: *J Neurol Neurosurg Psychiatry* 67:688–689, 1999.
Opalski A: *Paris Med* 1:214–220, 1946.

OPHTHALMOPLEGIA

If extraocular muscle testing reveals misalignment of the visual axes, first determine whether this is due to nerve palsy or some other causes of impaired motility.

I. Causes of impaired ocular motility other than nerve palsy.
   A. Concomitant strabismus.
   B. Graves' ophthalmopathy.
   C. Myasthenia gravis (and other pharmacologic or toxic causes of neuromuscular blockade).
   D. Convergence spasm.
   E. Blowout fracture of the orbit with entrapment myopathy.
   F. Restrictive ophthalmopathy (*Brown's superior oblique tendon sheath syndrome*).
   G. Orbital inflammatory disease (orbital pseudotumor).
   H. Orbital masses, neoplasms.
   I. Orbital infections.
   J. Brainstem disorders causing abnormal prenuclear inputs (internuclear ophthalmoplegia, skew deviation).

O

OPHTHALMOPLEGIA

    K. Ocular myopathies.

    L. Chronic progressive external ophthalmoplegia (*Kearns-Sayre and related mitochondrial syndromes*).

    M. Congenital syndromes.

II. Causes of abducens (VI) nerve palsies.

    A. Nuclear (associated with ipsilateral horizontal gaze palsy).

       1. Developmental anomalies (Möbius, Duane's syndromes).

       2. Infarction.

       3. Tumor (pontine glioma, cerebellar tumors).

       4. Wernicke-Korsakoff.

    B. Fascicular.

       1. Infarction.

       2. Demyelination.

       3. Tumor.

    C. Subarachnoid space lesions.

       1. Aneurysm or anomalous vessels (anterior inferior cerebellar artery, basilar artery).

       2. Subarachnoid hemorrhage.

       3. Meningitis (infectious, neoplastic).

       4. Sarcoidosis.

       5. Cerebellopontine angle tumor (acoustic neuroma, meningioma).

       6. Clivus tumor (chordoma, nasopharyngeal carcinoma).

       7. Trauma.

       8. Surgical complication.

       9. Postinfectious.

    D. Petrous.

       1. Infection or inflammation of mastoid or petrous tip.

       2. Trauma (petrous fracture).

       3. Thrombosis of inferior petrosal sinus.

       4. Increased intracranial pressure (pseudotumor cerebri, supratentorial mass).

       5. Following lumbar puncture.

       6. Aneurysm.

       7. Persistent trigeminal artery.

       8. Trigeminal schwannoma.

    E. Cavernous sinus and superior orbital fissure.

       1. Aneurysm.

       2. Cavernous sinus thrombosis.

       3. Carotid cavernous fistula.

       4. Dural arteriovenous malformation.

       5. Tumor (pituitary adenoma, meningioma, nasopharyngeal carcinoma).

       6. Pituitary apoplexy.

       7. Sphenoid sinusitis (mucormycosis).

       8. Herpes zoster.

       9. Granulomatous inflammation (sarcoidosis, Tolosa-Hunt syndrome).

F. Orbital.
1. Tumor.
2. Infection.
3. Trauma.
G. Uncertain localization.
1. Nerve infarction (diabetes, hypertension, arteritis).
2. Migraine.
III. Causes of trochlear (IV) nerve palsies.
A. Nuclear and fascicular.
1. Developmental anomalies.
2. Hemorrhage.
3. Infarction.
4. Trauma.
5. Demyelination.
6. Surgical complications.
B. Subarachnoid.
1. Trauma.
2. Tumor (pineal, tentorial meningioma, trochlear schwannoma, ependymoma, metastases).
3. Surgical complication.
4. Meningitis (infectious, neoplastic).
5. Mastoiditis.
C. Cavernous sinus and superior orbital fissure.
1. As for cranial nerve VI palsies.
D. Orbital.
1. Trauma.
2. Ethmoiditis.
3. Ethmoidectomy.
E. Uncertain localization.
1. Infarction (diabetes, hypertension, arteritis).
IV. Causes of oculomotor (III) nerve palsies.
A. Nuclear and fascicular.
1. Developmental anomaly.
2. Infarction.
3. Tumor.
B. Subarachnoid.
1. Aneurysm (posterior communicating artery).
2. Meningitis (infectious, syphilitic, neoplastic).
3. Infarction.
4. Tumor.
5. Surgical complication.
C. Tentorial edge.
1. Increased intracranial pressure (uncal herniation, pseudotumor cerebri).
2. Trauma.
D. Cavernous sinus and superior orbital fissure.

  1. As for VI nerve palsies.
  2. Infarction.
  E. Orbital.
    1. Trauma.
    2. Tumor.
    3. Infection.
  F. Uncertain localization.
    1. Mononucleosis and other viral infections.
    2. Following immunization.
    3. Migraine.
    4. Cyclic oculomotor palsy of childhood.
    5. Guillain-Barré and Miller Fisher syndromes.
    6. Sjögren's and Behçet's syndromes.

Combined ophthalmoparesis: Third, fourth, and sixth nerve involvement; most commonly occur with *base of skull infiltrations, cavernous sinus or superior orbital fissure lesions, and generalized neuropathies.* Proptosis, chemosis, and vascular engorgement suggest orbital or cavernous sinus involvement. Base of skull problems include extension of nasopharyngeal carcinoma, sarcoidosis, lymphoma, clivus chordoma, pituitary apoplexy, meningeal carcinoma, and cavernous sinus thrombosis.

Chronic progressive external ophthalmoplegia (CPEO) is a slowly progressive, painless, symmetric ophthalmoplegia, without fluctuations or remissions. Saccades are slow, usually with no diplopia. Ptosis and orbicularis oculi weakness usually accompany the external ophthalmoplegia. The pupils are spared, and there are no orbital signs. Fibrotic changes of the extraocular muscles may occur over time, causing a superimposed restrictive ophthalmopathy. CPEO has multiple causes. *Kearns-Sayre syndrome* is one of the causes, due to a mitochondrial cytopathy. It has a childhood or adolescent onset without a family history (no male-to-male transmission), cerebellar ataxia, atypical retinal pigmentary degeneration, short stature, hearing loss, cardiac conduction defects often leading to Stokes-Adams attacks, increased cerebrospinal fluid protein, spongiform changes of the cerebrum and brainstem, and muscle mitochondrial abnormalities. Both cardiac and endocrine complications may be life threatening.

Painful ophthalmoplegias may be due to diabetes, aneurysm, tumors (primary and metastatic), *Tolosa-Hunt syndrome* (granulomatous inflammatory process affecting the cavernous sinus and surrounding structures), herpes zoster, cavernous sinus thrombosis, carotid cavernous fistula, ophthalmoplegic migraine, arteritis, carcinomatous meningitis, or fungal infection.

Internuclear ophthalmoplegia (INO) is characterized by (1) slow, incomplete adduction or complete inability to adduct past midline (*convergence movements may be preserved*) and (2) dissociated nystagmus of the opposite abducting eye. Skew deviation (hypertropia on the lesion site) is often present. INO is caused by a lesion of the medial longitudinal fasciculus (MLF) between mid-pons and the oculomotor nucleus ipsilateral to the side of impaired adduction. Subtle defects are best solicited by observing the fast phases of optokinetic nystagmus. In bilateral INOs, gaze-evoked vertical nystagmus, impaired vertical pursuit, and decrease vertical vestibular responses are often present. *The most frequent cause of INO in young adults (especially when bilateral) is multiple sclerosis.* Vascular causes tend to be more common in older patients. Other causes include intra or extra-axial brainstem tumors, hydrocephalus, subdural hematoma, infection, nutritional and metabolic disorders, and drug intoxication. Myasthenia gravis and Miller Fisher syndrome could cause similar appearing "pseudo INO."

One-and-a-half syndrome refers to ipsilateral horizontal gaze palsy and INO (see Gaze palsy). This results from combined lesions of the MLF and the more ventral, ipsilateral abducens nucleus or paramedian pontine reticular formation (PPRF). The only intact horizontal movement is abduction of the contralateral eye. Acutely, the patient may appear exotropic, with nystagmus in the deviated eye. Vergence and vertical movements may be spared. Causes include brainstem ischemia (most common), multiple sclerosis, tumor, or hemorrhage. As with INO, myasthenia must be considered if there are no long tract or sensory signs. There is also a vertical one-and-a-half syndrome that has been described with a dorsal midbrain lesion.

REFERENCE

Leigh RJ, Zee D: Neurology of eye movements, ed 3, Philadelphia, FA Davis, 1999.

OPTIC NERVE

Anatomically, the optic nerve has four major portions: (1) intraocular (1 mm); (2) intraorbital (~25 mm); (3) intracanalicular (~9 mm); and (4) intracranial (~16 mm). *The signs and symptoms of optic nerve dysfunction include* a decreased sense of brightness, diminished visual acuity, afferent pupillary defects, color desaturation, and *characteristic visual field defects*—central, centrocecal, arcuate, or altitudinal scotomas; these findings may accompany all the disorders described below except acute papilledema. Disc swelling may be present (papilledema, "anterior" optic neuropathy, or "papillitis" in the case of optic neuritis) or absent ("posterior" or "retrobulbar" neuropathy or neuritis) in optic nerve disease. Optic atrophy indicates optic nerve fiber loss resulting from chronic or past optic nerve disease.

Papilledema is disc swelling caused by increased intracranial pressure. Funduscopic manifestations include disc hyperemia, venous dilation, blurred disc margins with haziness of the retinal vessels, peripapillary hemorrhages, retinal and choroidal folds, and absent venous pulsations (these are absent in 20% of individuals and their presence aids only in excluding papilledema), and nerve fiber layer infarcts. Papilledema is usually bilateral; unilateral papilledema associated with contralateral optic atrophy sometimes

O

OPTIC NERVE

occurs with subfrontal masses such as meningioma (*Foster Kennedy syndrome*). In acute papilledema, visual acuity and pupillary response are usually normal unless the macula is involved by exudates, edema, or hemorrhage. Chronic papilledema may cause visual loss or blindness, with constriction of the visual fields and nerve bundle defects.

Optic neuritis refers to the inflammation of the optic nerve. In two thirds of the patients the site of inflammation is *retrobulbar*. It is most common between 15 and 45 years of age, seen more commonly in women, and presents as an acute unilateral visual loss, with increased periorbital pain with eye movement. Disc swelling occurs in 50% of affected adults. Visual acuity usually returns to near normal levels within several months. Most cases are associated with demyelinating disorder (multiple sclerosis) or are idiopathic. The risk of developing multiple sclerosis after isolated optic neuritis is more than 60% if patients are followed up for more than 10 years. Other causes include viral or postviral syndromes, contiguous inflammation (such as sinusitis or meningitis), sarcoidosis, tuberculosis, syphilis, "autoimmune" neuritis, and paraneoplastic optic neuritis.

Treatment: IV methylprednisolone (1 g/day 3 days) followed by oral prednisone (1 mg/kg/day 11 days) hastens recovery, but a regimen of oral prednisone alone may increase the risk of recurrence or increase the risk of subsequently developing multiple sclerosis.

Ischemic optic neuropathy: Infarction of the optic nerve. There is acute unilateral visual loss and disc swelling (retrobulbar form is rare) in the elderly; recovery rate is poor. The common "idiopathic" form is associated with hypertension and diabetes mellitus, a normal erythrocyte sedimentation rate (ESR), and steroid unresponsiveness. The rarer "arteritic" form is associated with headaches, weight loss, fever, arthralgias, myalgias, jaw claudication, and scalp tenderness; an elevated ESR; and steroid responsiveness (see vasculitis).

Toxic and nutritional optic neuropathies: Slowly progressive bilateral visual loss. They are usually retrobulbar. Causes include drugs (e.g., ethambutol, isoniazid, chloramphenicol, streptomycin), toxins (lead and methanol), vitamin deficiencies (B_{12}, thiamine, niacin, and riboflavin), and *tobacco-alcohol amblyopia* seen with heavy tobacco and alcohol use (probably nutritional and responds to vitamin supplementation).

Neoplastic optic neuropathies include *compressive lesions* such as primary optic nerve tumors (gliomas and perioptic meningiomas) and *infiltrative lesions* such as found in leukemia, lymphoma, plasmacytomas and histiocytosis, and carcinomatous meningitis.

Others: Radiation (may be delayed for years), inflammatory (SLE, vasculitis, and sarcoidosis), Leber's hereditary optic neuropathy (mitochondrial mutation) and trauma.

REFERENCES

American Academy of Ophthalmology: *Basic and clinical science course: section 5—neuro-ophthalmology,* 1997–1998, 54–55.

Beck RW: *Neurology* 42:1133–1135, 1992.
Gass A, Moseley IF: *J Neurol Sci* 172(Suppl 1):S17–S22, 2000.
Kaufman DI, et al: *Neurology* 54:2039–2044, 2000.
Miller NR, Newman NJ: *Walsh and Hoyt's clinical neuro-ophthalmology*, ed 5,
    Baltimore, Williams and Wilkins, 1999.

OPTOKINETIC NYSTAGMUS

The optokinetic system is an ocular motor subsystem that enhances the ability to stabilize images on the retina, thus allowing adequate visual acuity. When the head moves for an extended period, the vestibular response decays because of the mechanical properties of the labyrinthine sense organs. Only retinal information remains as the input resulting in compensatory eye movements. When the proper conditions are reproduced in the laboratory with movement of the entire visual surround, *optokinetic nystagmus* (OKN) is generated: slow components of nystagmus that match eye velocity with visual surround velocity, and fast components that reset eye position.

At the bedside a true optokinetic stimulus is usually not possible. Stimulation with hand-held moving stripes induces nystagmus reflecting smooth-pursuit eye movement function (slow components) and saccadic system integrity (fast components). The examiner looks for the presence of both components of nystagmus and for symmetry in both horizontal and vertical directions. Some clinical conditions are well demonstrated by observation of the bedside OKN response, as follows:

1. Presence of optokinetic nystagmus proves that visual function is at least partially intact and is relevant in examining infants and in patients with suspected psychogenic blindness or complex visual impairment (parietal and occipital lesions).
2. Frontal lobe lesions often produce abnormalities of saccades but spare pursuit. The eyes tonically deviate in the direction of the moving target, and the fast phases may be absent or impaired when the target moves toward the side of the lesion.
3. Deep parietal lesions may impair pursuit toward the side of the lesion, causing an abnormal slow component of OKN when the target moves toward the side of the lesion. There may be an amplitude asymmetry between the two directions.
4. Extensive hemispheric lesions may impair both pursuit and saccades. Movement of the target toward the side of the lesion may produce deficits in both slow and fast components.
5. Occipital or temporal lesions usually spare OKN. If the OKN response is asymmetric, deep parietal involvement is probable.
6. Moving the OKN target away from the field of action of an individual eye muscle prompts saccades in the appropriate direction and may help define a muscle paresis. Look for differences between paired

muscles, for example, the left lateral rectus and the right medial rectus: the paretic eye moves more slowly and lags behind.

7. Internuclear ophthalmoplegia may be demonstrated by horizontal movement of the target, resulting in dysconjugate saccades when fast components of OKN require action of the affected medial rectus muscle.

8. Downward movement of the OKN target may help demonstrate convergence retraction nystagmus (see Nystagmus).

9. Congenital nystagmus may be accompanied by "inverted" OKN, in which the fast components are in the direction of target movement.

REFERENCE

Leigh RJ, Zee DS: *The neurology of eye movements*, ed 3, Philadelphia, FA Davis, 1999.

PAGET'S DISEASE

Paget's disease, a disorder of local bone remodeling, usually develops after 40 years of age and becomes evident as pain at rest or motion. Back pain may occur as a result of the bony changes, but compression fracture is also possible. The bony changes may lead to lumbar stenosis or thoracic cord compression. Skull involvement can lead to headache or cranial nerve abnormalities (hearing loss, vision loss, diplopia, or facial weakness). With more severe skull involvement, basilar invagination and odontoid process dislocation may occur, with resultant brainstem compression or obstructive hydrocephalus. Diagnosis is based on typical radiographic changes and increased 24-hour urine hydroxyproline excretion. Alkaline phosphatase level is often elevated. Therapy includes calcitonin, biphosphonates, and plicamycin. Nonsteroidal anti-inflammatory medications can reduce bone pain.

PAIN

Pain is produced by the stimulation of peripheral nocicepters or afferent nerve fibers. The perception of pain is modulated by many factors, including previous behavioral experiences, emotions, drugs, and hypnosis. This modulation suggests a neural mechanism that modifies either the transmission of pain or the emotional reaction to it, or both.

Cutaneous afferent nociceptive fibers enter the dorsal horn of the spinal cord, where they may ascend or descend 1 to 2 segments as Lissauer's tract. Primary afferents terminate in the superficial layers of the dorsal horn in an area known as the substantia gelatinosa. Second-order neurons decussate and ascend rostrally as the lateral and anterior spinothalamic tracts. The spinothalamic tract projects to the ventral posterolateral nucleus of the thalamus, which then sends its projections to other diencephalic structures, brainstem reticular activating system, limbic system, and the primary somatosensory cortex. In addition to the ascending pain system, there is a descending modulation system with origins in the brainstem peri-aqueductal gray and projections to the raphe nucleus. Projections from the raphe nucleus project directly to the ventral and dorsal horns of the spinal cord, including the substantia gelatinosa, and act to inhibit nociception. Serotonin is the main transmitter in this system. The locus ceruleus also acts as a descending modulating system, using norepinephrine as its trans-mitter. Prominent within the pain-modulating systems is the opiate receptor system and endogenous opioid peptides, which exist throughout the nervous system, particularly in the periaqueductal gray and raphenucleus.

Acute pain follows an injury and generally resolves with healing. It has a well-defined temporal onset and is often associated with objective physi-cal signs of autonomic activity such as tachycardia, hypertension, and diaphoresis.

Chronic pain persists beyond expected healing time and often cannot be related to a specific injury. It may not have a well-defined onset, does not respond to treatments aimed at the presumed origin or cause, and is not associated with signs of autonomic activity; the patients do not "look" like they are in pain.

Reflex sympathetic dystrophy (complex regional pain syndrome) and *phantom limb pain* are unique chronic pain syndromes. Reflex sympathetic dystrophy is characterized by burning pain, hyperesthesia, swelling, hyper-hidrosis, and trophic skin and bone changes. It is treated with sympathetic denervation and aggressive physical therapy. Phantom limb pain differs from the usual nonpainful sensory illusion that the lost limb is still present. Phantom limb pain is refractory to most treatments, although local anesthetic injections have limited success.

Chronic (noncancer) pain requires an integrated multidisciplinary approach directed at both physical and psychologic rehabilitation. The goal is to control the factors that increase pain. All therapies, especially drugs, should be given on a time-contingent basis, not as necessary (prn). The patient thus is not rewarded for having pain by getting medication. This approach serves to reduce the total amount of drug required daily. Each drug must be given an adequate trial. Start with simple analgesics, increase the dose or frequency before changing drugs, and when chang-ing, use equianalgesic doses. Avoid excessive sedation.

Pharmacologic management of pain utilizes treatment directed at specific sites along the pain pathways. Peripherally, aspirin and nons-teroidal anti-inflammatory agents produce analgesia by preventing the formation of prostaglandin from arachidonic acid metabolism (inhibition of cyclo-oxygenase). Prostaglandin sensitizes tissues to the pain-producing effects of bradykinin and other substances resulting from tissue injury. These medications are effective in treatment of mild to moderate pain, especially bone pain. These substances also potentiate the effects of nar-cotic analgesics. Capsaicin, a derivative of hot peppers, acts by depleting nociceptors of substance P, rendering the skin insensitive to pain. A treatment trial requires 2 to 4 weeks of daily topical application, three to four times per day, to the affected area.

Tricyclic antidepressants (TCAs) act via influencing the biogenic amine system, affecting levels of serotonin, norepinephrine, and dopamine. Patients with pain are often locked into a pain-depression-insomnia cycle, and TCAs can affect each of these aspects of pain. The TCAs are effective in a variety of chronic pain conditions, including chronic low back pain, headache, neuropathy, and neuralgias. Anticonvulsants act to suppress spontaneous neuronal firing. They are useful in the management of chronic pain states such as trigeminal neuralgia, postherpetic neuralgia, diabetic neuropathy, and post-amputation pain. Venlafaxine, which increases both levels of serotonin and norepinephrine is emerging as a relatively non-sedating but effective medication for treating neuropathic pain.

Narcotic analgesics are used to treat severe, acute pain and chronic pain. When using narcotics, start with the lowest dose needed to obtain analgesia and titrate to pain relief or to the appearance of unacceptable side effects. Whereas prn dosing for several days allows for the determination of total daily dose, thereafter give narcotic analgesics on a fixed dosing schedule. Add nonnarcotic drugs to increase analgesia. Tolerance to narcotics usually becomes evident as a reduction in duration of analgesia and the need for higher doses. Treat this situation by increasing the dose or by using an alternative drug (start with one half of the equianalgesic dose).

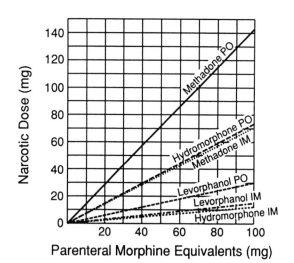

FIGURE 27

Narcotic conversion nomogram: high-potency narcotics. (From Grossman SA, Scheidler VR: *World Health Forum* 8:525, 1987.)

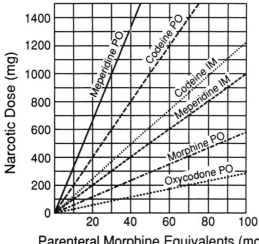

FIGURE 28

Narcotic conversion nomogram: low-potency narcotics. (From Grossman SA, Scheidler VR: *World Health Forum* 8:525, 1987.)

The narcotic conversion nomogams can guide conversion between narcotics (Figures 27 and 28). For example, 30 mg of oral methadone is equivalent to approximately 20 mg of parenteral morphine. Physical dependence occurs if the patient receives prolonged therapy in high doses, and patients experience withdrawal symptoms with abrupt narcotic cessation. Physical dependence is not to be confused with psychological dependence, which is a behavioral syndrome of drug craving.

Other pharmacologic interventions include the use of corticosteroids in the treatment of cancer, especially when cancer is due to bony metastasis, neuroleptics, venlafaxine or Gabapentin in dysesthetic pain; and dextroamphetamine for potentiating narcotic analgesia and reducing narcotic-induced sedation. Antihistamines (hydroxyzine) and neuroleptics can also be used to decrease nausea associated with narcotic use.

Other treatment modalities used in pain management include trigger-point injections; epidural, intrathecal, and sympathetic blockade; ganglionolysis; cordotomy; transcutaneous and percutaneous electrical stimulation; dorsal column stimulation; and relaxation techniques, including biofeedback and hypnosis.

REFERENCES

Bach S et al: *Pain* 33:297, 1988.
Portenoy RK: *CA Cancer J Clin* 1988; 38:327–392.
Schwartzmann RJ, McLellan TL: *Arch Neurol* 44:555, 1987.

PARANEOPLASTIC SYNDROMES

Paraneoplastic syndromes (PS) are autoimmune remote effects of cancer that are not caused by metastatic complications of a systemic cancer. Autoantibodies have been identified in several types of PS and summarized in Table 60. Neurologic symptoms precede the identification of cancer in 50% of cases.

Clinical features which suggest a PS include (1) subacute onset, (2) severe neurologic disability, (3) inflammatory CSF with increased cells, elevated protein, and oligoclonal bands, (4) clinical syndrome that predominantly affects one specific portion of the nervous system, and (5) stereotypical presentation. There are two main groups: (1) "classic" PS, that when present, strongly suggest an underlying cancer (Lambert-Eaton myasthenic syndromes [LEMS], subacute cerebellar degneration [SACD] opsoclonus/myoclonus in children) and (2) PS that sometimes are associated with cancer but more often appear in the absence of a neoplasm (polymyositis, amyotrophic lateral sclerosis [ALS], polyneuropathy). Injury to the nervous system is mediated by the immune system, which directs a response at the tumor and against the shared antigens in the nervous system (onconeural antigens). This is the basis for antibody testing in PS. The presence of autoantibodies helps to confirm the clinical diagnosis and to focus the search for an underlying malignancy. Furthermore, it is associated with a more indolent course than the same tumor in a patient without paraneoplastic syndrome. With the exception of myasthenia gravis, LEMS, neuromyotonia, dermatomyositis, carcinoid myopathy, and peripheral neuropathies associated with osteosclerotic myeloma, treatment of paraneoplastic syndromes is generally unsatisfactory. The PS may progress regardless of the underlying cancer, and only rarely does treatment of the primary disorder affect the course of the syndrome.

The paraneoplastic syndromes include the following:

I. *Brain and cranial nerves*: SACD, opsoclonus-myoclonus, limbic encephalitis and other dementias, brainstem encephalitis, optic neuritis, photoreceptor degeneration.
II. *Spinal cord and dorsal root ganglia*: Myelitis, necrotizing myelopathy, sensory neuronopathy, subacute motor neuronopathy, motor neuron disease.
III. *Peripheral nerves*: Subacute or chronic sensorimotor peripheral neuropathy, Guillian-Barré, mononeuritis-multiplex and vasculitic neuropathy, brachial neuritis, autonomic neuropathy, peripheral neuropathy with islet-cell tumors or paraproteinemias.
IV. *Neuromuscular junction and muscle*: LEMS, myasthenia gravis, dermatomyositis or polymyositis, acute necrotizing myopathy, carcinoid myopathy, myotonia, cachectic myopathy, neuromyopathy.
V. *Multiple levels of central and peripheral nervous system or unknown site*: Encephalomyelitis, neuromyopathy, stiff-person syndrome.

TABLE 60

ANTINEURONAL ANTIBODY-ASSOCIATED PARANEOPLASTIC DISORDERS

Antibody	Associated Cancer	Syndrome	Antigen	Onconeuronal Antigen
Anti-Hu	SCLC, neuroblastoma	Encephalomyelitis, Sensory neuronopathy	All neuronal nuclei	HuD, HuC, and Hel-N1
Anti-Yo	Gynecologic, breast	Cerebellar degeneration	Cytoplasm Purkinje cells	CDR34, CDR62-1, and CDR62-2
Anti-Ri	Breast, gynecologic, SCLC	Cerebellar ataxia, opsoclonus	Neuronal nuclei CNS	NOVA1 and NOVA2
Anti-amphiphysin	Breast	Stiff-person, encephalomyelitis	Synaptic vesicles	Amphiphysin
Anti-VGCC	SCLC	LEMS	Presynaptic VGCC	A1-subunit
Anti-MYsB	SCLC	LEMS	Presynaptic VGCC	B-Subunit VGCC
Anti-Ma	Multiple	Cerebellar, brainstem dysfunction	Neuronal nuclei and cytoplasm	Ma1 and Ma2
Anti-Ta	Testicular	Limbic encephalitis, brainstem dysfunction	Neuronal nuclei and cytoplasm	Ma2
Anti-Tr	Hodgkin's lymphoma	Cerebellar degeneration	Cytoplasm neurons, Purkinje cells, spiny dendrites	In progress
Anti-CAR	SCLC, others	Photoreceptor degeneration	Retinal photoreceptor	Recoverin
Anti-CV2	SCLC, others	Encephalomyelitis, cerebellar degeneration	Glia	POP66

LEMS, Lambert Eaton myasthenic syndrome; SCLC, Small cell lung cancer; VGCC, Voltage gated calcium channels.

P

PARANEOPLASTIC SYNDROMES

REFERENCES

Dalmau JO, Posner JB: *Arch Neurol* 1999, 56:405–408.

Posner JB, ed: *Neurologic complications of cancer,* ed 2, Philadelphia, FA Davis, 1995, 353–385.

PARIETAL LOBE

The parietal lobe contains the primary somatosensory and parietal association cortices (Brodmann's area 1, 2, 3) dealing with integration of multiple sensory modalities. It mainly receives fibers from the ventral posterior nucleus of the thalamus. It also contributes fibers to the corticospinal tracts. Parietal lobe syndromes depend on the laterality of the lesion.

Hemisphere-independent parietal syndromes include contralateral cortical sensory loss, incongruent homonymous hemianopsia, contralateral hemiparesis (associated with hemiatrophy if onset is in childhood), impaired ipsilateral optokinetic saccades with compensatory nystagmus, sensory hallucinations, and simple sensory seizures.

Dominant parietal lobe syndromes include aphasia, alexia, Gerstmann's syndrome, tactile agnosia, and apraxia (ideomotor and ideational).

Nondominant parietal lobe syndromes include neglect, anosognosia, topographic memory loss, constructional apraxia, "dressing apraxia," and acute confusional states.

Bilateral parietal lesions are associated with visual agnosia, Balint's syndrome, Anton's syndrome, color agnosia, and catatonia.

PARKINSONISM

The cardinal symptoms of Parkinson's disease occur in other akinetic rigid syndromes. These disorders are distinguished from Parkinson's disease by the presence of additional neurologic symptoms, (supranuclear palsy, cerebellar signs, severe dementia, spasticity, symmetry, orthostatic hypotension, etc.) and are sometimes called "Parkinson's plus syndromes." Parkinson's-plus syndromes have a transient or absent response to L-dopa, insidious onset, and rapidly progressive course to disability.

These syndromes include the following:

1. Progressive supranuclear palsy (PSP) is characterized by supranuclear ophthalmoplegia, pseudobulbar palsy, axial rigidity, and mild dementia. Patients present with complaints of postural instability and frequent falls (patients characteristically fall backwards). Dysphagia and dysarthria are frequently noted by family and patient. Slow saccades may be the earliest sign. Ophthalmoplegia is vertical in most patients at presentation and upward gaze is affected more than downward, although *downward is much more specific* because upward gaze

restriction is more common in the elderly. PSP has been linked to mutation on chromosome 17 in the tau gene (hence the term *tauopathies*).

2. Multiple system atrophy (MSA) has a few recognized variants: sporadic olivopontocerebellar atrophy (OPCA), Shy-Drager syndrome, and striatonigral degeneration (SND). Patients have significant dysautonomia, with prominent symptoms of orthostatic hypotension and sphincter dysfunction. Early postural instability and gait disability, dysarthria, and dysphagia are also indicative of MSA variant. Patients may manifest bradyphrenia, but dementia is not common. The SND variant has predominantly akinetic rigid symptoms; a linear hyperintense signal abnormality can be seen on MRI between the claustrum and the putamen. Patients with the OPCA variant manifest cerebellar signs with prominent degeneration of cerebellum and pons on MRI.

3. Corticobasal ganglionic degeneration (CBGD) is distinguished from Parkinson's disease by the presence of asymmetric cortical symptoms and signs. Severe ideational and ideomotor apraxia is prominent and alien hand syndrome is unique to this akinetic rigid syndrome. MRI reveals asymmetric perirolandic frontal temporal atrophy. This disorder, similar to PSP, has been linked to mutation on chromosome 17 in the tau gene.

4. Others: Dementia syndrome (Alzheimer's, diffuse Lewy body disease, frontotemporal), Lytico-Bodig, progressive pallidal atrophy may have akinesia as part of their clinical expression.

There are few current therapeutic options for the syndromes mentioned above. Patients do not respond well or for long term to anti-Parkinson's medication or surgical interventions. Symptomatic support of blood pressure in MSA and trial of dopaminergic agents are warranted, however, because a minority of patients may respond to dopamine therapy in the early stages.

Secondary parkinsonism: Refers to those disorders that are secondarily associated with the akinetic rigid syndromes, i.e., neuroleptics, postencephalitic, vascular insults to the midbrain, or multiple subcortical lacunes associated with lower body Parkinson's disease, hydrocephalus, hypoxia, trauma, metabolic (parathyroid), and toxins (Mn, CO, MPTP, cyanide, lithium, methyldopa, metoclopramide). Treatment for secondary Parkinson's disease is symptomatic and aimed at elimination of primary cause.

Others: Hallervorden-Spatz disease, Huntington disease, Lubag disease, Wilson's disease, neuroacanthocytosis, and mitochondrial cytopathies with striatal necrosis.

REFERENCES

Gilman S, Low PA et al: *J Neurol Sci* 163:94–98, 1999.
Rowland LP: *Merritt's neurology*, Philadelphia, Lippincott Williams & Wilkins, 2000.

PARKINSON'S DISEASE

Parkinson's disease (paralysis agitans, idiopathic Parkinson's disease) is a neurodegenerative disorder. *The cardinal symptoms* are bradykinesia (slowness or fatiguing of movement), rigidity (cogwheel or lead pipe), resting tremor (4 to 6 Hz) and, in the late stages, postural instability. *Classic signs* and symptoms include micrographia (small tapering writing), masked facies, hypophonia, stooped posture, and shuffling gait accompanied by poor or absent arm swing. Parkinson's patients characteristically present with masked facies and diminished blink rate in the unmedicated state. Studies have found a correlation between central dopamine levels and spontaneous blink rate. Depression may precede the diagnosis of Parkinson's disease by several years, and cognitive deficits are commonly observed (30% to 60%).

Although the loss of multiple neurotransmitters is recognized in Parkinson's disease, the loss of dopaminergic pigmented neurons in the substantia nigra evidenced in early pathologic studies predicted the therapeutic effects of L-dopa. L-dopa is the biochemical precursor to dopamine, which unlike dopamine, crosses the blood-brain barrier. Thus, dopamine replenishment therapy dominates the therapeutic strategies available for Parkinson's patients.

Dopaminergic agents: All anti-Parkinson's medications are designed to ameliorate symptoms rather than change the course of the disease. Thus dosage and intervals should be titrated to the individual patient's symptomatic need.

1. *Ergot-derived dopaminergic agents* include bromocriptine (Parlodel), pergolide (Permax), lisuride, and cabergoline. Most of these agents were initially investigated as adjunct therapy for L-dopa and subsequently found to be effective monotherapy in newly diagnosed patients. Effectiveness was assessed as a comparable level of anti-Parkinson effects with a decrease in the "supplemental" L-dopa dosage required and a delay of the development of motor fluctuations. Cognitive deficits and hallucination tendencies may be exacerbated, and adverse GI symptoms and hypotension are not uncommon.
2. *Nonergot-derived dopaminergic agonists* include pramipexole (Mirapex) and ropinirole (Requip). These agents appear to be better tolerated with less adverse effects than the ergot derivatives. A unique adverse effect of pramipexole is increased somnolence. Patients should be instructed to avoid driving immediately after a dose of pramipexole. As monotherapy, these agents are also found to be effective in decreasing the required dose of L-dopa and delaying the adverse motor fluctuations. Comparison studies reveal these agents to be more effective than bromocriptine (Parlodel).

MAO inhibitors, i.e. Selegiline (deprenyl), inhibits monoamine oxidase B. Selegiline was found to delay and decrease the need for L-dopa in de novo patients. Controversy surrounds its use, secondary to the recognition of its metabolism to amphetamine and an early study that documented a higher mortality rate (later refuted). Avoid meperidine in patients taking Selegiline because it may precipitate severe complications. Selective serotonin reuptake inhibitors or triptans may precipitate a hypertensive crisis if taken with Selegiline.

COMT inhibitors include entacapone (Coptan) and tolcapone (Tasmar). These medications are recommended only as adjunctive therapy to L-dopa and should be given with each dose. They are primarily recommended in advanced Parkinson's patients who require greater than 600 mg of L-dopa daily. Adverse effects include worsening of L-dopa failure syndrome.

Amantadine (Symmetrel) was discovered serendipitously to be an effective therapy in Parkinson's disease. It was subsequently found to have antiglutaminergic (NMDA antagonist) effects as well as dopamine reuptake inhibitory activity. It is occasionally effective in alleviating the severe dyskinetic symptoms of the levodopa failure syndrome. Adverse effects are predominantly cognitive in nature and thus lower doses (bid—last dose before 3 PM) are recommended in the elderly.

Anticholinergic agents: Benztropine (Cogentin) and Trihexyphenidyl (Artane). Their usage in Parkinson's disease predates the administration of L-dopa. They are utilized mainly for refractory tremor and sialorrhea. The anticholinergic effects exacerbate cognitive symptoms and are therefore not recommended in the elderly or demented individuals or those with a predisposition to adverse cognitive effects.

L-dopa/carbidopa remains the standard therapy for progressive symptoms of Parkinson's disease. It has been found to be effective in alleviating symptoms of bradykinesia, rigidity, and tremor (although the initial response may be exacerbation). It is less effective on the akinetic symptoms involving gait and is ineffective and may exacerbate postural instability and gait freezing (this is true for all the dopaminergic agents). The levodopa failure syndrome is described as progressive symptoms of *on-off fluctuations, wearing off phenomenon, worsening hyperkinetic dyskinesia, and dystonia*. Patients with stable blood levels of L-dopa, i.e., undergoing intravenous infusion of L-dopa, do not experience these severe fluctuations. Thus, it has been hypothesized that the pulsatile concentrations of L-dopa exacerbates the motor fluctuations. Controlled release (CR) L-dopa/carbidopa preparations (50/200, 25/100) have been designed to prevent pulsatile stimulation of the receptors. The bioavailability of these preparations are significantly (30% to 70%) decreased, therefore increased doses of L-dopa are required.

Stereotactic surgical intervention predates the discovery of L-dopa therapy. The resurgence of stereotactic surgery for Parkinson's disease followed the development of brain imaging systems, which allowed access to discrete basal ganglia nuclei. The increasing prevalence of levodopa failure syndrome further promoted surgical interventions because dyskinesia, on-off fluctuations, and wearing off phenomenon are quite susceptible to stereotactic lesions.

1. *Posteroventral pallidotomy* is effective in alleviating symptoms of bradykinesia, akinesia, rigidity, and tremor, although it alleviates tremor to a lesser degree than thalamotomy or combined thalamotomy-pallidotomy. It is particularly effective in the long-term improvement of dyskinesia, on-off fluctuations, and the wearing off phenomenon. Improvement in postural instability and gait disorders has been found, although reports on the long-term effects on these symptoms are conflicting.

2. Ventroinferomedial thalamotomy and thalamic stimulation are effective in the attenuation of resting tremor, dyskinesia, dystonia, and rigidity. It is less effective for treating akinesia and may worsen it.

3. *Subthalamic nucleus stimulation or lesioning* are also effective in the akinetic symptoms of Parkinson's disease as well as those of the levodopa failure syndrome. The advantage over pallidotomy appears to be the considerable attenuation of levodopa required by the patient. Dyskinesia may continue to occur in patients despite stimulation requiring a decrement in L-dopa dose. This may indicate less alleviation of dyskinesia than pallidotomy in Parkinson's patients.

Clinical pearls in managing PD are as follows:

1. Most patients continue to require short acting L-dopa for optimal therapeutic management and shorter intervals (of up to q 2 to 3 hr) are often effective in treating severe motor fluctuations. Concomitant intake of large amino acid loads (protein load particularly in dairy products) will competitively inhibit the transport of L-dopa into the brain.

2. Early morning dystonia usually can be treated with starting the L-dopa earlier.

3. Patients may also present with acute confusion and hallucinations. Recent changes or additions to medications should be investigated and discontinued. Anticholinergics, amantadine, and the ergot agonists, and COMT inhibitors should be early suspects. The atypical antipsychotics utilized for patients with Parkinson's disease are olanzapine (Zyprexa), quetiapine (Seroquel), clozapine (Clozaril) (remember to check blood for dyscrasias), and risperidone (Risperdal). Recent studies suggest risperidone should be reserved as a last resort because it does precipitate extrapyramidal effects similar to those experienced with phenothiazines and haloperidol which should be avoided.

4. Patients who manifest significant dyskinetic symptoms should have their medication dosage decreased and the interval between the doses decreased as well, to prevent motor fluctuations as stated earlier. *Peak dose dyskinesia* may be treated with reducing each dose of L-dopa or increasing the frequency if decreasing the dose results in more wearing off. Slow release L-dopa or selegiline may be added. *Diphasic dyskinesia* is treated with increasing the dose of L-dopa or switching to a dopamine agonist with a lower dose of L-dopa. Amantadine may also be helpful in alleviating dyskinesia. Long term, stereotactic surgical interventions appear to be the most effective.

REFERENCES

Hallett M, Litvan I: *Neurology* 53:1910–1921, 1999.
Poewe W: *Curr Opin Neurol* 12:411–415, 1999.

PERIODIC PARALYSIS (see *Myotonia*)

Periodic paralysis refers to remitting and relapsing episodes of flaccid, painless weakness traditionally categorized according to the serum potassium level during the attack. However, the episodes are better classified by sensitivity to potassium and changes in its level rather than by its absolute value. They can be primary familiar (autosomal dominant) forms or can result from other causes. Genetic forms of periodic paralysis associated with mutations in the α subunit of the skeletal muscle sodium-channel protein include hyperkalemic periodic paralysis and paramyotonia congenita. Table 61 reviews clinical features of the primary familial kalemic periodic paralysis.

TABLE 61
PRIMARY FAMILIAL KALEMIC PERIODIC PARALYSIS

Characteristic	Hypokalemic	Hyperkalemic
Age of onset	10–20 yr, worse during third and fourth decades	Infancy/childhood
Inheritance	Autosomal dominant, 3 male:1 female, often not expressed in female	Autosomal dominant, male = female
Duration of attacks	Hours to days	Usually <1 hr
Frequency of attacks	Several per week to years between attacks	Several per day to months between attacks
Clinical signs	Often occurs in early morning, begins with hip weakness and spreads over 1 hr from proximal to distal; can totally paralyze patient, ↓ DTRs, spares face, eyes, and respiratory muscles	Proximal > distal weakness, spreads over minutes, associated with myotonia of face, eyes, hands; respiratory muscles may be involved
Laboratory findings	K^+ 1.5–3 mEq ECG changes of ↓ K^+ EMG silent during attack	K ↑ in 80%, ± ↑ CK ECG changes of ↑ K^+ EMG silent during attack
Precipitating factors	Heavy exercise followed by rest or sleep, cold, emotion, heavy meal, alcohol, trauma, epinephrine, corticosteroids	Rest after exercise, cold, anesthesia, sleep, pregnancy
Provocative tests	Glucose ± insulin	Oral KCl
Treatment	KCl, acetazolamide, spironolactone	Acetazolamide, calcium gluconate

Secondary hypokalemic periodic paralysis occurs in illnesses with potassium depletion, including hyperaldosteronism, chronic diarrhea, or chronic use of potassium-depleting diuretics. A high incidence of hypokalemic periodic paralysis is associated with thyrotoxicosis in Oriental men.

Secondary hyperkalemic periodic paralysis is seen only with very high potassium levels, and cardiac abnormalities usually predominate. Causes include renal insufficiency, potassium-sparing diuretics, and adrenal insufficiency.

Normokalemic periodic paralysis has not been established as a distinct clinical entity. On clinical study it resembles hyperkalemic periodic paralysis and probably represents the approximately 20% of patients with normal potassium levels.

All forms of periodic paralysis may respond to acetazolamide therapy. Its mode of action includes kaliuresis but also induces metabolic acidosis, which may explain its benefit with hypokalemic periodic paralysis. Other kaliuretic diuretics (such as thiazides) may also be effective.

REFERENCE

Ebers GC et al: *Ann Neurol* 30:810–816, 1991.

PERIPHERAL NERVE

CLINICAL CLUES IN THE DIAGNOSIS OF FOCAL PERIPHERAL NERVE DISEASE

I. Upper extremity.
   A. With marked differences in strength between BICEPS and BRACHIORADIALIS (both innervated by C5–6 roots via *upper trunk*), think of:
      1. A lesion of the *lateral cord* or *musculocutaneous nerve* (if BICEPS is *weaker*).
      2. A lesion of the *posterior cord* or *radial nerve* (if BRACHIORADIALIS is *weaker*).
   B. With marked differences in strength between BICEPS and DELTOID, think of:
      1. A lesion of the *lateral cord* or *musculocutaneous nerve* (if BICEPS is *weaker*).
      2. A lesion of the *posterior cord* or *axillary nerve* (if DELTOID is *weaker*).
   C. The *median nerve* sensory fibers to the hand pass via the upper brachial plexus, originating from:
      1. The C6 root to the thumb.
      2. The C6 and C7 roots to the index finger.
      3. The C7 root to the middle finger.
   D. It is not possible to differentiate C8 from T1 radiculopathy because all INTRINSIC MUSCLES of the hand are innervated by C8 and T1 roots.

E. With an *ulnar nerve* lesion of the arm, elbow, or upper forearm, sensory loss usually involves palmar and dorsal aspects of the little and ring fingers. With an *ulnar nerve lesion* of the distal forearm or wrist, sensory loss involves only the palmar aspect of these fingers (due to sparing of the *dorsal ulnar sensory branch* that arises 6 to 7 cm above the wrist).

F. With *ulnar neuropathy*, sensory loss should not ascend above the wrist. With C8–T1 radiculopathy or *lower trunk plexopathy*, sensory loss can ascend to the entire medial aspect of the upper limb, following the distribution of the *medial cutaneous nerves* of the forearm and arm (both arising from the *lower trunk*).

G. With weakness and/or atrophy of the THENAR and HYPOTHENAR eminences, think of:
1. C8–T1 radiculopathy.
2. A *lower trunk* brachial plexopathy.
3. Concomitant *ulnar* and *median* mononeuropathy (for example, carpal tunnel syndrome and ulnar neuropathy at the elbow). In this case, FLEXOR POLLICIS LONGUS should be intact (flexor of the distal phalanx of the thumb, located in the forearm and innervated by the *anterior interosseus branch of the median nerve*).

H. If there is suspicion of a *lower trunk* brachial plexopathy and/or C8–T1 radiculopathy, the presence of a second-order-neuron Horner's syndrome is supportive evidence.

I. When evaluating wrist drop, correct the wrist angle to the neutral position before testing finger flexors and extensors:
1. If the BRACHIORADIALIS and TRICEPS are spared, the lesion is an isolated *posterior interosseous* mononeuropathy. In such cases there is no sensory loss.
2. If only the TRICEPS is spared, the *radial nerve* lesion is at the spiral groove.
3. If the TRICEPS is weak, the *radial nerve* lesion is at the axilla.
4. If, in addition to the TRICEPS, the DELTOID is weak, the lesion is not radial nerve, but rather a *posterior cord* brachial plexopathy (supplying *radial* and *axillary* nerves).

J. In the case of scapular winging,* the winging is caused by:
1. SERRATUS ANTERIOR weakness if:
   a. There is considerable winging at rest.
   b. There is medial translocation of the scapula (vertebral border closer to the midline).
   c. The shoulder appears lower on the affected side.
   d. Winging is accentuated by forward flexion of the humerus.

P

PERIPHERAL NERVE

---

* Note that scaptular winging can be falsely diagnosed in patients with poor posture or skeletal deformity. In addition, proximal weakness (such as myopathy or spinal muscular atrophy) can cause generalized shoulder girdle atrophy and "pseudowinging."

2. TRAPEZIUS weakness is:
   a. There is less winging at rest.
   b. There is lateral translocation of the scapula.
   c. The shoulder is definitely lower on the affected side.
   d. Winging is decreased by forward flexion of the humerus.
   e. Winging is increased by abduction of the humerus.

II. Lower extremity.
   A. The *only L4-innervated* muscle below the knee is TIBIALIS ANTERIOR (L4–5, dorxiflexor of the ankle).
   B. When evaluating foot drop (complete or incomplete), testing inversion of the ankle (TIBIALIS POSTERIOR) and flexion of the toes (FLEXOR DIGITORUM LONGUS) is very important. These muscles are innervated by L5 (and to a lesser extent S1) nerve roots via the *tibial nerve*. They are spared with *peroneal neuropathy* but are weak with L5 radiculopathy. Remember to correct the angle of the foot back to 90 degrees before testing eversion and inversion.
   C. It is not possible to differentiate L2 from L3 radiculopathy because QUADRICEPS, ILIOPSOAS, and ADDUCTOR muscles are innervated by L2 and L3 roots.
   D. The testing of THIGH ADDUCTORS (L2–4, *obturator nerve*) is essential in differentiating "pure" *femoral neuropathy* from root or lumbar plexus involvement (THIGH ADDUCTORS are not involved in *femoral* neuropathy).
   E. In proximal weakness of the lower extremity(ies), compare QUADRICEPS and THIGH ADDUCTORS with THIGH ABDUCTORS (GLUTEUS MEDIUS). If the weakness is significantly different, think of a selective root-plexus involvement rather than a myopathy (QUADRICEPS and THIGH ADDUCTORS are L2–4 and GLUTEUS MEDIUS is L5–S1).

Peripheral innervation is shown in Figures 29 to 36.

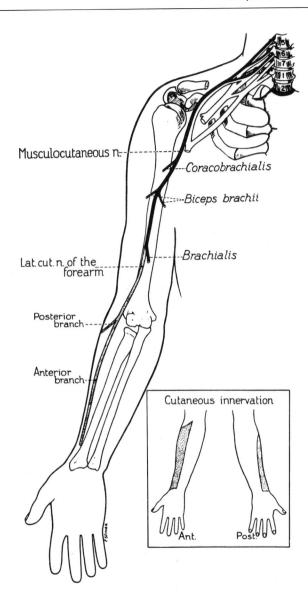

FIGURE 29

Musculocutaneous nerve. (From Haymaker W, Woodhall B: *Peripheral nerve injuries: Principles of diagnosis,* Philadelphia, WB Saunders, 1953.)

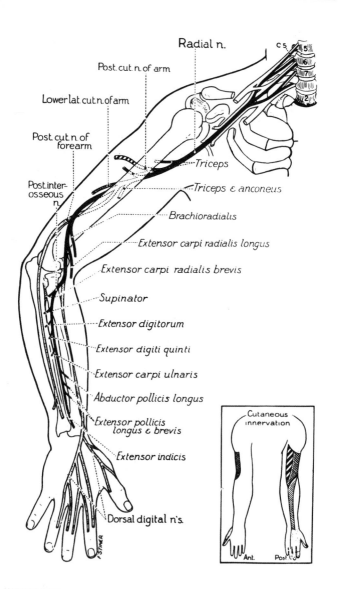

FIGURE 30

Radial nerve. (From Haymaker W, Woodhall B: *Peripheral nerve injuries: Principles of diagnosis*, Philadelphia, WB Saunders, 1953.)

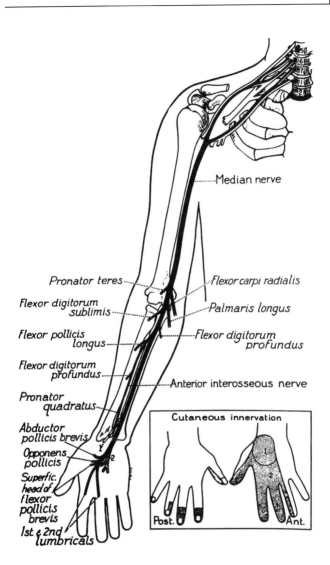

FIGURE 31

Median nerve. (From Haymaker W, Woodhall B: *Peripheral nerve injuries: Principles of diagnosis*, Philadelphia, WB Saunders, 1953.)

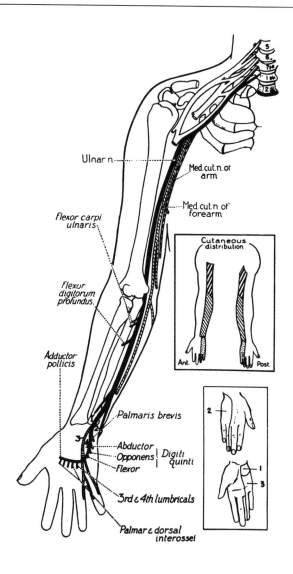

Ulnar n

Med.cut.n. of arm

Med.cut.n. of forearm

Flexor carpi ulnaris

Flexor digitorum profundus

Adductor pollicis

Cutaneous distribution

Ant.

Post.

Palmaris brevis

Abductor
Opponens
Flexor

Digiti quinti

3rd & 4th lumbricals

Palmar & dorsal interossei

FIGURE 32

Ulnar and medial cutaneous nerves. (From Haymaker W, Woodhall B: *Peripheral nerve injuries: Principles of diagnosis*, Philadelphia, WB Saunders, 1953.)

P

PERIPHERAL NERVE

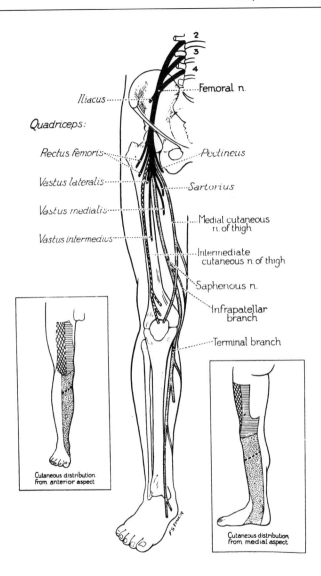

FIGURE 33

Femoral nerve. (From Haymaker W, Woodhall B: *Peripheral nerve injuries: Principles of diagnosis*, Philadelphia, WB Saunders, 1953.)

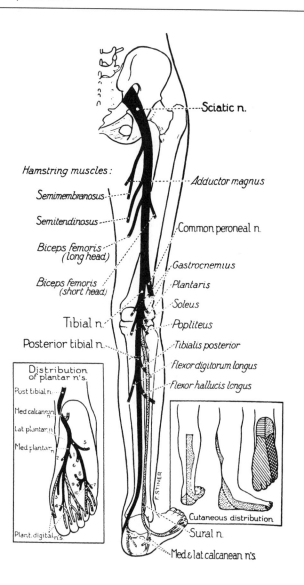

Sciatic n.

Hamstring muscles:
Semimembranosus
Semitendinosus
Biceps femoris (long head)
Biceps femoris (short head)
Tibial n.
Posterior tibial n.

Adductor magnus
Common peroneal n.
Gastrocnemius
Plantaris
Soleus
Popliteus
Tibialis posterior
flexor digitorum longus
flexor hallucis longus

Distribution of plantar n's.
Post tibial n.
Med calcanean n.
Lat plantar n.
Med plantar n.
Plant. digital n's.

Cutaneous distribution
Sural n.
Med & lat calcanean n's.

F. STINER

FIGURE 34

Sciatic, tibial, posterior tibial, and plantar nerves. (From Haymaker W, Woodhall B: *Peripheral nerve injuries: Principles of diagnosis*, Philadelphia, WB Saunders, 1953.)

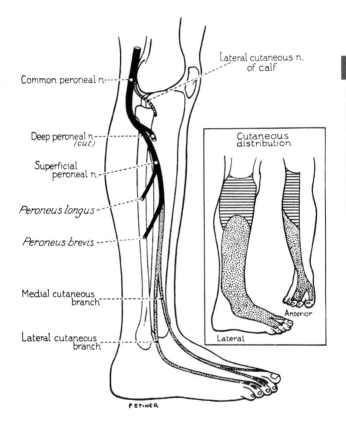

FIGURE 35

Superficial peroneal nerve. (From Haymaker W, Woodhall B: *Peripheral nerve injuries: Principles of diagnosis*, Philadelphia, WB Saunders, 1953.)

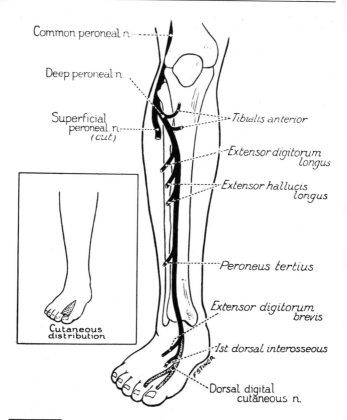

FIGURE 36

Deep peroneal nerve. (From Haymaker W, Woodhall B: *Peripheral nerve injuries: Principles of diagnosis*, Philadelphia, WB Saunders, 1953.)

PET AND SPECT

Both positron emission homography (PET) and single photon emission computed tomography (SPECT) are based on transaxial reconstruction of images derived from the distribution of administered radionuclides. A series of tomographic images are reconstructed by computer. Spatial resolution is significantly lower than that obtained with CT or MRI. PET methodology provides both qualitative and quantitative data (the latter require an arterial line for serial blood sampling), whereas SPECT provides only qualitative data. Both methods are safe, and actual radiation exposure is less than or equal to that received in many other routine radiologic procedures.

PET uses positron-emitting nuclides such as oxygen-15, fluorine-18, carbon-11, and nitrogen-13, which must be produced in a cyclotron. They have a short half-life, enabling administration of relatively high doses of radioactivity but remaining within safe limits of radiation exposure. These radionuclides can be incorporated into biologically active compounds to measure biochemical, pharmacologic, and metabolic processes. Deoxyglucose labeled with fluorine-18 (FDG) is used to measure brain glucose metabolism. Compounds labeled with oxygen-15 are used to measure regional cerebral blood flow and volume and cerebral metabolic rates. Specific receptors such as dopamine or serotonin can be targeted with positron-emitting analogues of those monoamines.

In clinical situations PET has utility in the evaluation of patients with refractory seizures of presumed focal origin. Detection of unilateral temporal hypometabolism using FDG is considered a highly specific procedure for localizing the epileptic focus. Gliomas can also be evaluated for malignant potential, and FDG uptake patterns can differentiate necrosis from tumor recurrence. PET is also being used in ischemia and dementia. In Alzheimer's disease, biparietal hypometabolism is characteristic. Other uses for PET have been limited to research studies by the high cost, invasiveness, and need for extremely sophisticated technology.

SPECT utilizes gamma emitters, such as iodine-123 or technetium-99, attached to highly lipophilic substances that easily pass the blood-brain barrier by simple diffusion. Thus uptake, as measured by gamma camera, is proportional to regional blood flow. Gamma emitters have also been successfully labeled to various neurotransmitter analogues, allowing for localization and evaluation of receptor densities. Indications for studies are similar to those for PET. In contrast to PET, however, SPECT technology is widely available.

REFERENCES

Alavi A, Hirsch LJ: *Semin Nucl Med* 21:58–81, 1991.
American Academy of Neurology: *Neurology* 41:163–167, 1991.

PITUITARY

Mass lesions occurring within the sella include pituitary adenomas, arachnoid cysts, and rarely, tumors of the neurohypophysis. Meningiomas, metastases, dermoids, teratomas, arachnoid cysts, and cholesteatomas may occur in any of several locations around the sella. Suprasellar masses include craniopharyngiomas, optic gliomas, chondromas, hypothalamic gliomas, supraclinoid carotid artery aneurysms, choroid plexus papillomas, and colloid cysts of the third ventricle. Parasellar lesions include cavernous carotid aneurysms, temporal lobe neoplasms, and gasserian ganglion neuromas. Chordomas and basilar artery aneurysms are seen in the retrosellar region. Infrasellar lesions include sphenoid sinus mucoceles, carcinomas, granulomas, and other nasopharyngeal tumors.

Pituitary adenomas may cause only endocrine symptoms if less than 10 mm in diameter (microadenoma). Larger tumors usually produce visual symptoms or headache, or both, with or without endocrine abnormalities, including variable hypopituitarism. Pituitary adenomas are usually classified on histologic study on the basis of immunoperoxidase stains used to identify specific hormones. Prolactin-secreting and nonfunctional adenomas (usually chromophobe adenomas) are the most common. The most common of these, the prolactinomas, usually become evident as amenorrhea or galactorrhea, or both, in females and decreased libido and impotence in males. Glycoprotein hormone-secreting tumors typically produce only symptoms of local mass effect and make up the majority of nonfunctioning adenomas.

The less common growth hormone-secreting and adrenocorticotropic hormone (ACTH)-secreting adenomas become evident as acromegaly and Cushing's syndrome, respectively, usually while small in size. Acromegaly may also be associated with entrapment neuropathies, such as carpal tunnel syndrome, and with diabetes. Cushing's syndrome may be associated with mental status changes, personality changes, and myopathy. Rarely, pituitary tumors secrete follicle-stimulating hormone (FSH) and, even less commonly, thyroid-stimulating hormone (TSH) or luteinizing hormone (LH).

Prolactinomas may rapidly expand during pregnancy. The differential diagnosis of hyperprolactinemia includes hypothalamic and infundibular lesions (loss of inhibitory control of prolactin secretion), renal failure, *Chiari-Frommel syndrome* (amenorrhea-galactorrhea syndrome following pregnancy), and drugs (phenothiazines, butyrophenones, benzodiazepines, reserpine, morphine, alpha methyldopa, and isoniazid). Serum prolactin levels >100 ng/ml (normal level, <15 ng/ml) are almost always due to tumor. Levels from 15 to 100 ng/ml may be due to tumor but are more commonly due to the other disorders listed previously, particularly drugs. MRI scan with gadolinium enhancement is the imaging test of choice. However, since microadenomas are sometimes undetected by MRI, endocrinologic testing is needed to confirm the diagnosis of small, hormone-secreting pituitary tumors if they are suspected on clinical examination. Treatment of symptomatic prolactinomas often consists of bromocriptine because of the risk of tumor recurrence after surgical resection. Occasionally microadenomas resolve with medical treatment. Visual symptoms resulting from macroadenomas usually remit with bromocriptine use. Transsphenoidal microsurgical resection is required when medical therapy is inefficacious or symptoms progress quickly.

Extension into brain parenchyma requires an intracranial approach. Corticosteroid coverage should be provided during surgery. Visual and endocrine function may improve after surgery and must be followed up regularly after surgery. Postoperative radiation therapy is used only for macroadenomas that do not respond to medical or surgical management. Transsphenoidal microsurgical resection is the primary treatment in growth hormone-secreting and ACTH-secreting tumors and in symptomatic glycoprotein hormone-secreting tumors. Craniopharyngiomas, which may be distinguished from pituitary adenomas by the presence of calcifications (see later discussion), are treated by surgical removal and postoperative radiation therapy. Intracavitary irradiation using stereotactically placed yttrium-90 or phosphorous-32 is highly effective in the treatment of cystic craniopharyngiomas, if applied as initial treatment in patients with solitary cysts. There is a fairly high recurrence rate, even if resection seems complete. Stereotactic decompression of recurrent fluid-filled cysts may obviate the need for craniotomy in some cases.

Pituitary apoplexy refers to the sudden expansion of the pituitary gland, usually the result of hemorrhage into a preexisting adenoma. Sudden severe headache, variable ocular motor palsies, rapid loss of vision (chiasmal or optic nerve), evidence of hypopituitarism, and subarachnoid hemorrhage with associated changes in mental status including coma may be present. Features helpful in the difficult clinical distinction from aneurysmal subarachnoid hemorrhage are the presence of mixed oculomotor palsies or bilateral ophthalmoplegias and the presence of an afferent pupillary defect or chiasmal patterns of field loss. Diagnostic procedures include CT and MRI, which may show a pituitary mass containing blood; angiography to exclude an intracavernous aneurysm; and lumbar puncture. Baseline hormonal levels should be obtained before treatment, for subsequent determination of endocrine dysfunction. Treatment includes immediate high-dose IV corticosteroid therapy and prompt transsphenoidal decompression to prevent further vision loss.

Empty sella syndrome is the major cause of asymptomatic sellar enlargement. The subarachnoid space extends into the sella through an incompetent diaphragm with flattening of the gland inferiorly and posteriorly. Empty sella syndrome may also follow pseudotumor cerebri, spontaneous regressive changes of pituitary adenomas, and surgery. Although usually asymptomatic, symptoms may occur, including headache, occasional mild endocrine abnormalities, CSF rhinorrhea, and rarely, visual disturbances. If symptoms are present, pituitary tumor should be excluded with endocrine and neuro-ophthalmic evaluations and MRI. Differential diagnosis of an enlarged sella turcica in the absence of endocrinopathy includes nonsecreting adenoma, empty sella syndrome, and craniopharyngioma. Hypopituitarism, diabetes insipidus, and visual field defects are much less common in empty sella syndrome. A ballooned sella without erosion is more characteristic of craniopharyngioma.

Cerebral salt wasting syndrome: Some patients with hyponatremia do not have syndrome of inappropriate ADH secretion (SIADH) (with resultant free water retention); instead they have inappropriate natriuresis. Hyponatremia in the setting of hypovolemia and renal sodium wasting occurs in patients with primary cerebral tumors, carcinomatous meningitis, subarachnoid hemorrhage, and head trauma following intracranial surgery and pituitary surgery. The pathophysiology is considered to be either by alteration of atrial natriuretic peptide or of the neural input to the kidney. It is important to recognize this syndrome because the treatment is different from SIADH. It responds to vigorous sodium and water replacement. Differentiation is done by careful assessment of volume status. If there is any doubt regarding the diagnosis, fluid restriction should be instituted. Then, if the natriuresis persists, cerebral salt wasting should be suspected and treated appropriately.

REFERENCES

Chung SM: *Neurosurg Clin N Am* 10:717–729, 1999.
Klibanski A, Zervas NT: *N Engl J Med* 324:822–831, 1991.

PORPHYRIA

The porphyrias are rare disorders of heme biosynthesis with neurologic, cutaneous, and other organ manifestations. They are classified as hepatic and erythropoietic. Neurologic symptoms occur in the *hepatic porphyrias*: acute intermittent porphyria (AIP), variegate porphyria (VP), hereditary coproporphyria (HC), and Doss porphyria (DP). These disorders (except DP, which is inherited as an autosomal recessive) are autosomal dominant enzymatic defects of the pathways of heme biosynthesis in the liver, resulting in elevations and excess excretion of the porphyrins and the porphyrin precursors (see Figure 37). Although the enzymatic defects are well charac-

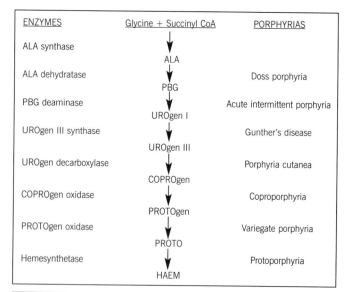

FIGURE 37

The Heme synthesis pathway. Enzymes involved in porphyrias: ALA, delta aminolevulinic acid; COPROgen, coproporphyrinogen; PBG, porphobilinogen; PROTO, protoporphyrin; PROTOgen, protoporphyrinogen; URO, uroporphyrin; UROgen, uroporphyrinogen.

terized, the pathogenesis of neurologic dysfunction is not known. It has been postulated that the delta-aminolevulinic acid (ALA) and porphobilinogen (PBG) are directly neurotoxic. Other possibilities include abnormalities of heme metabolism in neurons or interference with serotonergic metabolism.

The first step in the pathway catalyzed by ALA synthase results in the formation of ALA and it is the rate-limiting step. Heme exerts control at this step via three different mechanisms: (1) repression of synthesis of new enzyme, (2) interference of transfer of the enzyme from cytosol to mitochondria, and (3) direct inhibition of enzyme activity. Processes that deplete the regulatory pool of heme by inducing cytochrome p450 or increasing the turnover of hemoglobin will drive the heme synthesis pathway. For example, dilantin induces the cytochrome p450 system, and starvation increases the turnover of hemoglobin. Both processes deplete the heme pool, thereby removing repression of ALA synthetase.

Depending on the specific enzyme deficiency, there will be an excess of intermediates from preceding steps in the pathway excreted in urine and stool; it is the pattern of porphyrin precursors in the urine, feces, and serum that characterizes the type of porphyria. Diagnosis is complicated by the variable intensity of porphyrin excretion in affected individuals and drug-induced porphyrinuria in some normal individuals leading to occasional false-positive results (see Table 62). Lead poisoning can lead to elevation of ALA and porphyrins. Special handling of specimens obtained for porphyria is necessary. Twenty-four–hour urine collections should be kept refrigerated in a dark container. Twenty-four–hour stool collections must be kept frozen and in a light-free container.

The most common one of these rare disorders is AIP. Prevalence is estimated at 5 to 10 per 100,000 in the United States. Up to 90% of people with the enzyme deficiency (50% of normal activity) are asymptomatic. During the acute attacks, large amounts of PBG and ALA (20- to 200-fold elevated above normal levels) are excreted. About one-third of clinically asymptomatic carriers show an abnormal excretion of PBG (two- to fivefold

---

TABLE 62

HEPATIC PORPHYRIAS: BIOCHEMICAL FEATURES

Type of Porphyria	Enzyme Defect	Erythrocyte Porphyrins	Urine	Feces
Acute intermittent porphyria	PBG deaminase	None	↑ ALA, PBG	None
Variegate porphyria	Protoporphyrinogen oxidase	None	↑ ALA, PBG, COPRO	↑ COPRO, PROTO
Hereditary coproporphyria	Coproporphyrinogen oxidase	None	↑↑ COPRO	↑↑ COPRO
ALA dehydratase deficiency	ALA dehydratase	Protoporphyrin	ALA	None

ALA = Aminolevulinic acid; COPRO = coproporphyrin; PRE = precursor; PROTO = protoporphyrin; URO = uroporphyrin.

above the normal level), whereas the rest show normal excretion of this precursor. AIP lacks cutaneous manifestations, since the PBG is not a porphyrin.

Variegate porphyria occurs mainly in South Africa but has occurred worldwide; hereditary coproporphyria and Doss porphyria are very rare. HC and VP have neurologic and cutaneous manifestations such as photosensitive skin and blistering with excessive sun exposure or mild trauma.

Clinical manifestations include the following:

1. Dysautonomia presenting as abdominal pain (95%) out of proportion to clinical findings, nausea, vomiting (90%), diarrhea or constipation (85%), tachycardia (70%), orthostatic hypotension, hypertension (36%), diaphoresis, and urinary retention.
2. A motor more than sensory polyneuropathy often occurs (50%); rare cases have mononeuritis multiplex as well as ascending flaccid paralysis (2%) resembling Guillain-Barré syndrome, which may result in fatal respiratory failure. Cranial nerves may be involved.

TABLE 63

DRUGS AND ACUTE PORPHYRIA

Drugs That May Precipitate an Attack of Acute Intermittent Porphyria

Alcohol	Meprobamate
Barbiturates	Methsuximide
Carisoprodol	Methyldopa
Chloramphenicol	Methyprylon
Chlordiazepoxide	Pentazocine
Chloroquine	Phenylbutazone
Dichloralphenazone	Phenytoin
Ergots	Progesterones
Estrogens	Pyralones
Eucalyptol	Sulfonamides
Glutethimide	Sylfonal
Griseofulvin	Testosterones
Imipramine	Tolbutamide
	Trional

Drugs That Do Not Exacerbate Acute Intermittent Prophyria

Ascorbic acid	Nitrofurantoin
Aspirin	Opiates
Atropine	Penicillins
B vitamins	Phenothiazines
Chloral hydrate	Promethazine
Corticosteroids	Propranolol
Digoxin	Rauwolfia alkaloids
Diphenhydramine	Scopolamine
Guanethidine	Streptomycin
Methanamine mandelate	Tetracyclines
Meclizine	Tetraethylammonium bromide
Neostigmine	

3. Headaches.
4. Seizures: (15%) in adults, (30%) in children.
5. Psychiatric symptoms (25%): depression, delirium, psychosis, or agitation.
6. Myalgia (72%).

Definitive diagnosis requires measuring PBG deaminase activity in erythrocytes. Screening for the porphyrias is accomplished by measuring stool porphyrins and urinary ALA and PBG concentration.

Treatment consists of avoiding precipitating factors, such as drugs that activate heme biosynthesis (see Table 63), weight loss, or skipping meals. Other prophylactic measures include high carbohydrate diet and propranolol. Acute attacks are treated initially with IV glucose 10 to 20 g/hr; severe attacks may require IV hematin 3 to 4 mg/kg/24 hr, usually during the first 4 days. Urinary ALA and PBG decrease dramatically after 2 to 3 days of therapy. Hematin should not be used in conjunction with anticoagulant therapy because of its side effects, such as coagulopathy and phlebitis (the vein for infusion has to be changed each day). Women with cyclical perimenstrual acute attacks have benefited from luteinizing hormone-releasing hormone (LHRH) agonists. Psychiatric symptoms may be treated with phenothiazines. Abdominal symptoms respond to chlorpromazine. Opiates are used for treatment of pain. Treatment of seizures is perplexing because many anticonvulsants are porphyrinogenic, although benzodiazepines may be less likely to induce porphyria. Gabapentin, which is not metabolized by the liver, may be useful in this clinical setting. The safety of other new antiepileptic drugs is unknown.

REFERENCES

Gordon N: *Brain Dev* 21:373–377, 1999.
Nordmann et al: *J Hepatol* 30:12–16, 1999.

PREGNANCY

A variety of neurologic disorders may begin during or be modified by pregnancy. Conversely, the course and outcome of pregnancy can be affected by the presence of a neurologic disorder. These are best considered by disease category, as follows.

I. *Peripheral Nerve Disorders and Muscle Disease.*
   A. Mononeuropathies: Endometrial implants may occur along the cauda equina, roots, lumbosacral plexus, or sciatic nerve.
      1. *Bell's palsy:* Incidence increases threefold during pregnancy, with the majority of cases occurring in the third trimester and the first 2 puerperal weeks.
      2. *Carpal tunnel syndrome:* May occur transiently during pregnancy, regressing after delivery. Weakness and wasting are unusual.
      3. *Meralgia paresthetica:* Due to the entrapment of the lateral femoral cutaneous nerve of the thigh. Presents with mid-lateral

thigh numbness, tingling, or stinging pain, which is exacerbated by extending the hip when standing and relieved by sitting down. Although self-limited, usually resolving 3 months after delivery, treatment is occasionally necessary. This includes avoidance of excessive weight gain and, if severe, local anesthetic infiltration; more recently, 5% lidocaine patch has been used.

B. Plexopathies.

1. *Recurrent brachial plexopathy:* May be familial and presents as severe, persistent pain, and rapid onset of weakness in the arm and shoulder. As the pain diminishes, weakness increases and wasting of the shoulder girdle ensues. Improvement begins in 4 to 8 weeks; functional recovery occurs in 90% of patients at 4 years.

C. Polyneuropathies.

1. *Guillain-Barré syndrome:* Incidence and course unaffected by pregnancy. Pregnancy is not complicated except possibly increased premature labor in third trimester in severe cases.

2. *Chronic inflammatory demyelinating polyradiculopathy:* (CIDP) May begin during pregnancy; the relapse rate is three times greater during pregnancy, mostly occurring during the third trimester and postpartum period.

3. *Gestational distal polyneuropathy:* A symmetric axonal neuropathy associated with malnutrition consequent to hyperemesis.

4. *Acute intermittent porphyria:* Pregnancy may induce crisis in some patients. Most relapses occur early; more serious are those (15%) that occur in the second and third trimester or are complicated by hypertension, hyperemesis, eclampsia, and pre-existing renal disease. These cases are associated with prematurity and high fetal and maternal mortality.

5. *Charcot-Marie-Tooth disease:* May worsen during pregnancy.

D. Obstetrical palsies: Compression of a peripheral nerve or nerve trunk may be caused by the fetal head, forceps, trauma, hematoma during cesarean section, or improper positioning in leg holders. The most common maternal obstetrical palsy is peroneal compression, followed by femoral neuropathy, obturator neuropathy, and rarely sciatic neuropathy or lumbosacral trunk compression. The risk of permanent weakness with recurrent maternal obstetrical palsies is unknown, but requires recognition of underlying cephalopelvic disproportion and assessment of severity of the first neuropathy.

E. Myotonic dystrophy disability remains the same or worsens during pregnancy, especially the third trimester. *Regional anesthesia is preferred and depolarizing muscle relaxants are contraindicated.* Polyhydramnios suggests fetal myotonia.

II. *Movement disorders.*

A. Chorea gravidarum: >1/100,000 pregnancies. Most chorea occurs during the first trimester and dramatically disappears after childbirth. It may recur with subsequent pregnancies. Approximately one third have had Sydenham's chorea in the past. Differential diagnosis includes acute rheumatic fever, Wilson's disease, lupus, polycythemia, hyperthyroidism, and idiopathic hypoparathyroidism.

B. Wilson's disease: The infants are healthy, although penicillamine may be hazardous to the fetus. Pyridoxine, 50 to 100 mg/day, is recommended, and a reduction in penicillamine dosage to 250 mg/day for the last 6 weeks of pregnancy is recommended if cesarean section is to be performed.

III. *Autoimmune disorders.*

A. Multiple sclerosis (MS): The course during pregnancy is variable. Gestation, labor, and delivery may be normal in MS. MS exacerbations tend to occur less during pregnancy; when they do occur, they tend to be mild. In the first 3 to 6 months postpartum, 20% to 30% of women with MS will experience exacerbations and there is a two-to threefold increase in exacerbations compared to the pre-pregnancy year. Breast-feeding does not preclude the use of interferon-beta and glatiramer. Beta-interferon is contraindicated in pregnancy.

B. Myasthenia gravis may improve, stabilize, or worsen in about equal proportions during pregnancy, but there is frequent immediate postpartum exacerbation. Pregnancy-associated exacerbation is less frequent following thymectomy. Myasthenia may present during pregnancy or the postpartum period. Magnesium sulfate, scopolamine, and large amounts of procaine are contraindicated. Care must be taken in the use of anesthesia and sedative drugs. Newborns should be observed carefully for 72 hours for neonatal myasthenia due to passive transfer of the acetylcholine receptor antibodies from the maternal circulation. There is no contraindication to breast-feeding because of anticholinesterase drugs or prednisone.

IV. *Cerebrovascular disease.*

Age-adjusted relative risk of any hemorrhagic stroke is at least 2.5 times higher during pregnancy and increases to 28 times the nonpregnant risk in the first 6 weeks postpartum.

A. Subarachnoid hemorrhage incidence during pregnancy is estimated to range from 1 to 5 per 10,000 pregnancies. Cerebral arteriovenous malformations (AVMs) and aneurysms are the most common causes. Other causes include placental abruption, disseminated intravascular coagulation (DIC), anticoagulants, endocarditis and mycotic aneurysm, metastatic choriocarcinoma, eclampsia, postpartum cerebral phlebothrombosis, and spinal cord AVMs. AVMs tend to bleed during the second trimester and during childbirth. Aneurysms rupture most commonly during the third trimester, with the greatest risk of rebleeding occurring in the first few weeks after the initial hemorrhage or in the postpartum period. The decision to operate should be based on the same criteria used in nonpregnant patients. The natural history of both AVMs and aneurysms shows that both can rebleed during childbirth with fatal results.

Hyperventilation, hypothermia, and steroids have been safely used during pregnancy, *but mannitol should be restricted*. An untreated aneurysm is a relative contraindication to future pregnancies.

B. Cerebral ischemia: The relative risk of ischemic stroke is not increased during pregnancy but is almost nine times that of the nonpregnant state during the first 6 weeks postpartum. Eclampsia is the most commonly identified cause of ischemic stroke in pregnancy. Arterial occlusion accounts for 60% to 80%, cerebral venous thrombosis for 20% to 40% of strokes, and arterial dissection is less common. Mortality with cerebral venous thrombosis is around 30%, with residual disability varying with extent and site of the lesion. The assessment of the pregnant patient with transient ischemic attacks or stroke is the same as that of stroke in a young person. *Current guidelines suggest that no adverse fetal affects are associated with MRI*. At present, recombinant tissue plasminogen activator (rtPA) should be utilized during pregnancy only in women with significant neurologic deficits and with great caution. *Warfarin and aspirin are both contraindicated in pregnancy*.

C. Others: *Sheehan's syndrome* of postpartum hypopituitarism is secondary to pituitary infarction (usually the anterior pituitary) due to severe shock at the time of delivery. Failure to lactate is followed by amenorrhea, hypothyroidism, and hypoadrenocorticism. *Carotid-cavernous sinus fistula* has also been reported during the second half of pregnancy. *Reversible segmental cerebral vasoconstriction* is a rare syndrome presenting with headache and focal deficits, frequently in the early postpartum period.

V. *Neoplasms.*

Excluding pituitary tumors, primary intracranial tumors do not have an increased incidence during pregnancy. Most primary brain tumors will enlarge during pregnancy and shrink again postpartum. This appears to be secondary to the intrapartum increase in intravascular volume or tumor hormone dependence. Therefore, symptoms or signs may be more apparent during the second half of pregnancy. Although slow-growing tumors can be resected postpartum, *malignant gliomas and many posterior fossa tumors require prompt surgery*. Choriocarcinomas frequently metastasize (usually hemorrhagic) to the brain.

VI. *Headaches.*

Headaches are frequent during pregnancy; extensive evaluation, including neuroimaging, is often required because aneurysms and AVMs may present during this period. Episodic or chronic tension headache is most common. *Migraines* may first manifest during pregnancy, usually during the first trimester. Approximately 75% of migraineurs will improve or be free of headaches during pregnancy, especially during the second and third trimester, with the remainder failing to improve or worsening. *Treatment* is limited to acetaminophen and avoidance of precipitants during pregnancy. Low-dose narcotics may be used, including demerol and morphine, but not nonsteroidal anti-inflammatory agents. Preventive therapy should be avoided. Biofeedback is a safe adjunctive therapy. *Pseudotumor cerebri* has the same incidence as the nonpregnant, age-matched population. Symptoms will commonly begin in the first half of pregnancy.

VII. *Epilepsy.*

It is estimated that 0.3% to 0.5% of all births involve women with epilepsy. Pregnant women during epilepsy can be divided into two subtypes.

A. Gestational epilepsy constitutes seizures occurring only during pregnancy. Half of these women will have epilepsy during their first pregnancy. Only 25% have recurrent seizures during subsequent pregnancies. Seizures tend to occur in the sixth or seventh month of gestation. Most patients have no identifiable lesions; a few have underlying pathology, such as tumors or vascular malformations.

B. In chronic seizure disorder, the onset of seizure is before pregnancy. Most women experience no change in seizure frequency. In 15% of women, the seizures are more frequent. Less than 1% of all epileptic women experience status epilepticus during pregnancy. Multiple factors are responsible for exacerbation of seizures, including decreased antiepileptic drug (AED) levels, hormonal changes, stress, sleep deprivation, and medication noncompliance.

Pregnant women with epilepsy have been reported to be at increased risk for a number of complications such as vaginal bleeding, premature labor or delivery, abruptio placenta, fetal loss, and premature eclampsia. The rate of spontaneous abortions is comparable to the general population. Perinatal mortality is increased 1.2- to 3-fold. A convulsive seizure occurs during labor in 1% to 2% of women with epilepsy and in another 1% to 2% within 24 hours postpartum. Total AED concentration declines as pregnancy progresses due to dynamic changes in plasma protein binding. Therefore, *it is recommended to measure free AED concentration* and make appropriate dose adjustments on the basis of patient clinical condition, seizure frequency, and free AED concentration. The reversal of pregnancy-induced physiologic changes postpartum may cause drug toxicity, so that *drug levels should be checked periodically for at least the first 2 months after delivery*.

C. Epilepsy and birth defects: More than 90% of women with epilepsy who receive AEDs will deliver normal children free of birth defects. Major malformations and minor anomalies occur in a small but significant percentage of fetuses (6% to 8%), exposed in utero to AEDs. These children have been reported to be at increased risk for low birth weight, low Apgar scores, prematurity, microcephaly, prenatal and infant mortality, mental deficiency, development delay, and epilepsy. Risks to the fetus are probably higher when AEDs are used in combination and when there is a family history of birth defects. It is advisable to give *folate supplementation before conception and to treat with monotherapy* adjusted to the lowest effective level to avoid unnecessary fetal exposure.

VIII. *Eclampsia.*

Unique to pregnancy, eclampsia is heralded by the onset of hypertension, proteinuria, and edema, occurring after 20 weeks gestation, usually in a young primigravida. It may be complicated by oliguria or multiorgan failure. Eclampsia is also associated with chronic hypertension and renal disease. Maternal mortality ranges from 0% to 14%. There is now compelling scientific evidence in favor of magnesium sulfate rather than diazepam or phenytoin for treating eclamptic seizures. Hypertension control and fluid management are required. Delivery of the fetus and placenta is the definitive treatment for eclampsia occurring prepartum or intrapartum.

REFERENCES

Abramsky O: *Ann Neurol* 36:S38–S41, 1994.
American Academy of Neurology, Quality Standards Subcommittee: *Neurology* 51:944–948, 1998.
Delgado-Escueta AV et al: *Neurology*, 42(suppl 5):8–11, 1992.
Donaldson JO: *Neurology of pregnancy*, Philadelphia, WB Saunders, 1989.
Goldstein PJ et al: *Neurological disorders of pregnancy*, Mount Kisco, Futura, 1992.
Hiilesmaa VK: *Neurology* 42(suppl 5):149–160, 1992.
Kittner SJ et al: *N Engl J Med* 335:768–774, 1996.

PSEUDOBULBAR PALSY

Most lower brainstem nuclei are bilaterally innervated. Unilateral involvement of supranuclear pathways, therefore, may not produce symptoms. Bilateral involvement of corticobulbar fibers and frontal efferents subserving emotional expression, which pass through the genu of the internal capsule and the medial cerebral peduncles, results in pseudobulbar palsy. This should be distinguished from nuclear involvement (see Bulbar Palsy). In pseudobulbar palsy, there is decreased voluntary movement and spastic hyperreflexia of the involved muscles. Thus, gag and jaw jerk reflexes may be hyperactive, even though the patient is unable to swallow or chew. Frequently, there is a spontaneous release of emotional responses such as crying or laughing with little or no provocation (*labile emotion*). Frontal release signs (grasp, palmomental, suck, snout, rooting, and glabellar reflexes) may be prominent. These should be interpreted with caution, because many normal elderly persons (over age 80 years) exhibit palmomental and snout reflexes. Dementia is frequently present in patients with pseudobulbar palsy, except those with motor neuron disease.

Although a variety of lesions (demyelinating disease, motor neuron disease) can interrupt the corticobulbar and anterior fronto-ponto-medullary fibers, infarction is most common.

A syndrome similar to pseudobulbar palsy may occur with bilateral involvement of the opercular cortex, producing the anterior operculum syndrome (*Foix-Chavany-Marie syndrome*). It differs from classical pseudobulbar palsy in that emotional symptoms are rare, and there is loss of voluntary control of facial, pharyngeal, lingual, masticatory, or ocular muscles, with retention of reflexive and automatic movements in these muscle groups. This syndrome may be acquired or congenital as in *Worster-Drought syndrome*.

Successful treatment of pseudobulbar palsy, especially the emotional lability, has been reported with SSRIs, amitriptyline, levodopa, and amantadine.

REFERENCE

Christen HJ et al: *Dev Med Child Neurol* 42:122–132, 2000.

PSEUDOTUMOR CEREBRI

Pseudotumor cerebri (PTC) is characterized by clinical signs and symptoms of increased intracranial pressure (ICP) without evidence of intracranial mass, infection, hydrocephalus, or other apparent structural CNS pathology on neuroimaging studies and CSF exam.

Clinical features: More than 90% of PTC patients are obese and more than 90% are women. Mean age at diagnosis is about 30 years. Symptoms of PTC include increased ICP, headache (most frequent), nausea/vomiting, dizziness, tinnitus, "sounds in head," and also visual complaints and changes in visual acuity that may lead to total vision loss, diplopia, and pain on eye movements. Signs include optic disc swelling, CN VI palsy, contrast sensitivity deficits, color vision loss, constricted visual fields, and visual loss late in the course. Blind spot enlargement is always present with papilledema.

The *etiology* of PTC is unknown. Disorders associated with PTC are obesity and hypertension; rarely, PTC is associated with endocrinopathies, hyper/hypovitaminosis A, anemia, recent use of medications (tetracycline, indomethacin, nalidixic acid, nitrofurantoin, oral contraceptives, lithium), and prolonged use of corticosteroids. Systemic disorders linked with PTC include systemic lupus, hyperthyroidism, iron deficiency, and venous sinus thrombosis. An increased incidence of PTC is seen during pregnancy.

Diagnosis is made by exclusion of other causes of headache, papilledema, and increased ICP. This may require MRI and LP.

General principles of *management* include baseline and follow-up visual field and neuro-ophthalmological evaluation for perimetry, optic disc stereophotographs, visual acuity, and contrast sensitivity testing. Initial treatment is often with acetazolamide (250 to 1000 mg PO qd–tid). This is generally well tolerated, but side effects include metabolic alkalosis, paresthesias of the extremities, liver dysfunction, and allergic reactions. Furosemide has also been used. Weight loss is also essential. Repeated lumbar punctures may provide relief, and some cases may remit after LPs, necessitating ventriculoperitoneal shunting in rapidly progressing visual loss. Steroids provide symptomatic relief but increase weight and are not often useful for prolonged treatment. Acute visual loss may also be treated by optic nerve sheath decompression in patients who have failed medical therapy.

REFERENCE

Friedman DI: *Neurosurg Clin N Am* 10:609–621, 1999.

PTOSIS

DIFFERENTIAL DIAGNOSIS OF PTOSIS

I. Congenital ptosis.
   A. Isolated.
   B. With double elevator palsy.
   C. Anomalous synkinesis (including Gunn jaw winking).
   D. Lid or orbital tumor (hemangioma, dermoid).
   E. Neurofibromatosis.
   F. Blepharophimosis syndromes.
   G. First branchial arch syndromes (*Hallerman-Streiff*, *Treacher Collins*).
   H. Neonatal myasthenia.
II. Ptosis resulting from myopathy neuromuscular junction disease.
   A. Myasthenia gravis—ptosis may be variable and asymmetric. May see Cogan's lid twitch sign. Improves with edrophonium.
   B. Myopathy restricted to levator palpebrae superioris or including external ophthalmoplegia.
   C. Oculopharyngeal muscular dystrophy.
   D. Myotonic dystrophy.
   E. Polymyositis.
   F. Aplastic levator muscle.
   G. Dysthyroidism.
   H. Chronic progressive external ophthalmoplegia.
   I. Topical corticosteroid eye drops.
   J. Levator dehiscence-disinsertion syndrome. Resulting from aging, inflammation, surgery, trauma, or ocular allergy.
III. Ptosis resulting from sympathetic denervation (see Horner's syndrome).
IV. Ptosis resulting from third-nerve lesions.
   A. Nuclear lesions involving the levator subnucleus produce severe bilateral ptosis, medial rectus weakness, skew deviation if the IV nerve is involved, or upgaze paresis and pupillary dilatation if entire third-nerve nucleus is involved.
   B. Peripheral third-nerve lesions produce unilateral ptosis with mydriasis and ophthalmoplegia. Isolated ptosis is rare.
V. Pseudoptosis.
   A. Trachoma.
   B. Ptosis adiposis.
   C. Blepharochalasis.
   D. Plexiform neuroma.
   E. Amyloid infiltration.
   F. Inflammation resulting from allergy, chalazion, blepharitis, conjunctivitis.
   G. Hemangioma.

H. Duane's retraction syndrome.
I. Microphthalmos phthisis bulbi.
J. Enopthalmos.
K. Pathologic lid retraction on opposite side.
L. Chronic Bell's palsy.
M. Hypertropia.
N. Decreased mental status.
O. Hysterical.

REFERENCE

Glaser JS: *Neuro-ophthalmology*, Philadelphia, Lippincott, 1990.

PUPIL

Pupils are examined in both light and darkness, with attention to size, shape, and reactivity to light.

Bilateral dilation (mydriasis) may be produced by the following:

1. Drugs (see Table 64).
2. Emotional state.
3. Thyrotoxicosis.
4. Ciliospinal reflex.
5. Bilateral blindness resulting from severe visual system involvement anterior to the chiasm.
6. Parinaud's syndrome.
7. Seizures.
8. During rostro-caudal herniation caused by supratentorial mass lesions.

Bilateral constriction (miosis) may be produced by the following:

1. Near triad (accommodation, convergence, miosis).
2. Old age.
3. Drugs (see Table 64).
4. Pontine lesions.
5. Argyll Robertson pupils.

Anisocoria, or unequal pupil size, can be an important localizing sign. A difference of <1 mm exists in approximately 20% of the normal population; >1 mm, in as much as 5%. The asymmetry remains constant in light and dark. Drugs and toxins, including eye drops, may cause constriction or dilation of pupils, which is usually symmetric unless agents are applied locally in one eye. Causes of significant anisocoria may be determined on a clinical and pharmacologic basis using Table 65.

Causes of *episodic anisocoria* include the following:

1. Parasympathetic paresis (incipient uncal herniation, seizure, migraine).
2. Parasympathetic hyperactivity (cyclic oculomotor paresis).

TABLE 64

DRUG EFFECTS ON THE PUPILS

Constriction (Miosis)	Dilation (Mydriasis)
Systemic	
Narcotics	Anticholinergics
Morphine and opium alkaloids	Atropine
Meperidine	Belladonna
Methadone	Scopolamine
Propoxyphene	Propantheline
Barbiturates	Jimsonweed
Diphenoxylate	Nightshade
Chloral hydrate	Tricyclic antidepressants
Phenoxybenzamine	Trihexyphenidyl
Dibenzyline	Benztropine
Phentolamine	Antihistamines
Tolazoline	Diphenydramine
Guanethidine	Chlorpheniramine
Bretylium	Phenothiazines
Reserpine	Glutethimide
MAO inhibitors	Amphetamines
Alpha-methyldopa	Cocaine
Bethanidine	Ephedrine
Thymoxamine	Epinephrine
Indoramin	Norepinephrine
Meprobamate	Ethanol
Cholinergics	Botulinum toxin
Edrophonium	Snake venom
Neostigmine	Barracuda poisoning
Pyridostigmine	Tyramine
Cholinesterase inhibitor pesticides	Hemicholinium
Phencyclidine	Hypermagnesemia
Thallium	Thiopental
Lidocaine and related agents	Lysergic acid diethylamide
Marijuana	Fenfluramine (patients receiving reserpine)
Phenothiazines	
Local	
Miotics	Mydriatics and cycloplegics
Pilocarpine	Phenylephrine
Carbachol	Hydroxyamphetamine
Methacholine	Epinephrine
Physostigmine	Cocaine
Neostigmine	Eucatropine
Isoflurophate	Atropine
Echothiophate	Homatropine
Demecarium	Scopolamine
Aceclidine	Cyclopentolate
	Tropicamide
	Oxyphenonium

Adapted from Thurston SE, Leigh RJ: In Henning RJ, Jackson DL, eds: *Handbook of critical care neurology and neurosurgery,* New York, Praeger, 1985.

TABLE 65

CHARACTERISTICS OF PUPILS ENCOUNTERED IN NEURO-OPHTHALMOLOGY

	General Characteristics	Responses to Light and Near Stimuli	Room Condition in Which Anisocoria is Greater	Response to Mydriatics	Response to Miotics	Response to Pharmacologic Agents
Essential anisocoria	Round, regular	Both brisk	No change	Dilates	Constricts	Normal and rarely needed
Horner's syndrome	Small, round, unilateral	Both brisk	Darkness	Dilates	Constricts	Cocaine 4%, poor dilation; paredrine 1%, no dilation if third-order neuron damage
Tonic pupil syndrome (Holmes-Adie syndrome)	Usually larger* in bright light; sector pupil palsy, vermiform movement; unilateral or, less often, bilateral	Absent to light, tonic to near; tonic redilation	Light	Dilates	Constricts	Pilocarpine 0.1% or 0.125% constricts; mecholyl 2.5% constricts
Argyll Robertson pupils	Small, irregular, bilateral	Poor to light, better to near	No change	Poor	Constricts	
Midbrain pupils	Mid-dilated; may be oval; bilateral	Poor to light, better to near (or fixed to both)	No change	Dilates	Constricts	
Pharmacologically dilated pupils	Very large†, round, unilateral	Fixed†	Light		No‡	Pilocarpine 1% does not constrict
Oculomotor palsy (nonvascular)	Mid-dilated (6–7 mm), unilateral (rarely bilateral)	Fixed	Light	Dilates	Constricts	

From Glaser JS: *Neuro-ophthalmology,* Philadelphia, Lippincott, 1989.

*Tonic pupil may appear smaller following prolonged near-effort or in dim illumination; affected pupil is initially large, but with passing time gradually becomes smaller.

† Atropinized pupils have diameters of 8 to 9 mm. No tonic, midbrain, or oculomotor palsy pupil ever is this large.

‡ Pupils may be weakly reactive, depending on interim after instillation.

3. Sympathetic paresis (cluster headache [paratrigeminal neuralgia]).
4. Sympathetic hyperactivity (*Claude-Bernard syndrome* following neck trauma).
5. Sympathetic dysfunction with alternating anisocoria (cervical spinal cord lesions).
6. Benign unilateral pupillary dilation (involved pupil has normal light and near responses).

Relative afferent pupillary defect (RAPD) (see Figure 38), also called *Marcus-Gunn pupil*, results from a lesion of the optic nerve. Resting pupil sizes are normal. Both direct and consensual pupillary responses are

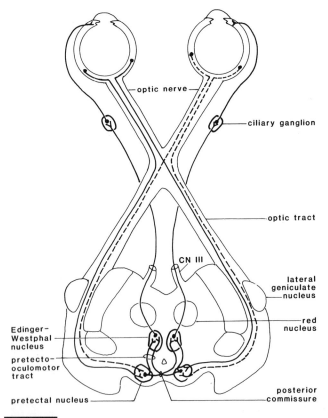

FIGURE 38

Pupillary light reflex pathways.

decreased with bright illumination of the involved side, whereas both responses are normal with illumination of the normal side. When alternately stimulating each eye ("swinging flashlight test"), both pupils dilate with stimulation on the abnormal side, and both constrict with the stimulation on the normal side.

The near reflex should be tested whenever pupils react poorly to light. Have the patient fixate a distant target, then quickly fixate his own fingertip held immediately in front of his nose.

Light-near dissociation may occur in the following:

1. Severe anterior visual dysfunction (such as severe glaucoma, bilateral optic neuropathy).
2. Neurosyphilis (*Argyll Robertson pupil*).
3. Adie's tonic pupil: *Holmes-Adie's syndrome* in which nearly 90% of the people have diminished deep tendon reflexes and orthostatic hypotension. Seventy percent are females. In 80% of patients, there is unilateral involvement, although the second pupil may become involved later.
4. Rostral dorsal midbrain syndrome (*Parinaud's syndrome*).
5. Aberrant III nerve regeneration.
6. Diabetes (out of proportion to any retinopathy).
7. Amyloidosis.
8. Myotonic dystrophy.

Lesions of the midbrain.
Efferent pupillary defects may occur with lesions involving the oculomotor nucleus or the fascicles of the third nerve coursing ventrally to exit the brainstem. Generally other signs of brainstem involvement or third-nerve palsy will also be apparent.

Three syndromes are clinically important:

1. *Argyll Robertson pupil:* Some patients have tertiary syphilis involving the central nervous system. Affected patients have small irregular pupils less than ~2 mm, which do not react to light with normal near response (light-near dissociation) and visual acuity. Similar pupils are seen in diabetes mellitus, chronic alcoholism, and encephalitis.
2. *Parinaud dorsal midbrain syndrome:* Seen in pineal tumors. Pupils are midposition with light-near dissociation. Afferent pupillary pathways in the pretectum are usually affected. Dorsal midbrain syndrome also causes paresis of conjugate up gaze (occasionally down), convergence retraction nystagmus, lid lag, and *Collier's sign* (lid retraction).
3. *Pretectal afferent pupillary defects:* Occasionally a pretectal lesion will be predominantly unilateral and hence produce RAPD.

REFERENCE

Loewenfield IE: *The pupil: anatomy, physiology and clinical applications*, vol 1, Ames, IA, Iowa State University, 1993.

R

RADIATION INJURY

Injury to the nervous system occurs either as a result of treatment of CNS tumors or when nervous tissue falls into the field of treatment of another organ system. The five major manifestations of radiation injury are outlined as follows.

I. Cerebral injury.
   A. *Acute encephalopathy* occurs during the first few days of radiotherapy with headache, fever, nausea, depressed sensorium, and worsening of previous focal deficits. It is more frequent and severe in patients with large brain masses or those receiving daily dose fractions greater than 300 cGy of whole-brain irradiation. It is probably caused by increases in preexisting cerebral edema and responds well to increased corticosteroid dose. It may be prevented by use of corticosteroid 24 to 72 hours before radiotherapy.
   B. *Early delayed encephalopathy* occurs 1 to 4 months after irradiation, becomes evident as headache, somnolence, nausea, irritability, fever, and transient papilledema, and usually resolves after several weeks. It occurs in 40% to 60% of pediatric patients with leukemia who are receiving 1800 to 2400 cGy of prophylactic whole brain irradiation. Corticosteroids may be beneficial. This syndrome may be due to damaged myelin and glia.
   C. *Focal cerebral necrosis* may develop several months to 10 years after focal or whole brain irradiation and becomes evident as a subacutely evolving mass lesion. Frequency is 3% to 5% after receiving 5000 cGy of radiation. "Tolerable" dose estimates vary (up to 6500 to 7000 cGy), but above the critical exposure level the frequency increases markedly. Peritumoral edema may predispose to injury, and corticosteroids may be protective. CT or MRI show edema and a patchy or ring-enhancing mass lesion. PET scanning may help differentiate cerebral necrosis from tumor recurrence. Corticosteroids frequently cause improvement, albeit temporary. Radiation necrosis occurs around the tumor and primarily involves the white matter, mostly sparing of cortex and deep gray structures, with demyelination, loss of oligodendrocytes, axonal loss and swelling, calcification, fibrillary gliosis, and mononuclear perivascular infiltrate with extensive vascular injury.
   D. *Diffuse cerebral injury*, the most frequent (2% to 19%) delayed effect of radiation therapy, occurs in adults with primary brain tumors receiving 4000 to 6000 cGy of whole brain irradiation and becomes evident as moderate to severe cortical dysfunction, progressive dementia, and gait disturbance. On pathologic study cerebral atrophy, diffuse demyelination, and spongiform changes with sparing of axons and blood vessels are present.

E. *Leukoencephalopathy* occurs 4 to 24 months after CNS irradiation, primarily in children who have received radiation therapy and chemotherapy (especially high dose methotrexate). Initial signs include memory, attentional, and visuospatial difficulties (especially in children younger than 4 or 5 years of age); ataxia; and focal motor deficits. CT or MRI shows enlarged ventricles, widened sulci, areas of calcification (especially basal ganglia), and areas of decreased density or signal. Pathologic study shows multifocal white matter destruction, especially in the centrum semiovale and periventricular white matter, dystrophic calcification of the lenticular nuclei, and mineralizing microangiopathy.

II. Spinal cord injury

A. *Transient myelopathy*, the most common radiation-induced spinal injury, usually occurs 1 to 30 months after completion of radiotherapy, with peak onset at 4 to 6 months. There is a positive correlation with radiation dose greater than 3500 to 4400 cGy. Lhermitte's sign (paresthesias radiating down the spine and limbs, precipitated by neck flexion) is often present. Myelopathic signs are usually absent. CT, MRI, and myelography results are normal. The syndrome resolves gradually over 1 to 9 months without risk of delayed, severe radiation myelopathy.

B. *Delayed progressive myelopathy* has a peak time of onset of 9 to 18 months after radiotherapy and a reported frequency of 1% to 2%. Risk is mostly correlated with the dose and dose schedule; risk is less than 5% with total doses of 4500 cGy in daily fractions of 180 cGy. Delayed progressive myelopathy usually begins with hypoesthesias or dysesthesias in lower extremities, then weakness and sphincter dysfunction. The level of dysfunction ascends up to the area irradiated. Symptoms progress over weeks to months, with paraplegia or quadriplegia in about 50% of those affected by this syndrome. Results of imaging studies are usually normal but may show focal or diffuse fusiform spinal cord enlargement. CSF is usually normal but may show increased levels of protein or white blood cells. The clinical picture may stabilize spontaneously or improve temporarily with corticosteroid therapy. Pathologic study shows coalescing foci of demyelination and axonal degeneration more severe in white than in gray matter, especially in the posterior columns and superficial lateral tracts.

C. *Motor neuron syndrome*. Beginning 4 to 14 months after radiotherapy, this rare syndrome becomes evident as subacute, diffuse leg weakness, atrophy, fasciculations, depressed deep tendon reflexes, and flexor planter responses without sensory or sphincter involvement. Symptoms gradually progress over several months, then stabilize without improvement. Results of EMG show diffuse denervation. CSF may be normal or have slight increase in protein level. This syndrome may result from damage to lumbosacral anterior horn cells, motor axons, or nerve roots.

III. Peripheral nerve. Radiation plexopathy of the brachial or lumbosacral plexuses must be distinguished from recurrent tumor. Radiation plexopathies tend to have less pain, more weakness, and myokymia on EMG. Contrast-enhanced CT or MRI also helps differentiate these conditions.

IV. Cerebrovascular disease. Extracranial carotid disease, with transient ischemic attacks or strokes, may develop 6 months to many years (median, 19 years) after radiation therapy. Occlusive disease of the intracranial arteries follows irradiation of optic gliomas, pituitary, or suprasellar tumors (2 to 20 years later; median, 5 years later). The most frequent finding on arteriography is narrowing or occlusion of the supraclinoid internal carotid artery, and two-thirds of patients may show a "moyamoya" pattern.

V. Radiation-induced tumors. In order of decreasing frequency, meningiomas, sarcomas, and gliomas may occur after radiation therapy. Meningiomas have a latency of 15 to 50 years after irradiation, and gliomas may develop around 10 years after irradiation. Diagnosis of a radiation-induced malignancy depends on the following:

1. The second tumor should occur within the field of radiation.
2. There should be a significant delay between end of irradiation and appearance of the secondary tumor.
3. The primary and secondary tumors must have different histologic features.
4. There should be no family history of neurocutaneous syndromes.

REFERENCES

Dropcho EJ: *Neuro Clin* 9(4):969–988, 1991.
Duffner PK, Cohen ME: *Neuro Clin* 9(2):479–495, 1991.
Gutin PH, Leibel SA, Sheline GE, eds: *Radiation injury to the nervous system*, New York, Raven, 1991.

RADICULOPATHY

Radiculopathy is usually manifested by radiating pain, weakness, loss of deep tendon reflexes, and sensory changes in a segmental distribution. Neck or lower back pain and stiffness are common in cervical and lumbar radiculopathies, respectively. Symptoms may be aggravated by sneezing, coughing, straining with defecation, or neck or trunk movement. Bed rest usually offers relief. On examination, straight leg raising sign may be present in cases of lumbar radiculopathy. Crossed straight leg raising usually indicates a larger lesion. An isolated root lesion may result in a smaller area of sensory disturbance than expected by standard dermatomal maps due to cutaneous nerve overlap. Hyporeflexia is restricted to the involved root level. Weaknesses may occur in the appropriate myotomal distribution and may indicate a larger lesion with greater anterior root involvement. Central lumbar lesions may result in a cauda equina syndrome. Central disc herniation is relatively uncommon as a cause of radiculopathy.

Differential diagnosis: Although herniated intervertebral disc material is the most common cause of radiculopathy, other mass lesions and structural abnormalities should be excluded. These may include tumors, epidural abscess, spondylosis, brachial or lumbar plexopathy, and peripheral neuropathy.

Diagnostic studies should include plain x-rays with oblique views. Nerve conduction studies and EMG may identify evidence of denervation in a root distribution and exclude more peripheral lesions. Myelogram followed by CT is being supplanted in many centers by MRI.

Treatment of disc disease should begin conservatively with bed rest (acutely), traction, and nonsteroidal anti-inflammatory agents. *The majority of patients improve with time regardless of the type of intervention.* Surgical decompression is indicated when symptoms are unresponsive to conservative therapy, there is progressive weakness, or when central herniation results in myelopathy or a cauda equina syndrome.

COMMON CERVICAL ROOT SYNDROMES

1. *C5 radiculopathy* (C4-5 disc space): Pain and sensory loss in the shoulder and anterior and lateral arm. Hyporeflexia in biceps and brachioradialis. Weakness of the deltoid, external rotators of arm, and forearm flexors. Diaphragmatic paresis may occur rarely, owing to C5 fibers within the phrenic nerve.
2. *C6 radiculopathy* (C5-C6 disc space, the second most common level of cervical radiculopathy): Pain and sensory loss in the lateral arm and forearm and first and second digits. Hyporeflexia of biceps and brachioradialis. Weakness of forearm flexion, arm pronation, and finger and wrist extension.
3. *C7 radiculopathy* (C6-7 disc space, most common level of disc herniation): Pain and sensory loss in the posterior arm and third and fourth digits. Hyporeflexia in triceps. Weakness of triceps and wrist extensors.
4. *C8 radiculopathy* (C7-T1 disc space): Pain and sensory loss in the medial forearm and hand and fifth digit. Hyporeflexia in finger flexors. Weakness of the intrinsic hand muscles. Ipsilateral Horner's may be present.

COMMON LUMBAR ROOT SYNDROMES

1. *L4 radiculopathy* (L3-4 disc space): Pain and sensory loss in the hip and anterolateral thigh, knee, anteromedial leg, medial foot, and possibly great toe diminished patellar reflex weakness of quadriceps, anterior tibialis, and sartorius.

2. *L5 radiculopathy* (L4-5 disc space): Pain and sensory loss in the hip and lateral thigh (mainly pain), anterolateral leg, dorsum of foot, and medial toes (including great toe). Patellar and Achilles reflexes are spared. Weakness of peroneus, toe extensors, anterior tibialis, and gluteus medius and minimus.

3. *S1 radiculopathy* (L5-S1 disc space): Pain and sensory loss in buttock and posterior thigh (mainly pain), posterolateral leg, lateral foot, lateral toes, and heel. Hyporeflexia in ankle (Achilles). Weakness of hamstrings, gluteus maximus, and plantar flexors of foot and toes. S1-5 radiculopathies (see Cauda Equina).

REFERENCES

Argoff CA et al: *Neurol Clin* 16:833–850, 1998.
Brazis PW, Masdeu JC, Biller J: *Localization in clinical neurology*, Boston, Little Brown, 1996.
Yonenobu K: *Eur Spine J* 9:1–7, 2000.

REFLEX SYMPATHETIC DYSTROPHY (*see Complex Regional Pain Syndrome*)

REFLEXES

Evaluate latency of response, degree of activity, and duration of the contraction. Reflexes should be both observed and palpated. Compare right and left sides. In general, reflexes are not pathologic if they are symmetric unless they are absent or 4+ (see Table 66).

Hyporeflexia results from dysfunction of any part of the reflex arc. Conditions include neuropathy, radiculopathy, tabes dorsalis, syringomyelia, intramedullary tumors, and spinal motor neuron dysfunction. Bilateral hyporeflexia is the hallmark of neuropathies. Isolated, unilateral absent reflexes suggest radiculopathy. Hyporeflexia may occur in late stages of primary muscle diseases because of loss of muscle mass. Areflexia with rapidly progressive weakness and only mild sensory loss is the hallmark of Guillain-Barré syndrome. Hyporeflexia is seen transiently in acute upper motor neuron lesions such as cerebral infarction or spinal cord compression (spinal shock). Prolongation of both the contraction and relax-

TABLE 66
GRADING OF MUSCLE STRETCH REFLEXES

0	Absent, abnormal
1+	Diminished, may or may not be abnormal
2+	Normal
3+	Increased, may or may not be abnormal
4+	Markedly increased, abnormal. May be associated with clonus

ation times ("hung-up" reflex) is seen with hypothyroidism. This prolongation is most evident in the knee jerks. Areflexia may be a component of Adie's syndrome (see Pupil) (see also Hypotonic Infant).

Hyperreflexia usually results from an upper motor neuron lesion with loss of corticospinal inhibition. The extrapyramidal system may also play a role. Involvement may occur anywhere from the cortical Betz cell to just proximal to the spinal cord motor neuron. Unilateral hyperreflexia results from a unilateral lesion anywhere along the corticospinal tract, most commonly in the cerebral hemispheres or brainstem. Bilateral hyperreflexia occurs more commonly with myelopathy but also occurs with bilateral cerebral hemisphere or brainstem involvement. Symmetric, 3 + reflexes in the absence of clonus, Babinski, Tromner's, or Hoffmann's signs, or weakness and with a normal result of neurologic examination is usually benign. Reflexes are variable (usually normal) with extrapyramidal system dysfunction. Reflexes are normal, slightly decreased, or pendular with cerebellar tract dysfunction (see also Rigidity, Spasticity).

"Pathologic reflexes" (pyramidal tract reflexes) indicate upper motor neuron dysfunction. The extensor plantar response (Babinski's sign) consists

R

REFLEXES

TABLE 67

SEGMENTAL MUSCLE STRETCH AND CUTANEOUS REFLEXES

Reflex	Level	Nerve
Muscle Stretch ("Deep Tendon") Reflexes		
Jaw (masseter and temporal muscle)	CN V	Mandibular branch
Biceps	C5, 6	Musculocutaneous
Brachioradialis	C5, 6	Radial
Pectoral major	C5, 6, 7	Lateral pectoral
Triceps	C6, 7, 8	Radial
Finger flexors	C8	Medial (ulnar)
Adductor	L2, 3, 4	Obturator
Quadriceps (patellar knee jerks)	L2, 3, 4	Femoral
Internal hamstring	L4, 5, S1	Sciatic
External hamstring	L5, S1	Sciatic
Gastrocnemius-soleus (Achilles, ankle jerks)	L5, S1, 2	Tibial
Cutaneous ("Superficial") Reflexes		
Corneal	Pons	CN V (afferent), VII (efferent)
Pharyngeal Gag reflex	Medulla	CN IX (afferent), X (efferent)
Upper abdominal	T6–9	
Middle abdominal	T9–11	
Lower abdominal	T11–L1	
Cremasteric	L1, 2	Femoral (afferent), genitofemoral (efferent)
Plantar	L5, S1, 2	Tibial
Anal	S3, 4, 5	Pudendal
Bulbocavernosus	S3, 4	Puendal, pelvic autonomics

of dorsiflexion of the great toe and fanning of the remaining toes on stimulating the plantar surface of the foot. Hoffmann and Tromner signs are elicited by "flicking" the index or middle finger down or up, respectively, producing flexion of the thumb; they may be normal if present bilaterally, especially if reflexes are 3 + and symmetric. Ankle clonus is the continuing rapid flexion and extension of the foot elicited by forcibly and quickly dorsiflexing the foot. Pyramidal tract reflexes are normally present in infants (see Child Neurology).

Segmental muscle stretch and cutaneous reflexes are listed in Table 67.

RESTLESS LEGS SYNDROME (Ekbom Syndrome)

Restless legs syndrome is characterized by ill-defined, deep, "crawling" paresthesias in the lower legs, thighs, and occasionally, the arms; it is usually bilateral and occurs especially while at rest or during drowsiness, resulting in insomnia. There is a strong impulse to move or walk, to avoid the sensations. It is usually intermittent and lasts from minutes to hours. There is frequently an overlap between the restless legs syndrome and periodic movements of sleep (nocturnal myoclonic movements consisting of discrete, brief, repetitive flexion at the hips, knees, and thighs during light sleep). There may be a familial predisposition. Some similarities exist between this syndrome and growing pains in children.

A variety of conditions have been described in association with restless legs syndrome, including the following.

Uremia.
Pregnancy.
Iron deficiency anemia.
Exposure to cold.
Parkinson's disease.
Vitamin deficiencies.
Hyperlipidemia.
Prochlorperazine.

Chronic obstructive pulmonary disease.
Carcinoma.
Diabetes.
Acute intermittent porphyria.
Amyloidosis.
Caffeine.
Barbiturate withdrawal.

Treatment involves correcting the underlying condition. Diazepam, clonazepam, baclofen, dopamine agonists (levodopa and bromocriptine), carbamazepine, propoxyphene, and amitriptyline have been used with varying success. Recently, Pramipexole has been shown to be quite effective, Its tendency to cause paroxysmal sedation may be obviated if it is given only at bedtime.

REFERENCES

Ekbom KA: Neurology 10:388, 1960.
Mahowald MW, Ettinger MG: J Clin Neurophysiol 7:119–143, 1990.
Montplaisir J, et al: Neurology 52(5):938–943, 1999.
Walters AS, Hening WA, Chokroverty S: Mov Disord 6:105–110, 1991.

RETINA AND UVEAL TRACT

I. Systemic and neurologic disorders associated with retinal pigmentary degeneration.

A. Typical retinitis pigmentosa changes include early-onset nyctalopia, progressive visual loss, bone spicules, narrowing of retinal arterioles, and electroretinogram (ERG) changes. They may be associated with the following:

1. Myotonic dystrophy (rarely).
2. Leber's congenital amaurosis.
3. Senear-Loken disease (Leber's + juvenile nephronophthisis).
4. Friedreich's ataxia (may also rarely be associated with optic atrophy and deafness).
5. Spielmeyer-Vogt disease.
6. Neonatal and childhood adrenoleukodystrophy.
7. Usher's syndrome (vestibulocochlear dysfunction, mutism).
8. Pelizaeus-Merzbacher disease (mental retardation, ataxia).
9. Hallgren's disease (mental retardation, ataxia, deafness).

B. Atypical central and peripheral retinal pigmentary changes with variable degrees of visual impairment. The presumed mechanism in storage diseases is disruption of pigment epithelial function by accumulated metabolic material with secondary retinal receptor degeneration. Primary rod or cone dystrophy may exist in the first four of the following syndromes.

1. Laurence-Moon-Biedl (hypogenitalism, mental retardation, polydactyly).
2. Biemond (hypogenitalism, mental retardation, iris coloboma).
3. Alström (hypogenitalism, deafness, diabetes mellitus).
4. Bassen-Kornzweig (abetalipoproteinemia, ataxia, acanthocytosis).
5. Refsum's disease (polyneuropathy, ataxia).
6. Sjögren-Larsson syndrome (ichthyosis, spastic paresis, mental retardation).
7. Amalric-Dialinos syndrome (deafness).
8. Cockayne's syndrome (dwarfism, neuropathy, deafness).
9. Hallervorden-Spatz syndrome (neuropathy, basal ganglia degeneration).
10. Alport's syndrome (nephritis, hearing loss).
11. Hurler's (mucopolysaccharidosis [MPS]1), Hunter's (MPS II), Sanfilippo's (MPS III), and Scheie's disease (MPS V).

C. Postinflammatory.

1. Congenital and acquired syphilis.
2. Congenital rubella (German measles)—"salt and pepper fundus."
3. Congenital rubeola (measles).

D. Avitaminoses and vitamin metabolism disorders.

1. Pellagra.
2. Vitamin B_{12} metabolism disorder associated with aminoaciduria.

     E. Toxic.
       1. Chlorpromazine.
       2. Thioridazine.
       3. Indomethacin.
  II. Hereditary cerebromacular dystrophies.
     A. With cherry red spot of the macula.
       1. Sphingolipidoses—Tay-Sachs, Niemann-Pick, Gaucher's, metachromatic leukodystrophy (infantile form), Sandhoff's.
       2. Mucolipidoses—GM_1 gangliosidosis, Farber's syndrome.
       3. Mucolipidosis I.
       4. Mucopolysaccharidoses—Hurler's (MPS I), MPS VII.
       5. Goldberg's disease.
     B. Without cherry red spot.
       1. Ceroid lipofuscinoses—Jansky-Bielschowsky disease.
       2. Batten-Mayou, Spielmyer-Vogt disease.
       3. Kufs-Hallervorden.
  III. CNS vasculitides.
     All vasculitides may involve the retinal circulation with variable manifestations (arterial occlusive retinopathy, hemorrhages, retinal infiltrates).
  IV. Phakomatoses.
     A. Vascular malformations of the choroid or retina and the CNS.
       1. Von Hippel-Lindau syndrome (retinal angiomas and cerebellar hemangioblastomas).
       2. Sturge-Weber syndrome (choroidal hemangioma, parieto-occipital arteriovenous malformations [AVMs]).
       3. Wyburn-Mason syndrome (AVMs in the retina and brainstem).
       4. Retinal cavernous hemangioma (unclassified phakomatosis, rarely associated with intracranial AVMs).
     B. Retinal and intracranial tumors.
       1. Tuberous sclerosis.
       2. Neurofibromatosis.
  V. Dystrophies of the uvea.
     A. Angioid streaks (ruptures of Bruch's membrane) occur in the following diseases, which may be associated with neurologic dysfunction.
       1. Francois dyscephalic syndrome.
       2. Paget's disease.
       3. Acromegaly.
       4. Sickle cell anemia.
     B. Gillespie's syndrome (aniridia, ataxia, psychomotor retardation).
  VI. Retinovitreal syndromes and vitreal involvement.
     A. Wagner's vitreoretinopathy (rarely associated with encephaloceles).
     B. Dominant familial amyloidosis (diffuse vitreous opacification)
       Table 68 summarizes the diseases that affect retinal and uveal tract and CNS.

TABLE 68

DISEASES THAT MAY INVOLVE THE UVEAL TRACT AND CENTRAL NERVOUS SYSTEM

Infections

Bacterial
Meningococcus
Syphilis
Tuberculosis
Whipple's disease
Brucellosis
Leptospirosis
Listeriosis
Borrelia—Lyme disease

Parasitic
Trypanosomiasis
Toxoplasmosis
Ameliosis
Malaria

Viral
Cytomegalovirus
Herpes simplex
Herpes zoster
Varicella
Mumps
Rubella
Rubeola
Subacute sclerosing panencephalitis
Variola

Fungal
Aspergillosis
Candidiasis
Cryptococcosis
Histoplasmosis
Mucormycosis

Granulomatous Disease
Sarcoidosis
Wegener's granulomatosis

Collagen Vascular Disease
Systemic lupus erythematosus
Temporal arteritis
Polyarteritis

Neoplasms
Leukemia
Metastatic carcinoma
Reticulum cell sarcoma

Other
Behçet's syndrome
Multiple sclerosis
Sympathetic ophthalmia
Trauma
Uveal effusion
Vogt-Koyanagi-Harada
  (uveomeningoencephalitic)
  syndrome
Bing's syndrome (chorioretinitis,
  ophthalmoplegia,
  macroglobulinemia)
Romberg's syndrome (posterior
  uveitis, ophthalmoplegia,
  trigeminal neuralgia, seizures,
  unilateral facial atrophy)

Adapted from Finelli PF et al: *Ann Neurol* 1:247–252, 1977

REFERENCE

Nussenblatt RB, Palestine AG: *Uveitis*, St. Louis, Mosby, 1989.

RHEUMATOID ARTHRITIS

Neurologic complications usually occur in patients with moderate to severe rheumatoid arthritis (RA) and consist of neuropathy, myopathy, myelopathy, and involvement of the brain and meninges; subclinical involvement may occur earlier.

Peripheral neuropathy is the most frequent complication of RA and has three main types:

1. Most common are entrapment neuropathies, resulting from inflammation around the joints causing nerve compression. Carpal tunnel

syndrome is the most common. Other nerves involved include ulnar (at wrist or elbow), posterior interosseous (at elbow), posterior tibial (at popliteal fossa or tarsal tunnel), peroneal (at popliteal fossa), and medial and lateral plantar.

2. Distal sensory neuropathy may be asymptomatic or can cause dysesthesias. Vibration is most frequently involved, but all sensory modalities are affected. Segmental demyelination is the presumed cause.

3. Mononeuritis multiplex is usually of sudden onset from ischemic injury, causing both demyelination and axonal loss. It may be severe and may result in quadriparesis. Autonomic dysfunction can also occur.

Myelopathy from subluxation of the cervical spine is frequently observed in severe RA. Atlantoaxial subluxation, separation of the anterior arch of the atlas from the dens by greater than 3 mm, is most frequent. Lateral cervical spine films during *active* flexion and extension are usually sufficient for diagnosis. MRI, CT, myelography, and vertebral angiography may be needed in selected cases. Vertical upward subluxation of the odontoid process from lack of lateral support of the atlas usually occurs on the background of atlantoaxial subluxation. Atlantoaxial subluxation may cause myelopathy, headaches, hydrocephalus, or lead to brainstem deficits from direct medullary compression or vertebral artery involvement. Sensory loss in the trigeminal and C2 distributions, nystagmus, and pyramidal tract signs can result. Basilar invagination, the penetration of the odontoid through the foramen magnum with compression of ventral medulla, is occasionally seen.

Complications affecting *muscle* include disuse atrophy, focal myositis (usually adjacent to actively involved joints), disseminated nodular myositis (non-necrotizing lymphocytic and plasma cell perivascular infiltrates), steroid myopathy, polymyositis (rare, more malignant course), and ischemia due to vasculitis.

CNS complications of RA include temporal arteritis, vasculitis (systemic vasculitis or isolated CNS angiitis), cranial neuropathies, infarction, hemorrhage, and encephalopathy, dural nodules (often asymptomatic), rheumatoid pachymeningitis (seizures and encephalopathy), and hyperviscosity syndrome (rare).

Neurologic symptoms may also be caused by drugs used to treat RA, such as gold (myokymia and peripheral neuropathy with rapid onset suggestive of Guillain-Barré syndrome), steroids (myopathy), chloroquine (neuropathy, myopathy or retinopathy), and penicillamine (reversible form of myasthenia gravis or inflammatory myopathy).

REFERENCES

Bekkelund SI et al: *J Rheumatol* 26:2348–2351, 1999.
Brick JE et al: *Neurol Clin* 7:629–639, 1989.
Dreyer SJ et al: *Clin Orthop* 366:98–106, 1999.

RIGIDITY

Rigidity is a form of increased muscle tone that is present throughout the range of motion of a limb (compare Spasticity). When released, the right limb does not spring back to its original position. Rigidity is not associated with increased reflexes. EMG reveals persistent motor unit activity during apparent relaxation.

Forms of rigidity include the following:

1. Cogwheel rigidity: An increased resistance to stretch interrupted by rhythmic yielding (that is, variable resistance) seen in extrapyramidal disease.
2. Lead-pipe rigidity: Constant resistance to movement of a limb, which may maintain its position at the end of the displacement, may also be seen in catatonia.
3. Gegenhalten or paratonia: Refers to increasing tone equal in response to increasing effort to move a limb passively throughout its range of motion (that is, velocity and load-dependent resistance), seen in bilateral frontal lobe or mesial basal temporal lobe disease, encephalopathies, and dementias.

The following are not true rigidity:

1. Voluntary rigidity: Agonist-antagonist cocontraction associated with heightened emotional states.
2. Involuntary rigidity: For example, an acute condition in the abdomen.
3. Hysterical rigidity.
4. Reflex rigidity: Spasms in response to pain or cold.
5. Decorticate and decerebrate posturing are imprecise terms. Decorticate posturing is a slow, stereotyped flexion of arm, wrist, and fingers with adduction at the shoulder and leg extension with plantar flexion of the foot. It occurs with supratentorial processes compressing the diencephalon. Decerebrate posturing is pronation of the arm with adduction and internal rotation of the leg, along with plantar flexion of the foot. It occurs with more caudal compression of the midbrain and rostral pons. Extension in the arms with flexion or flaccidity in the legs is associated with lesions of the pontine tegmentum (see also Herniation).

ROMBERG SIGN

A test comparing the stability of a person standing with both feet together and eyes open to that with eyes closed. A normal response is a slight increase in sway. A marked increase in sway indicates proprioceptive sensory loss. Increased sway may also indicate cerebellar ataxia, vestibulopathy, frontal lobe impairment, or other motor impairment. Patients with cerebellar or vestibular dysfunction tend to fall toward the side of the lesion.

S

SARCOIDOSIS

Sarcoidosis is a multisystem disorder of unknown etiology characterized by noncaseating granulomas in affected tissues. The disease may affect any organ, and the nervous system is affected in 5% of cases of sarcoidosis. Generally it affects young adults and is more common in blacks. It usually begins with bilateral hilar adenopathy, pulmonary infiltrate, uveitis, or skin lesion. Hypercalcemia and hypercalciuria are common.

MANIFESTATIONS OF NEUROSARCOIDOSIS

1. Muscle: Slowly progressive myopathy with proximal weakness.
2. Peripheral nerve: Mononeuritis multiplex, polyneuropathy, Guillain-Barré syndrome, polyradiculopathy.
3. Cranial nerves: Peripheral facial nerve palsy of one or both sides is common. Other cranial nerves can be affected, but ophthalmoplegia is rare. A paralyzed pupil is an occasional finding. Deafness may occur.
4. Spinal cord: May be compressed by an extramedullary or intramedullary granuloma. Spinal block may occur.
5. Intracranial: Most common presentations relate to basilar meningitis with involvement of neighboring structures (cranial nerves, hypothalamus, pituitary), obstruction of CSF pathways, and hydrocephalus. Mass lesions are often found in the hypothalamic region. Infrequently neurosarcoidosis comes to medical attention as a mass lesion mistaken for a meningioma before surgery.
6. Opportunistic infections occur because of defective immune system or as treatment complication and may include tuberculous meningitis, progressive multifocal leukoencephalopathy, nocardiosis, herpes simplex encephalitis, and cryptococcal meningitis.

DIAGNOSTIC TESTS

Definitive diagnosis is based on biopsy demonstration of typical granulomas. CT and MRI are helpful in localizing CNS lesion. Gallium scan helps in detecting systemic involvement and is more sensitive than chest X-ray. CSF examination may show increased protein level, pleocytosis, and low glucose level. Oligoclonal bands and high IgG index may occur. Angiotensin-converting enzyme has 56% to 86% sensitivity in serum but is not specific. Its level in CSF is presumed to reflect CNS disease activity.

TREATMENT AND PROGNOSIS

A regimen of prednisone, 40 to 80 mg daily, is the mainstay of treatment. If treatment fails or if corticosteroids cannot be tapered, cytotoxic agents may be added. Most patients respond to treatment but one third relapse when treatment is discontinued. Prognosis is usually better when disease is limited to peripheral nerve. Effective response to radiotherapy for intracranial sarcoidosis has been reported.

REFERENCES

Belfer MH, Stevens RW. Am Fam Physician 58(9):2041–2050, 1998.
Scott TF: *Neurology* 43:8–12, 1993.

SEPSIS

Sepsis is the constellation of active infection and changes in respiratory rate, pulse, and fever. Neurologic complications most frequently include obtundation (up to 70%) and less commonly include paratonic rigidity, seizures, and asterixis. It is important to distinguish septic encephalopathy from disorders producing primary neurologic disease (for example, meningitis, stroke, brain abscess), other metabolic encephalopathies (for example, hypoxia, hypo- and hyperglycemia, thyrotoxicosis, adrenal failure, Reye's syndrome), drug reactions, hematologic conditions (such as hyperviscosity syndromes, primary disseminated intravascular coagulation, leukemia, sickle cell crises) and other disorders of thermoregulation.

Neuromuscular complications of sepsis include critical illness polyneuropathy, a pure axonal sensorimotor polyneuropathy presenting as respiratory failure, distal weakness, and reduced reflexes with relative sparing of cranial musculature. This condition has been associated with the use of high-dose corticosteroids, particularly in combination with neuromuscular blocking agents having a steroid structure (e.g., pancuronium). Prognosis for recovery is often poor.

Other syndromes include disuse atrophy and myositis. These conditions need to be distinguished from Guillain-Barré syndrome, nutritional deficiency neuropathies, paraneoplastic syndromes, and neuromuscular blockade from some antibiotics (such as aminoglycosides).

REFERENCES

Bolton CF et al: *Ann Neurol* 33:94–100, 1993.
Vincent JL: *Lancet* 351:922–923, 1998.
Wanze RP et al: *Clin Infect Dis* 22:407–412, 1996.

SHUNTS

Ventriculoperitoneal (VP) shunts are favored in infants and growing children because extra tubing can be left in the peritoneal cavity, allowing for growth and extending the time between shunt revisions. Ventriculojugular (VJ) shunts may be used after major growth is completed; complications (thrombi, endocarditis, septic or tubing emboli, and arrhythmias) are more frequent and serious than with VP shunts. Lumboperitoneal (LP) shunts are useful in communicating (especially "normal pressure") hydrocephalus. External ventriculostomy is useful immediately after cranial surgical procedures, when CSF protein level is very high or when there is debris in the CSF.

Mechanical malfunction can be due to disconnection, breakage or obstruction (ventricular catheter plugged with glia or choroid plexus; valve plugged with high-protein CSF or debris; distal catheter plugged with thrombus (VJ) or omentum (VP). Classic symptoms of shunt dysfunction in older children and adults are headache, lethargy, nausea, and vomiting. Gradual shunt malfunction may come to medical attention as impaired school performance, irritability, or personality change. Infants may have irritability, poor feeding, vomiting, and an abnormally shrill cry. Children

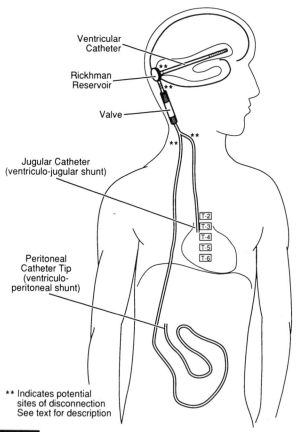

FIGURE 39

Typical shunt system (many variations exist).

with repeated episodes of shunt malfunction generally come to medical attention in a similar manner with each episode.

Begin the evaluation by pumping the valve. Difficulty compressing the valve ("pumps hard") suggests distal obstruction; slow refill suggests proximal obstruction or slit ventricles. Even if the shunt pumps, it may not be working properly. Palpate the shunt tubing for any interruption. Obtain a shunt series (plain x-rays of the entire shunt system; reservoirs and pumps may be radiolucent) to look for interruption and a non-contrasted head CT scan to assess ventricular size (old films are invaluable for comparing ventricular size). Tap the shunt (Huber needle only) for CSF pressure (if obstructed proximal to reservoir, measured pressure will not be elevated) and CSF examination.

A shunt tap is not always necessary when a fever develops in a child with a shunt. Upper respiratory infection, otitis media, pharyngitis, urinary tract infection, and gastroenteritis are frequent causes of febrile illness in any child, including those with shunts. A tap should be performed if the child is lethargic, unusually irritable, photophobic, or has neck stiffness. A shunt tap should also be considered if there is a history of similar presentation with a previous shunt infection or if there is unexplained fever or leukocytosis. Although intrathecal antibiotics may be successful, removal of an infected shunt is usually necessary for effective treatment.

CNS complications of shunts include meningitis, seizures, hematomas, and hygromas. Asymptomatic bilateral subdural effusions are common and require no treatment. Peritoneal complications include ascites and cyst formation, perforation of viscus or abdominal wall, infection with obstruction of the distal end of the catheter, and peritoneal metastases from CNS tumors (for example, medulloblastoma). Other complications include soft-tissue infection along the shunt tract and pressure necrosis of the skin.

Figure 39 shows the major components of typical shunt systems.

REFERENCES

Wilkins RH, Rengachary SS: *Neurosurgery update II*, New York, McGraw-Hill, 1991.
Youmans JR: *Neurological surgery*, ed 3, Philadelphia, WB Saunders, 1990.

SICKLE CELL DISEASE

Sickle cell anemia is due to a genetic defect in hemoglobin in which valine is substituted for glutamic acid at position six of the beta-hemoglobin chain, creating hemoglobin S (HbS). This leads to red cells that are rigid and easily damaged and results in a hemolytic anemia. Sickle cell trait is unlikely to produce neurologic manifestations.

Neurologic manifestations are seen in one-third of patients with sickle cell disease (SS for homozygous, SC for heterozygous, AS for trait only) and may be the presenting sign. The frequency of neurologic manifestations is proportional to the propensity for sickling: 6% to 35% in SS, 6% to 24% in SC disease, and 0% to 6% in sickle trait (AS).

S

SICKLE CELL DISEASE

Stroke, including thrombosis and hemorrhage, occurs in 13% to 17% of patients. About 75% have ischemia; the remainder have hemorrhage. Venous thrombosis may occur rarely. Cerebral infarcts occur at a mean age of 7 years, recurrence rates are as high as 67%, with a mean interstroke interval of 28 months. Eighty percent of recurrences occur within 36 months of the initial infarct. Intracranial hemorrhage occurs in 3% of sickle cell patients at a mean age of 25 years. Hemorrhages are more often subarachnoid in children and intraparenchymal in adults. They may occur in association with aneurysms, rupture of dilated vessels, hemorrhage into infarcted tissue, or "moyamoya". Angiography may precipitate sickling but may be safely performed after abnormal hemoglobin is reduced to less than 20% by transfusions.

Patients with SS disease have a higher stroke rate than patients with SC disease. The level of fetal hemoglobin (HbF) correlates inversely with stroke incidence. Three intrinsic mechanisms contribute to ischemia in sickle cell disease. (1) There may be large vessel endothelial injury because of the sickled cells, resulting in endothelial hyperplasia and vessel occlusion. Particularly common are middle cerebral artery infarcts and watershed infarcts. (2) There may be sludging of sickled cells during a sickle crises, with resultant ischemia in small vessels. (3) The chronic anemia leads to chronically increased cerebral perfusion and vasodilation and lack of cerebral autoregulatory reserve in meeting regional cerebral metabolic demands. These abnormal, dilated vessels may also rupture, with resultant hemorrhage.

Recurrence of stroke may be prevented by exchange transfusion to keep the percentage of sickle cells below 20%. Transfusions are typically repeated for approximately 2 years after a stroke (peak time for recurrences).

Acute or chronic *encephalopathy* may occur and possibly represents a manifestation of cerebrovascular disease.

Seizures occurs in 8% to 12% of patients and are usually generalized tonic-clonic. In SS disease, they can occur in the absence of recognized cerebrovascular involvement or intercurrent illness, although there may be precipitating factors such as medications, surgery, or anesthesia. In SC disease intercurrent illness is frequently responsible.

CNS infections with encapsulated organisms (such as *Streptococcus pneumoniae*) occur in patients with SS disease as a result of decreased phagocytic ability of the reticuloendothelial system (autosplenectomy).

Pain during sickle crisis is often severe and localizes to the affected organ. It is commonly treated with opiate analgesics. Idiopathic headache is common and may be related to increased cerebral blood flow.

Myelopathy resulting from vertebral body infarction, extramedullary hematopoiesis, and spinal cord infarction has been reported.

Visual disturbances are much more frequent in SC than in SS disease. About one-third of patients with SC disease first seek medical attention for visual impairment. Visual complications include vitreous, retinal, and sub-retinal hemorrhages; central retinal artery and vein occlusions; retinitis proliferans; and other retinal vascular changes.

REFERENCE

Pavlakis SG, Prohovnik I, Piomelli S, DeVivo DG: *Adv Pediatr* 36:247–276, 1989.

SLEEP DISORDERS

ABRIDGED CLASSIFICATION OF SLEEP DISORDERS

I. Disorders of initiating and maintaining sleep (insomnias).
   A. Associated with psychiatric disorders such as personality disorders, affective disorders, or psychoses.
   B. Associated with abuse of or withdrawal from drugs or alcohol.
   C. Sleep apnea syndromes.
   D. Alveolar hypoventilation, including Ondine's curse.
   E. Sleep-related myoclonus.
   F. Restless legs syndrome.
   G. Neurologic and medical disorders that interfere with sleep.
   H. "Pseudoinsomnia" (subjective symptoms without laboratory evidence of a sleep disturbance).
   I. Normal short sleeper.
   J. Rapid eye movement (REM) interruptions and other polysomno-graphic abnormalities.
II. Disorders of excessive somnolence.
   A through G, as listed above, are also associated with excessive somnolence.
   H. Narcolepsy.
   I. Idiopathic CNS hypersomnolence.
   J. Klein-Levin syndrome.
   K. Insufficient sleep.
   L. Normal long sleeper.
III. Disorders of the sleep-wake cycle.
   A. Jet lag.
   B. Shift work.
IV. Parasomnias.
   A. Sleepwalking (somnambulism).
   B. Sleep terror (pavor nocturnus).
   C. REM behavior disorder.
   D. Others.

Insomnia is the most common sleep disorder. Associated medical or psychiatric conditions should be treated. General management of insomnia includes optimizing the patient's "sleep hygiene" as follows: Wake and retire at the same time each day (including weekends); use the bed only for sleep and sex; leave the bed if not asleep within 10 minutes of retiring; avoid heavy exercise or large meals just before bedtime; avoid daytime napping; make sure the bedroom is not too warm or cold; exercise regularly; and discontinue use of alcohol, caffeine, cigarettes, and psychoactive drugs. Other treatments include biofeedback and sleep restriction therapy. Short-acting benzodiazepines may offer temporary adjunctive benefit, but their long-term use is not recommended. Other sedatives, including chloral hydrate, zolpidem, and diphenhydramine, may be used judiciously.

REFERENCE

Gillin JC, Byerley WF: *N Engl J Med* 322:239–248, 1990.

Sleep apnea syndrome is characterized by daytime somnolence and nighttime, or sleep-related, apnea resulting from either upper airway obstruction or central causes, or both. The typical patient is obese and snores loudly. Recurrent hypoxemia, hypercapnia, heart failure, arrhythmia, and sudden death may result. Diagnosis is made by polysomnography, including EEG, nasal and oral airflow recording, chest and abdominal respiratory movement, ECG, and pulse oximetry. Treatment consists of weight reduction, lateral sleep position, avoidance of sedatives or alcohol, and nasal continuous positive airway pressure (CPAP). Some patients may benefit from surgical correction of upper airway obstruction.

REFERENCE

Kaplan J, Staats BA: *Mayo Clin Proc* 65:1087–1094, 1990.

Narcolepsy is a disorder of excessive daytime somnolence characterized on clinical study by sleep attacks, cataplexy (sudden weakness or loss of tone elicited by emotional stimuli), hypnagogic hallucinations, and sleep paralysis. Polysomnographic confirmation includes absence of sleep apnea and daytime mean sleep latency of less than 5 minutes accompanied by REM sleep in at least two of five daytime naps on the multiple sleep latency test (MSLT). Ninety-eight percent of patients have HLA-DR2 and HLA-DQwl antigens. Treatment consists of a regimen of stimulants (such as methylphenidate, 10 to 60 mg daily, or dextroamphetamine, 5 to 50 mg daily) for sleepiness, tricyclic antidepressants (such as protriptyline, 15 to 40 mg daily) for cataplexy and sleep paralysis, and regular, brief daytime naps. Tolerance to stimulants may develop and is sometimes relieved by a "drug holiday." Abuse potential is high for stimulants. Monoamine oxidase (MAO) inhibitors are also useful but should not be used with tricyclics. Selegiline, a selective MAO-B inhibitor, improves daytime alertness and may have fewer side effects than amphetamines.

Modafinil (Provigil) is a CNS stimulant useful in treating narcolepsy. Its mechanism of action is unclear, but it appears to work like a sympathomimetic although its pharmacological profile is not exactly like those of sympathomimetic amines. In a large randomized trial, all aspects of narcolepsy were significantly improved by Modafinil compared with placebo. The most common side effect is headache and it has drug interactions with several medications including oral contraceptives, cyclosporine, and inducers and inhibitors of the cytochrome P450 CYP3A4 (some anticonvulsants, rifampin and ketoconazole). Doses range up to 400 mg per day.

REFERENCES

Aldrich MS: *N Engl J Med* 323:389–394, 1990.
US Modafinil in Narcolepsy Multicenter Study: *Neurology* 54(5):1166–1175, 2000.

Sleep terrors (pavor nocturnus) typically occur in the first third of sleep. Patients often arouse with a blood-curdling cry and cannot explain what is frightening them. In contrast to common nightmares, with sleep terrors the patient is amnestic for them the next morning. Sleep terrors occur almost exclusively in children and disappear by adolescence. Treatment usually consists of reassuring the parents; occasionally a regimen of benzodiazepines or imipramine is useful.

Restless legs syndrome (see Restless Legs Syndrome).

SPASTICITY

Spasticity is a velocity-dependent increase in muscle tone. It is one component of the upper motor neuron syndrome. Other components include flexor spasms, weakness, tonic flexor and extensor dystonia, increased stretch reflexes, extensor plantar response (Babinksi's sign), and loss of dexterity. It results from damage to various descending pathways. Isolated lesions of the pyramidal tract are not sufficient to produce spasticity or the complete syndrome.

Overall, no medication is particularly useful in relieving the disabling spasticity of cerebral lesions (tightly flexed and adducted upper extremities, extended and adducted lower extremities). Painful flexor spasms can be markedly reduced by administration of baclofen or diazepam. Dantrolene may be helpful but causes mild to moderate muscle weakness, sedation, and dizziness. Combinations may be more effective, with fewer side effects.

Baclofen is a gamma aminobutyric acid (GABA) agonist and also interferes with the release of excitatory transmitters. Starting dosage is 5 mg three times a day (tid), increased by 5 mg every three days to a maximum dosage of 80 mg per day in divided doses. Adverse effects are mood changes, hallucinations, gastrointestinal symptoms, hypotension, changes in accommodation and ocular motor function, and deterioration in seizure control. Care should be used if renal disease is present; avoid abrupt withdrawal of the drug. Continuous infusion of intrathecal baclofen by means of an implanted infusion pump at a rate of 15 to 450 µg per day is useful in spasticity caused by spinal cord lesions or demyelinating disease and may be useful in spasticity of cerebral origin in cerebral palsy.

Diazepam facilitates GABA-mediated presynaptic and postsynaptic inhibition. Starting dosage is 2 mg twice daily, increased slowly to a maximum dosage of 60 mg per day in divided doses.

Dantrolene sodium interferes with excitation-contraction coupling by decreasing the release of calcium at the sarcoplasmic reticulum. Starting dosage is 25 mg every day, increased by 25 mg every three to four days to a maximum dosage of 100 mg qid. Side effects are hepatotoxicity (follow liver enzymes) and diarrhea.

Drugs that bind to $\alpha2$ adrenergic receptors, and decrease sympathetic outflow along with inhibiting afferent inputs into the spinal reflex arc can be used to treat spasticity. Tizanidine starting at 2 mg BID and increasing up to 8 mg TID is generally well tolerated but may cause increased fatigue or sedation. Clonidine 0.2 to 1 mg per day in divided doses has similar effects but may cause sedation or orthostatic hypotension.

A regimen of chlorpromazine (25 to 75 mg per day) causes alpha adrenergic blockade and has been used to reduce spasticity, but sedation and fear of tardive dyskinesia have limited its use.

Phenytoin (100 to 400 mg per day) and carbamazepine (600 to 1200 mg per day) act on the Ia afferent muscle spindle to reduce spontaneous and stretch-evoked discharges.

Surgical intervention with selective posterior rhizotomy has been used in patients with cerebral palsy and severe spasticity. Longitudinal myelotomy has been used to control severe flexor spasms. Spinal cord and cerebellar stimulation act by stimulating inhibitory pathways.

Botulinum toxin is useful in managing spasticity locally in all conditions (cerebral palsy, multiple sclerosis, stroke, etc.) with spasticity. Side effects include flaccidity, development of neutralizing antibodies and rare systemic weakness. Doses take effect several days after injection and may last up to three months.

REFERENCES

Alonso PJ, Mancall EL: *Semin Neurol* 2(3):215–218, 1991.
National Institutes of Health: *Conn Med* 55:471–477, 1991.
Young RR, Wiegner AW: *Clin Orthop* 219:50, 1987.

SPINAL CORD

Relation of the spinal cord segments and roots to the vertebral column is depicted in Figure 40. Cross-sectional anatomy of the cervical cord is shown in Figure 41.

SPINAL CORD SYNDROMES

An acute *spinal cord* lesion causes "spinal shock," which becomes evident as paralysis, areflexia, anesthesia, and bowel or bladder dysfunction below the level of the lesion. Spinal shock may last weeks and may evolve into spasticity, exaggerated tendon and withdrawal reflexes, and Babinski's signs.

Anterior cord syndrome is characterized by paresis and impaired pain perception; proprioception is preserved below the lesion. The syndrome is usually caused by spinal cord compression or anterior spinal artery occlusion. Posterior cord syndrome consists of pain and parathesias out of proportion to motor impairment that are referable to the affected segments; the syndrome is commonly associated with demyelinating lesions. Central cord syndrome,

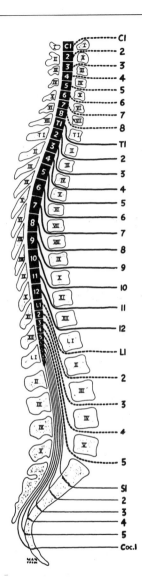

FIGURE 40

Relation of spinal segments and roots to the vertebral column. (From Haymaker W, Woodhall B: *Peripheral nerve injuries: principles of diagnosis,* Philadelphia, WB Saunders, 1953.)

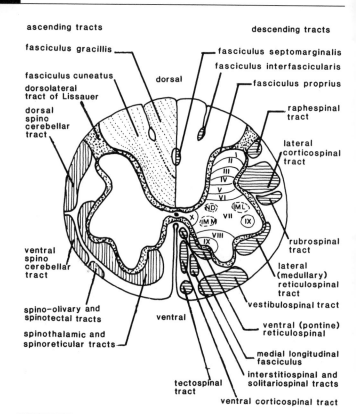

ascending tracts

fasciculus gracillis

fasciculus cuneatus

dorsolateral
tract of Lissauer

dorsal
spino
cerebellar
tract

ventral
spino
cerebellar
tract

spino-olivary and
spinotectal tracts

spinothalamic and
spinoreticular tracts

dorsal

descending tracts

fasciculus septomarginalis

fasciculus interfascicularis

fasciculus proprius

raphespinal
tract

lateral
corticospinal
tract

rubrospinal
tract

lateral
(medullary)
reticulospinal
tract

vestibulospinal tract

ventral (pontine)
reticulospinal

medial longitudinal
fasciculus

interstitiospinal and
solitariospinal tracts

ventral corticospinal tract

tectospinal
tract

ventral

FIGURE 41

Cervical spinal cord (cross section). Gray matter columns: *I–X*, Rexed's laminae: *IML*, interomediolateral column; *ND*, nucleus dorsalis (Clarke's column); *PM*, posteromedial column.

often seen with hyperextension injuries in the neck, results in patchy sensory loss, urinary retention, and weakness disproportionately affecting the legs.

Spinal cord hemisection produces the Brown-Sequard syndrome, consisting of (1) ipsilateral spastic paresis; (2) ipsilateral loss of touch and vibratory and joint position sense; and (3) contralateral loss of pain and temperature sensation below the level of the lesion.

CAUSES OF MYELOPATHY

Congenital or developmental: Spinal dysraphism (see Developmental Malformations), craniocervical junction abnormalities, syringomyelia, congenital cervical spinal stenosis, tethered-cord syndromes, diastatomyelia.

Degenerative: Spondylosis, motor neuron disease, spinocerebellar degeneration, hereditary spastic paraplegia.

Demyelinating: Multiple sclerosis, neuromyelitis optica (*Devic's disease*).

Infectious: Poliomyelitis, herpes zoster, rabies, viral encephalomyelitis, bacterial meningitis, epidural or subdural abscess, syphilis, tuberculosis, typhus, spotted fever, fungal infections, trichinosis, schistosomiasis, HTLV-1, human immunodeficiency virus (HIV), cytomegalovirus.

Inflammatory or immune response: Postinfectious, postvaccination, arachnoiditis, sarcoidosis, lupus erythematosus.

Metabolic or nutritional: Pernicious anemia (B_{12} deficiency), pellagra, chronic liver disease.

Neoplastic: Extramedullary or intramedullary tumors, meningeal carcinomatosis, paraneoplastic.

Toxic: Ethanol (direct effect and through hepatic cirrhosis and portocaval shunting), arsenic, cyanide, lathyrism, clioquinol, intrathecal contrast or chemotherapeutic agents.

Traumatic (see below): Vertebral subluxation or fracture, transection, contusion, concussion, hemorrhage, birth injury (particularly breech delivery), electrical injury.

Vascular (see below): Arterial and venous infarction, hemorrhage (epidural, subdural, intraparenchymal), vasculitis, vascular malformations, aneurysms, effects of radiation therapy (see Radiation).

DEGENERATIVE JOINT DISEASE

Degenerative joint disease of the spine occurs as a result of changes in the intervertebral disks (spondylosis) with aging. Spondylosis leads to osteophyte formation, meningeal fibrosis, and disk herniation.

Spondylosis in the cervical spine can cause progressive myelopathy, radiculopathy, or both. Thoracic lesions become evident mainly as paraparesis. Lumbar lesions cause radiculopathies, neurogenic claudication, or acute back pain syndromes. Neurogenic claudication, like vascular claudication, causes exertional pain, but it differs from vascular claudication as follows: (1) the pain may be felt in buttock or thigh with prolonged standing or walking; (2) the pulses are normal; (3) reflexes may be decreased while at peak pain; and (4) the pain is relieved with waist flexion or rest but generally takes several minutes or more to resolve.

Syringomyelia describes a condition in which there is an abnormal cavity or cyst in the spinal cord. Syrinxes are usually cervical but may extend rostrally (syringobulbia) or caudally. They are frequently associated with developmental malformations of the craniocervical junction (Arnold-Chiari malformations, platybasia), myelomeningocele, kyphoscoliosis, intramedullary tumors, vascular malformations, or trauma. Hand numbness is the usual initial complaint with cervical syrinxes. Loss of pain and temperature sensation in a capelike (suspended) distribution with sparing of vibratory and joint position sense (dissociated sensory loss) is due to destruction of crossing pain fibers at the lesion level. Segmental weakness, atrophy, fasciculations, spasticity, incontinence, and hyperreflexia occur frequently. The course is usually slowly progressive; a sudden decline may indicate development of hematomyelia or progression of an underlying condition. Management includes cyst drainage and scrupulous hand care to prevent painless cuts and wound infections.

TRAUMA

Initial management of spinal cord trauma should include maintenance of airway, breathing, and circulation; immobilization (spine board, collars); bladder catheterization; nasogastric intubation; administration of high-dose IV corticosteroids; and serial neurologic examinations. Radiographic studies are directed to the area of interest but generally include cross-table lateral and AP cervical views (all seven cervical vertebrae must be seen) and films of the thoracic and lumbar spine. An open-mouth odontoid film may be obtained in conscious patients. CT is sensitive for identification of fractures. Myelography or MRI can identify acute compressive lesions such as hematomas. High dose corticosteroids help improve clinical outcome in traumatic spinal cord injuries.

VASCULAR SYNDROMES

Anterior spinal artery infarctions typically affect the midthoracic region, causing severe local, radicular, and deep pain; paraparesis; sphincter disturbance; and dissociated distal sensory loss (pain and temperature sensation more affected than vibration, touch, and joint position sense). Sacral sensation may remain intact. Causes include systemic hypotension, aortic dissection, vasculitis, embolism, sickle cell disease, and extrinsic arterial compression by tumor, bone, or disk material. Posterior spinal artery infarction is less common and produces pain, loss of proprioception, and variable involvement of corticospinal and spinocerebellar tracts.

Spinal subdural and epidural hemorrhage most commonly occurs after trauma, lumbar puncture, or spinal or epidural anesthesia. Other causes include anticoagulant use, blood dyscrasias, thrombocytopenia, neoplasm, and vascular malformation. The initial symptom is severe back pain at the level of the bleed. Myelopathy or cauda equina syndrome with symptoms dependent on lesion level develop over hours to days. MRI is especially useful in determining lesion location. Laminectomy with clot evacuation should be performed as soon as possible, since prognosis for recovery is better when surgery is performed early and the preoperative deficits are not severe.

Spinal subarachnoid hemorrhage most commonly results from aneurysm rupture but may occur with vascular malformations. Other causes include aortic coarctation, spinal artery rupture, mycotic aneurysms, polyarteritis nodosa, spinal tumors, lumbar puncture, blood dyscrasias, and anticoagulants. Severe back pain followed by signs of meningeal irritation are usually the first manifestations. Multiple radiculopathies and myelopathy may develop. Headache, cranial neuropathies, and obtundation are associated with diffusion of blood above the foramen magnum. Cerebrospinal fluid is bloody and intracranial pressure may be elevated; treatment is directed at the underlying cause.

Hematomyelia: Intramedullary spinal hemorrhage is rare but occurs after trauma, spinal arteriovenous malformation rupture, hemorrhage into tumor or syrinx, or venous infarction or with clotting or bleeding disorders. Emergency surgical decompression is often indicated.

Spinal cord compression and tumors are discussed in the Tumors section.

SPINOCEREBELLAR DEGENERATION

Spinocerebellar degeneration is a general term used to describe a heterogeneous group of inherited disorders in which ataxia is a prominent manifestation.

CLASSIFICATION

I. Inherited disorders with known metabolic defects.
    A. Intermittent ataxia.
        1. Hyperammonemia: Ornithine transcarboxylase deficiency, argininosuccinate synthetase deficiency (citrullinemia), argininosuccinase deficiency (argininosuccinicaciduria), and arginase deficiency (hyperornithinemia).
        2. Aminoacidurias: Hartnup disease, intermittent branched-chain ketoaciduria, isovaleric acidemia.
        3. Disorders of pyruvate and lactate metabolism: Pyruvate dehydrogenase deficiency, pyruvate carboxylase deficiency, Leigh disease, and multiple carboxylase deficiencies, Acetazolamide responsive ataxia.
    B. Progressive ataxias.
        1. Abeta- and hypobetalipoproteinemia.
        2. Hexosaminidase deficiency.
        3. Cholestanolosis (cerebrotendinous xanthomatrosis).
        4. Leukodystrophies: Metachromatic, late-onset globoid cell, and adrenoleukodystrophy.
        5. Mitochondrial encephalomyopathies.
        6. Partial hypoxanthine guanine phosphoribosyl transferase deficiency.
        7. Wilson's disease.
        8. Ceroid lipofuscinosis.
        9. Sialidosis.
        10. Sphingomyelin storage disorders.
    C. Disorders associated with defective DNA repair.
        1. Ataxia telangiectasia.
        2. Xeroderma pigmentosum.
        3. Cockayne's syndrome.

II. Autosomal recessive ataxia (onset usually before 20 years of age).
  A. Friedreich's ataxia.
  B. Early-onset cerebellar ataxia with retained tendon reflexes, hypogonadism, myoclonus (progressive myoclonic ataxia, Ramsay Hunt syndrome), childhood deafness, congenital deafness, optic atrophy, cataracts, and mental retardation (Marinesco-Sjögren syndrome), and pigmentary retinopathy.
  C. Autosomal recessive late-onset ataxia.
III. Autosomal dominant cerebellar ataxias "ADCA" (onset usually after 20 years of age).
  A. ADCA I "SCA1, SCA2, SCA3, and SCA4": Ataxia with ophthalmoplegia, optic atrophy, dementia, or extrapyramidal features (including Machado-Joseph disease).
  B. ADCA II "SCA7": Ataxia with pigmentary maculopathy with or without ophthalmoplegia or extrapyramidal features.
  C. ADCA III "SCA5, SCA6, and SCA11": Pure ataxia.
  D. Periodic dominant ataxia episodic ataxia1 and 2.
IV. Ataxia associated with mitochondrial DNA defects.
  A. Sporadic: Kearns-Sayre syndrome (large deletion or duplication).
  B. Maternally inherited in many cases: MERRF (8344 mutation), some patients with MELAS (3243 mutation), and neurogenic muscle weakness, ataxia, and retinitis pigmentosa (8993 mutation).
V. Ataxia associated with toxic and deficiency disorders.
  A. Drug induced (antiepileptic drugs such as phenytoin, carbamazepine, or barbiturates; lithium; cytotoxic agents such as cytosine arabinoside; and 5-fluorouracil).
  B. Solvent (such as toluene).
  C. Heavy metals (inorganic mercury and thallium poisoning).
  D. Alcoholism and thiamine deficiency.
  E. Vitamin E deficiency.

Friedreich's ataxia is the most common type of spinocerebellar degeneration. It is inherited by an autosomal recessive pattern. It is caused by a triple nucleotide repeat (GAA) expansion at chromosome 9 that encodes the protein frataxin. Symptoms develop from 18 months to 24 years of age and consist of progressive limb and truncal ataxia, dysarthria, and areflexia in the lower extremities. Pyramidal signs and loss of position and vibration sense evolve gradually. Skeletal deformities (kyphoscoliosis and pes cavus) and cardiomyopathy are seen in more than two thirds of patients. Systemic involvement manifests by increased incidence of diabetes, blindness, and deafness. Ambulation is usually lost by age 25, and death frequently occurs in the fourth or fifth decade of life. Treatment is aimed at symptomatic management of the skeletal deformities, diabetes, and the cardiac disorders.

Pathologically, Friedreich's ataxia is characterized by an atrophic spinal cord with gliosis and cell loss affecting the posterior columns and the corticospinal and spinocerebellar tracts predominantly. Cranial nerve nuclei VIII, X, and XII are depleted, as are the dentate nuclei and superior cerebellar peduncles. Large, myelinated peripheral nerves are lost. Myocardial fibers are degenerated.

Early-onset cerebellar ataxia with retained reflexes is not uncommon and is often confused with Friedreich's ataxia. Reflexes are normal or brisk. Optic atrophy, cardiomyopathy, diabetes, and skeletal deformities are not seen. Life span is considerably longer than with Friedreich's ataxia. It is an autosomal recessive condition linked to chromosome 13q.

The adult forms of spinocerebellar degeneration occur less frequently than Friedreich's ataxia, and there may be several clinical manifestations within kindred. The condition tends to progress more rapidly in early-onset patients than in those with late-onset ataxia.

Olivopontocerebellar atrophy (OPCA) is a pathologic diagnosis applied to diverse clinical entities. Symptoms may include progressive ataxia, tremor, spasticity, involuntary movements, optic atrophy, and sensory abnormalities; it may be indistinguishable on clinical examination from the hereditary ataxias listed above.

The genetic diagnosis of SCA depends on triple repeat expansion. The exact number of the repeat varies between diseases. It tends to be greater than 40 for most SCA. Most diseases show evidence of anticipation. Supportive care should be provided for most patients, including physical therapy, speech therapy, and social organization. Genetic counseling is recommended for all patients of reproductive age.

REFERENCES

Bradley WG et al: *Neurology in clinical practice*, ed 3, Boston, Butterworth-Heinemann, 2000.
Harding AE, Deufel T, eds: *Adv Neurol* 61, 1993.
Martin JB: *N Engl J Med* 340(25):1970–1980,1999.

SYNCOPE

Syncope is brief loss of consciousness and postural tone resulting from decreased cerebral perfusion. It may occur after prodromal features, such as diaphoresis, pallor, nausea, and visual changes (blurring, dimming, constriction), or it may occur suddenly without prodrome; the generalization that the latter situation is more suggestive of an arrhythmogenic source does not preclude that an arrhythmia can also produce a prodrome. If cerebral hypoperfusion persists, as when the subject is held upright in a procedure chair, tonic-clonic jerks and urinary incontinence (convulsive syncope) may result. After a syncopal spell, some patients have transient generalized weakness, but confusion, headache, and drowsiness are uncommon.

Syncope can be classified by pathophysiologic mechanism as follows.

I. Vasovagal (vasodepressor, neurocardiogenic) syncope occurs either spontaneously or in response to stimuli that include prolonged standing, hot conditions, stress, pain, fear, or other strong emotional stimuli (such as the sight of blood). This common type of syncope is thought

S

SYNCOPE

to be mediated by the Bezold-Jarisch reflex: venous pooling in the lower extremities results in reduced cardiac output and blood pressure, thus activating aortic arch and carotid sinus baroreceptors with a resultant increase in sympathetic outflow that causes the poorly filled ventricle to contract vigorously. Mechanoreceptors (C-fibers) in the heart chambers and pulmonary artery are activated in some individuals; via projections to the dorsal vagal nucleus of the medulla, the mechanoreceptors produce an increase in vagal tone and a withdrawal of peripheral sympathetic tone, resulting in bradycardia, vasodilation, and consequently loss of consciousness. Vasovagal syncope is particularly common in young adults.

II. Impaired splanchnic and visceral vasoconstriction results in a defective vasopressor response to postural changes. Causes include medications (antihypertensives, tricyclic antidepressants, phenothiazines, levodopa, lithium), autonomic neuropathy (diabetes, amyloidosis, porphyria, Guillain-Barré syndrome, Riley-Day syndrome), idiopathic orthostatic hypotension, central dysautonomias, sympathectomy, and prolonged bedrest.

III. Hypovolemia occurs in the context of dehydration (as from strenuous exercise, hot environment, vomiting, diarrhea, or inadequate oral intake), hemorrhage, or another source of blood loss (hemodialysis, phlebotomy). In contrast to "benign" conditions such as vasovagal syncope, here loss of consciousness may indicate that the patient is going into circulatory shock and requires volume resuscitation.

IV. Reflex syncope is an inappropriate response to vagal stimuli. Syncope may thus occur in the context of micturition (mostly in men), the postprandial state (or after ingesting cold liquids), vagal irritation by esophageal diverticulae or mediastinal masses, carotid sinus stimulation (by a tight collar, head turning, or shaving), Valsalva (weightlifting, strain, defecation), coughing (classically in overweight smokers), or glossopharyngeal neuralgia.

V. Cardiac syncope is generally unrelated to posture and may be classified as follows:

   1. Arrhythmias that diminish cardiac output: Long QT syndrome, third-degree atrioventricular (AV) block (Stokes-Adams attack), sick sinus syndrome, profound sinus bradycardia and other bradyarrhythmias, supraventricular tachycardias, ventricular tachycardia and fibrillation, and pacemaker failure.
   2. Outflow obstruction: Aortic stenosis, hypertrophic obstructive cardiomyopathy, pulmonic stenosis, pulmonary embolism, pulmonary hypertension, tetralogy of Fallot.
   3. Pump failure: myocardial infarction, cardiac tamponade, severe congestive heart failure.

VI. Cerebrovascular disease is a very uncommon cause of syncope, but vertebrobasilar insufficiency and the subclavian steal syndrome have been associated with syncopal episodes. A history of acute severe headache preceding the loss of consciousness should prompt evaluation for subarachnoid hemorrhage.

VII. Metabolic derangement such as hypoxia, hypocapnia, and hypoglycemia frequently produce lightheadedness, rarely syncope.

Conditions that may mimic syncope include atonic seizures, cataplexy, acute vertigo, and conversion and factitious disorders. True syncope should not produce postictal confusion, and neither vertigo nor cataplexy is associated with loss of consciousness.

The most useful tools for evaluation of syncope are the clinical history (ask about precipitants, body position, prodrome, prior episodes, orientation on awakening, family history, seizure risk factors, cardiac and cerebrovascular disease, autonomic and neuropathic symptoms, and medications); physical exam (orthostatic vital signs, estimate of volume status, cardiac and cervical auscultation, and peripheral nerve and autonomic exam); and ECG (always check the corrected QT interval). More sophisticated (but lower yield) evaluation can be undertaken with echocardiogram, prolonged ambulatory ECG monitoring, and head-upright tilt test (the gold standard test for diagnosis of vasovagal syncope, with an estimated specificity of 90% in the absence of provocative agents such as isoproterenol). EEG, carotid ultrasound, and head CT have low diagnostic yield in the context of an unremarkable history and neurologic exam.

Treatment of vasovagal syncope may proceed in a stepwise fashion. First, patients are educated to avoid precipitants and dietary sodium intake is liberalized. Medications that may cause or exacerbate orthostasis or volume depletion are discontinued if possible. If these measures fail, beta-blockers are employed as first-line therapy. Should beta-blockers fail or be contraindicated, the patient may be tried on fludrocortisone or midodrine. If pharmacologic measures fail, pacemaker placement may be considered.

REFERENCES

Atiga WL et al: *J Cardiovasc Electrophysiol* 10:874–888, 1999.
Getchell WS et al: *JGIM* 14:677–687, 1999.

SYNDROME OF INAPPROPRIATE ANTIDIURETIC HORMONE (SIADH)

SIADH is due to antidiuretic hormone (ADH)-stimulated water conservation, resulting in hyponatremia with concentrated urine (osmolality >300 mmol/kg) and urine sodium excretion (>20 mEq/L). The diagnosis requires the patient to be *euvolemic*; have normal adrenal, renal, and thyroid function; and not be taking medications that stimulate ADH release.

Etiology: Neurologic causes include stroke, subdural hematoma, subarachnoid hemorrhage, head trauma, intracranial surgery, tumors, basal skull fractures, cerebral atrophy, acute encephalitis, tuberculous or purulent meningitis, Guillain-Barré syndrome, acute intermittent porphyria, and CNS lupus erythematosus. SIADH may also be caused by medications or by pulmonary disease. This syndrome must be differentiated from cerebral salt wasting (CSW) syndrome, which commonly occurs with SAH and following head trauma. In CSW, patients are usually hypovolemic.

Manifestations are due to the hyponatremia and include mental status changes, behavioral changes, weakness, anorexia, nausea, vomiting, muscle cramps, and extrapyramidal signs. Seizures, coma, and death may occur with severe hyponatremia.

Therapy involves treatment of the underlying cause and fluid restriction to 800 to 1000 mL daily. If hyponatremia is severe or the patient is symptomatic, correction with hypertonic saline is recommended. The rate of infusion should be no faster than 0.5 mEq per hour to avoid the possibility of inducing central pontine myelinolysis.

REFERENCE

Fall PJ: *Postgraduate Med* 107:75–82, 2000.

SYPHILIS

Neurosyphilis results from meningeal invasion by *Treponema pallidum*; parenchymal involvement occurs in later stages (that is general paresis and tabes dorsalis). Symptomatic neurosyphilis develops in only 4% to 9% of patients with syphilis who do not receive treatment. Clinical syndromes include the following:

1. *Asymptomatic neurosyphilis* refers to the presence of CSF abnormalities in the absence of neurologic signs and symptoms. The highest rate of abnormalities occurs early, 13 to 18 months after initial infection; the diagnosis is made on the basis of positive results of serum or CSF serologic tests and abnormal CSF, usually with mildly increased level of protein (40 to 200 mg/dl); normal glucose level; and a mild, lymphocytic pleocytosis (50 to 400 cells/mm^3). The level of CSF gammaglobulins may be increased. Normal CSF 5 years after infection reduces the risk of CNS syphilis to 1%. Ten percent to 25% of patients with asymptomatic neurosyphilis who do not receive treatment become symptomatic. Lumbar puncture, therefore, should be performed in all patients in whom a diagnosis of syphilis is made beyond the primary stage or in whom the dating of primary infection cannot be established.
2. *Acute syphilitic meningitis* usually occurs within the initial 2 years of infection and becomes evident as headache, nuchal rigidity, confusion, and cranial nerve (CN) palsies (especially, CN II, III, VI, and VIII).
3. *Meningovascular syphilis* usually occurs within 4 to 7 years after initial infection and results from an endarteritis, most commonly of the middle cerebral artery. Meningovascular syphilis becomes evident as a focal CNS ischemia that evolves acutely or over days and is often associated with a prodrome (weeks to months) of headache, dizziness, and psychiatric disturbances.

4. *General paresis (meningoencephalitis)* usually occurs 15 to 20 years after initial infection as a result of spirochete invasion of the cortex. Dementia is the initial manifestation. Seizures may occur. Untreated, the condition is fatal within 4 years.

5. *Tabes dorsalis* occurs 20 to 25 years after infection and results from inflammation of the posterior roots and posterior columns. Classic presentation includes triads of symptoms (lightning pain, dysuria, and ataxia) and signs (Argyll-Robertson pupils, areflexia, and proprioceptive loss). Later involvement includes visceral crises, optic atrophy, ocular motor palsies, Charcot joints, and foot ulcers. Early treatment usually arrests the progression and may reverse some of the symptoms.

6. Less common manifestations include optic neuropathy, eighth nerve neuropathy, spinal neurosyphilis (for example, meningomyelitis and meningovascular), and gumma (granulomatous mass lesions in brain or spinal cord).

7. Patients coinfected with human immunodeficiency virus (HIV) have a higher rate of early neurosyphilis (meningitis or meningovascular) and may be at an increased risk for neurologic relapse after treatment of primary and secondary syphilis with IM benzathine penicillin. This may indicate that the CNS is a "sheltered" site from which relapse may proceed.

Diagnosis depends on clinical findings, serum serology results, and CSF examination. Serum treponemal serologic tests (VDRL and RPR) become nonreactive with treatment and therefore can be used to assess therapeutic efficacy. However, their titers progressively decline, even during the course of untreated disease, becoming nonreactive in 25% of patients with late (neuro) syphilis. Serum treponemal tests (FTA-ABS, MHA-TP) are usually unaffected by treatment, their titers remaining elevated indefinitely. Therefore a nonreactive FTA-ABS result excludes neurosyphilis.

The CSF in neurosyphilis usually shows elevated protein level, normal glucose level, and lymphocytic pleocytosis (10 to 400 cells/mm^3). The CSF VDRL has very high specificity but low sensitivity (30% to 70%). Thus nonreactive CSF VDRL does not exclude neurosyphilis. The CSF FTA-ABS test has a high false-positive rate, and its role in diagnosis is unclear. As with all CSF serologic studies, a traumatic spinal fluid sample may also give misleading results.

Treatment of neurosyphilis consists of a regimen of aqueous penicillin G, 2 to 4 million units IV q 4 hr for 10 to 14 days. An alternative treatment is penicillin G procaine 2 to 4 million units IM qd with probenecid 500 mg po qid for 10 to 14 days. In cases of penicillin allergy, treatment options include penicillin desensitization followed by standard penicillin therapy; other regimens, such as tetracycline hydrochloride 500 mg PO qid for 30 days, erythromycin 500 mg PO qid for 30 days, or ceftriaxone 250 mg IM qd, are recommended for primary, secondary or latent syphilis but are of unproven value for tertiary neurosyphilis.

Follow-up CSF examination should be performed at 6 and 12 months. The CSF cell count is the earliest indicator of response and relapse and should normalize within 6 months. CSF protein level declines more slowly, taking as long as 2 years to normalize. CSF VDRL titers are the last to decline and may remain mildly elevated despite adequate treatment. Repeat treatment is indicated if the CSF pleocytosis persists after 6 months or is abnormal 2 years after treatment. Because CSF protein level and VDRL titers take much longer to normalize, treatment cannot be considered inadequate unless these values unequivocally increase.

REFERENCES

Hook EW, Marra CM: *N Engl J Med* 326:1060–1069, 1992.
Katz DA, Berger JR, Duncan RC: *Arch Neurol* 50:234–249, 1993.
Simon RP: *Arch Neurol* 42:606–613, 1985.

T

TASTE

Taste receptor cells are modified epithelial cells in the taste buds located in the anteroposterior aspect of the tongue, soft palate, pharynx, epiglottis, and proximal one third of the esophagus. The facial, glossopharyngeal, and vagus nerves mediate taste sensation. Proximal lesions of the facial nerve between the pons and facial canal where the chorda tympani joins the facial nerve result in the unilateral loss of taste on the anterior two thirds of the tongue. The greater superficial petrosal branch of the facial nerve carries taste from the soft palate. The lingual, tonsillar, and pharyngeal branches of the glossopharyngeal nerve carry taste from the posterior one third of the tongue and pharynx. The superior laryngeal branch of the vagus carries taste from the esophagus and epiglottis.

All afferent taste fibers project to the solitary tract nucleus. Fibers then project to the thalamus, ventral forebrain, lateral hypothalamus, and amygdala. From the thalamus, fibers mediating taste sensation project to the insular cortex.

Salt, sour, sweet, and bitter tastes can be perceived throughout the oral cavity. Taste depends on the adaptive state of the tongue. Even water can evoke a taste if the tongue is adapted to certain substances. When there is either a change in the flow rate or composition of saliva, there may be ageusia (absence of taste), dysgeusia (distortion of taste), or hypogeusia (diminished taste). Therefore when a change in taste sensation is being evaluated, one must rule out conditions affecting production of salivary fluids, for example, Sjögren's syndrome, pandysautonomia, post-radiation, and amyloidosis. Olfactory dysfunction must also be considered in disorders of taste.

Taste testing is accomplished with the use of a cotton applicator. Ideally, the patient should not speak but should point to cards with the words *sweet*, *salty*, *bitter*, and *sour* written on them. Causes of an alteration in taste sensation include an upper respiratory tract infection, nasal disorders, head injury with damage to either the lingual or chorda tympani, heavy smoking, hepatitis, following influenza, viral encephalitis, hypothyroidism, diabetes, hypogonadism (Kallmann's syndrome), neoplasm, and vitamin B_{12} deficiency. Medications that cause a change in taste include antirheumatic, antiproliferative drugs, calcium channel blockers; and drugs with sulfhydryl groups. Cerebellar pontine angle tumors occasionally cause a loss of taste.

Gustatory hallucinations may occur as an aura of partial epilepsy or in alcohol-induced delirium and are usually associated with olfactory hallucinations.

REFERENCE

Nelson GM: *Anat Rec* 253:70–78, 1998.

TEMPORAL LOBE

The temporal lobe is bordered superiorly by the sylvian fissure and merges with the parietal and occipital lobes. In addition to the neocortex, it contains the amygdala, hippocampus, and paleocortical areas, such as olfactory and entorhinal cortices. The primary auditory cortex (Brodmann's area 41, 42; Wernicke's area on dominant hemisphere) and auditory association area are within the superior temporal gyrus. Signs of temporal lobe dysfunction include partial complex seizures, memory difficulties (especially bilateral hippocampal involvement, but nonverbal memory may be impaired with nondominant hippocampal damage and verbal with dominant hemisphere lesions), Wernicke's aphasia with dominant temporal lesions, agnosias, visual field defects (superior quadrantanopsias), and behavioral and emotional disturbances. The *Klüver-Bucy syndrome* of placidity, apathy, hypersexuality, hyperorality, and visual and auditory agnosia occurs with bilateral anterior temporal lobe injury. Klüver-Bucy syndrome may occur in the setting of brain trauma, encephalitis, stroke, tumors or degenerative dementias.

THYROID

Both hyperthyroidism and hypothyroidism can have neurologic manifestations. Prompt recognition and treatment can result in good clinical outcomes.

HYPERTHYROIDISM

A. Thyrotoxic crisis is a medical emergency. *Manifestation:* High fever, tachycardia, hypotension, vomiting, diarrhea, and delirium. It may progress to coma and death if not treated promptly. Crisis may be precipitated by infection or inadequate preparation for thyroid surgery. *Management* includes thiourea agents, sodium iodide, adrenergic blockers, corticosteroids, sedatives, body cooling, and fluid/electrolyte maintenance. *Mortality* is as high as 30%.

B. Acute thyrotoxic encephalomyelopathy may occur, presenting as an acute bulbar palsy with associated encephalopathy. Brain swelling and focal hemorrhages are seen pathologically. Symptoms may resolve with achievement of a euthyroid state. Seizures, usually generalized, may develop or be exacerbated during thyrotoxicosis. EEG abnormalities (generalized slowing and increased alpha activity) are seen in 60% of patients with hyperthyroidism.

C. Psychological manifestations: Psychosis is also associated with hyperthyroidism. "Apathetic hyperthyroidism" is common in the elderly and may manifest as dementia with apathy and depression.

D. Tremor: An accentuation of physiologic tremor, due to increased sensitivity to sympathetic input, is very common in hyperthyroid patients and involves primarily the upper extremities. Treatment consists of correcting the thyroid abnormality; propranolol is also useful.

E. Other CNS syndromes: Chorea, resulting from hypersensitivity of dopaminergic receptors, which responds to neuroleptics. Stroke results from cerebral embolism in thyrotoxic atrial fibrillation. Acute anticoagulation may be appropriate.

F. Peripheral nervous system abnormalities associated with thyroid disease include a rare *chronic thyrotoxic myopathy*; however, complaints of nonspecific weakness are common. Creatine kinase (CK) is normal or decreased. EMG reveals short-duration polyphasic motor unit potentials. Muscle power normalizes as the patient becomes euthyroid. Thyrotoxic periodic paralysis that resembles hypokalemic periodic paralysis also occurs. Myasthenia gravis has an increased incidence in patients with hypo- or hyperthyroidism and hypo- or hyperthyroidism has an increased incidence in myasthenic patients. *Neuropathy* is very uncommon.

HYPOTHYROIDISM

Hypothyroidism may present in infancy with mental retardation and growth abnormalities, resulting in Cretinism. Fortunately, this is now rare, since many countries have instituted neonatal screening programs.

A. CNS manifestations: In the elderly, hypothyroidism may present with *cognitive dysfunction*, sometimes confused with a primary degenerative dementia. Associated signs of systemic hypothyroidism are variable and psychosis may occur. All new-onset dementia patients must be screened for hypothyroidism. *Coma* occurs rarely, usually in chronic, severe, undiagnosed disease. Seizures may occur. EEG changes include slowing of alpha activity and decreased driving response with high-frequency photic stimulation. Markedly reduced background amplitude may be seen in hypothermic states. CSF protein is elevated in 40% to 90% of hypothyroid patients, occasionally >100% mg/dL. Gamma globulin may also be increased in both CSF and serum for unknown reasons. *Emergency management* consists of thyroid replacement (PO or IV); corticosteroids; treatment of hypoglycemia, fluid/electrolyte abnormalities, and hypothermia; and ventilatory support as needed.

Cerebellar ataxia with impaired tandem gait and limb incoordination but often without nystagmus or dysarthria has also been reported.

B. Peripheral manifestations occur in a variety of forms. *Hypothyroid myopathy* has weakness (proximal > distal), cramps, pain, and stiffness as common complaints, but objective weakness is less common. Creatine phosphokinase (CPK) is often elevated. EMG findings are nonspecific. *Myoedema*, a percussion-induced local mounding of contracted muscle that relaxes slowly, may be elicited, but can also occur in emaciated patients and some normal subjects. The contraction is electrically silent on EMG. Muscle hypertrophy, known as *Hoffman's syndrome* in adults and *Kocher-Debre-Semelaigne syndrome* in children, is rare. Patients complain of stiffness and painful muscle cramps, and the movements are slow and weak. The muscles are large and firm. *Pseudomyotonia*, or delayed muscle relaxation after handshake or percussion, may be present and is differentiated from myotonia by its electrical silence on EMG.

Peripheral neuropathies are mostly entrapment neuropathies (carpal tunnel), resulting from mucoid infiltration of the nerve and the surrounding tissue. Eighty percent of patients complain of distal paresthesias. Polyneuropathies are less frequent. Deep tendon reflexes have slowed relaxation time, also seen in hypothermia, leg edema, diabetes, parkinsonism, drugs, and normal aging.

REFERENCES

Anagnos A, Ruff RL, Kaminski HJ: *Neurol Clin* 15:673–696, 1997.
Horak HA et al: *Neurol Clin* 18:203–213, 2000.

TOURETTE'S SYNDROME; GILLES DE LA TOURETTE'S SYNDROME (GTS)

The DSM-IV defines GTS as characterized by the following:

1. Both multiple motor tics and one or more vocal tics present at some time during the illness, although not necessarily concurrently.
2. Tics occur many times a day (usually in bouts), nearly every day or intermittently for more than 1 year, without a tic-free interval of more than 3 consecutive months.
3. Anatomic location, number, frequency, complexity, and severity of tics change over time.
4. Onset before 18 years of age.
5. Does not occur exclusively during psychoactive substance intoxication or known central nervous system disease.
6. Social, academic, or occupational functioning is impaired.

Tics are sudden, intermittent, and patterned involuntary movements. Motor tics may be simple, like eye blinking, or complex, like facial gestures, grooming behaviors, jumping, or obscene gestures (copropraxia).

Vocal tics include sniffing, snorting, throat clearing, or barking. More complex vocal tics include coprolalia (utterance of obscenities), echolalia, and palilalia. In contrast to public perception, coprolalia is quite rare. Tics may be exacerbated by anger or stress, may be diminished during sleep, and may become attenuated during some absorbing activity. They may be voluntarily suppressed for minutes to hours.

The onset of tics is most commonly between 5 and 10 years. Boys are affected three to four times more than girls. GTS lasts for life and frequently waxes and wanes in severity. Obsessive compulsive (OCD) and attention deficit hyperactivity disorders (ADHD) occur in 25% to 35% of patients with GTS.

Pathogenesis is unknown. Recent theories have focused on genetics and also on antecedent streptococcal infection. The term PANDAS refers to Pediatric and Adolescent Neuropsychiatric Disorders Associated with Streptococcus.

It is important to inform the patient and his family that GTS is not a psychological problem. A multidisciplinary therapeutic program must be established, in close collaboration with the parents and the child. Early treatment does not alter the natural history of the disease. Clonidine, an α_2-adrenergic agonist, may be started as a first choice to avoid or delay use of neuroleptic agents. Initial daily dose is 0.05 to 0.1 mg increased to 0.025 to 0.05 mg weekly, the usual effective dose being 0.3 mg daily. Patients presenting with associated OCD find some benefit from the use of clonidine. Other medications include pimozide, haloperidol, tetrabenazine, and anticholinergic agents. Haloperidol or clonidine are effective in 50% of cases. Stimulant drugs used for ADHD may unmask or exacerbate TS.

REFERENCE

Arzimanoglou AA: *J Neurol* 245:761–765, 1998.

TRANSIENT GLOBAL AMNESIA (TGA)

The syndrome occurs in middle aged or elderly individuals and recurs in 3%. An individual behaves in an apparently automatic fashion for minutes to hours (<24 hours) without recollection of those events and has retrograde amnesia that may be spotty. During the ictus, the patient repetitively asks questions about his or her plight, identity, and location in ways that indicated an acute awareness of the amnesia. Although the patient recovers, a permanent island of memory loss for the period encompassed by the TGA may remain. TGA attack can follow a wide variety of stresses, including strenuous exertion, sexual intercourse, immersion in water, pain, and emotional stress. The pathogenesis of TGA is unknown but may be a manifestation of migraine, transient vascular insufficiency, or complex partial seizure (transient epileptic amnesia). An investigation with diffusion weighted MR images revealed cellular edema in the anterior temporal lobe in TGA. Patients with TGA and their families require explanation and reassurance during and after the attack.

REFERENCE
Zeman AZ, Hodges JR: *Br J Hosp Med* 58(6):257–260, 1997.

TRANSPLANTATION—NEUROLOGIC ASPECTS

ORGAN HARVEST

The determination of death prior to organ harvest is based on neurologic criteria. At present, most jurisdictions require absence of function of the entire brain (see Brain Death).

CLINICAL SYNDROMES IN ORGAN RECIPIENTS

Organ recipients often present with complex syndromes and multiple possible etiologies. Following organ transplantation, 30% to 60% of patients develop neurologic complications. Some of the syndromes are due to preexisting deficits due to underlying illness; others can be classified as complications during surgery, metabolic encephalopathies, neurotoxicity of immunosuppressant agents, opportunistic CNS infections, secondary malignancies as a direct side effect of immunosuppression, and other specific neurologic complications seen mostly after certain organ transplantations.

Specific clinical syndromes include the following.

1. Complications related to transplantation procedures: Acquired nerve injuries: femoral or lateral cutaneous nerve injuries after kidney transplantation.
2. Effect of immunosuppressant agents—*Cyclosporine:* tremor (40%), leukoencephalopathy (5%), hemiparesis, paraparesis, tetraparesis, predominantly sensory neuropathy; *Corticosteroids:* proximal myopathy, anxiety and dysthymia, psychosis (3%), "steroid pseudorheumatism," headache, fever, lethargy on withdrawal; *OKT3 monoclonal antibody:* transient flu-like symptoms, aseptic meningitis (2% to 14%), encephalopathy (1% to 10%); *Tacrolimus* produces neurologic complications that are similar to cyclosporine, but less frequent.
3. Opportunistic CNS infection: Secondary to immunosuppression; occurs in up to 10% of recipients with high mortality; usually occurs 1 month or more after transplantation. Usually, infections in the first posttransplantation month are due to the surgical procedure itself, acquired from the donor kidney, or were present before transplantation. Infections from 1 to 6 months are at the peak of immunosuppression and mostly due to viruses (cytomegalovirus [CMV], Epstein-Barr virus [EBV]), opportunistic organisms (*Aspergillus fumigatus, Nocardia asteroides,* and *Listeria monocytogenes*). Beyond 6 months posttransplantation, infections are due to lingering effects of previously acquired infections.

Fungi: *Cryptococcus:* most common pathogen, usually presents after 6 months of immune suppression; *Aspergillus:* often presents as stroke or encephalopathy; *Candida*: usually presents as chronic meningitis; *Mucormycosis*: seen in diabetic recipients.

Bacteria: *Listeria*: most common bacterium, usually causing meningitis; *Nocardia*: usually causes abscess; *Tuberculosis*: uncommon.

Parasitic: *Toxoplasmosis*: presents after 1 to 4 months.

Viruses: *Cytomegalovirus*: may cause chorioretinitis; *Varicella*: new infection may cause encephalitis with high morbidity, reactivation produces shingles, either diffusely or in dermatomal distribution; *HTLV-I*: causes myelopathy after blood transfusion in heart, bone marrow, and kidney recipients; *JC virus*: progressive multifocal leukoencephalopathy (see Encephalitis).

4. Posttransplant lymphoproliferative disorders: Primary CNS lymphoma is 35-fold higher in the recipients of kidney transplants. It has a poor prognosis and poor response to chemotherapy and radiotherapy.

5. Other neurologic syndromes include the following:

Cerebellar dysfunction: Dysarthria, ataxia due to neurotoxicity of immunosuppressants.

Creutzfeldt-Jakob disease: Increased risk for patients receiving cadaveric dura transplantation.

Demyelination: Central pontine myelinolysis due to osmotic shifts, frequently during the perioperative period.

Guillian-Barré syndrome: Described following bone marrow transplantation.

Hearing loss: Due to cyclosporine-mediated thromboembolic process or antibiotic toxicity.

Language disorders: Reversible, due to Tacrolimus neurotoxicity or reversible demyelination.

Malignancy: Primary CNS lymphoma due to immunosuppression.

Mental status deterioration: With cyclosporine and accompanying diffuse changes on MRI; cognitive slowing, insomnia, delirium, perceptual disturbances seen with cyclosporine and Tacrolimus in liver recipients.

Metabolic acidosis: Can cause coma in kidney recipients.

Migraine: In bone marrow recipients, due to cyclosporine or hypothesized defect in donor-derived platelets.

Movement disorder: Chorea due to cyclosporine in liver transplantation for Wilson's disease.

Myopathy: In lung transplantation with cyclosporine, azathioprine, prednisone, with prolonged response to neuromuscular blockade; myositis is one manifestation of graft-versus-host disease.

Nerve injury: Recurrent laryngeal palsy in heart-lung recipient.

Neuromyotonia: Antibody-mediated channelopathy, seen in patients after bone marrow transplantation.

Neurocardiogenic symptoms: Angina and vasovagal syncope seen in heart recipients, presumed due to reinnervation.

Neuropathy: Reported in a pancreas transplant recipient.

Pain: Due to varicella zoster; due to local effects at operative sites; musculoskeletal pain due to direct cyclosporine effects in kidney recipients; due to oral mucositis in bone marrow recipients.

Seizures: Generalized tonic-clonic seizures occur in bone-marrow transplantation with a regimen of busulfan, cyclophosphamide, cyclosporine, methylprednisolone; seen with Tacrolimus; seen in liver recipients, often with neuropathologic lesions at autopsy.

Sleep disorder: Somnolence syndrome related to radiation in bone marrow recipient.

Stroke and cerebral ischemia: 44% to 59% of all neurologic complications of posttransplantation patients; less common with Tacrolimus than with cyclosporine in liver recipients; due to hypoperfusion in heart recipient.

Taste disturbance: In bone marrow recipients.

Visual disturbance: Side effect of cyclosporine.

REFERENCES

Burn DJ, Bates D: *J Neurol Neurosurg Psychiatry* 65:810–821, 1998.
Liguori R: *Neurology* 54:1390–1391, 2000.
Nakamura Y et al: *Neurology* 53:218–220, 1999.
Wen PY et al: *Neurology* 49:1711–1714, 1997.

TREMORS

Tremors are regular, rhythmic oscillations produced by alternating contraction of agonist and antagonist muscles. They usually affect the distal extremities (especially fingers and hands), head, tongue, jaw, and only rarely, the trunk. Tremors disappear during sleep. The frequency is usually consistent in all the affected parts, regardless of the size of muscles involved. It is important to observe the amplitude, frequency, and rhythm of the tremor, as well as the effects of physiologic (posture, limb movement, diurnal variation, and so forth) and psychologic factors.

CLASSIFICATION

1. *Action or postural tremor:* Present when the limbs and trunk are held in certain positions or during active movements.

   A. *Physiologic tremor:* Small-amplitude, high-frequency (6 to 12 Hz) tremor seen in normal individuals; exaggerated by stress, endocrine disorders (hyperthyroidism, hypoglycemia, and pheochromocytoma), or drugs (such as lithium, tricyclics, phenothiazines, epinephrine, theophylline, amphetamines, thyroid hormones, isoproterenol, corticosteroids, valproate, levodopa, and butyrophenones) and toxins (such as mercury, lead, arsenic, bismuth, and carbon monoxide). Dietary factors may contribute (caffeine, monosodium glutamate, and ethanol withdrawal). Management depends on the cause; relaxation methods and stress reduction may help if psychologic factors are involved. Beta blockers have been used with some success, particularly in performers with "stage fright."

B. *Essential tremor:* A postural tremor that often increases with action or intention. It has a frequency of 4 to 7 Hz and usually consists of flexion-extension of the fingers and hands initially, but may progress proximally; the head and neck, jaw, tongue, or voice may be involved. It is exacerbated by emotional and physical stress and diminished with rest, relaxation, and use of ethanol. It may be familial (dominant inheritance), sporadic, or associated with other movement disorders (Parkinson's disease, torsion dystonia, or torticollis). Propranolol is the drug of choice but is contraindicated in patients with asthma or diabetes and in older patients with heart failure. Start with doses of 10 to 20 mg three or four times a day, increasing dosage if necessary. Primidone therapy is also useful, starting at 50 mg. It may be increased up to 250 mg TID as tolerated. Sedation or GI complaints may limit its use. Benzodiazepines are also useful in treating essential tremor.

C. *Primary writing tremor:* Occurs only during writing. Electrophysiologic studies suggest that it may be a form of dystonia. It may respond to anticholinergic therapy.

D. *Rubral tremor:* A coarse tremor present at rest, increasing with postural maintenance and even more with movement. Suggests ipsilateral cerebellar outflow lesion.

II. Rest tremors.

A. *Parkinsonian tremor:* Frequency of 3 to 7 Hz with variable amplitude, sometimes asymmetric. It occurs at rest and disappears with movement and during sleep. It is prominent in the hands, with flexion-extension or adduction-abduction of the fingers. There is also pronation-supination of the hands. Movements of the feet, jaw, and lips may be present. It responds to anticholinergic therapy or dopaminergic drugs.

III. Intention tremor.

A. *Cerebellar tremor:* A tremor of 3 to 5 Hz occurring during the performance of an exact, projected movement and worsening as the action continues. There may be tremors of the lead or trunk (titubation). The oscillation begins proximally and occurs perpendicular to the line of movement. Causes include lesions of cerebellar pathways, cerebellar degeneration, Wilson's disease, and drugs or toxins (such as phenytoin, barbiturates, lithium, ethanol, mercury, and fluorouracil).

IV. Other tremors.

A. *Orthostatic tremor,* a tremor of the legs, is present only when standing and disappears with walking. As such, it may be considered a task-specific tremor. It responds to clonazepam therapy, 4 to 6 mg per day.

B. *Hysterical tremor* may be a symptom of conversion disorder. The tremor is often irregular in frequency and may diminish or disappear with distraction.

REFERENCES:

Findley LJ, Koller WC: *Neurology* 37:1194–1197, 1987.
Hallett M: *JAMA* 266:1115–1117, 1991.

TRIGEMINAL NEURALGIA (*Tic Douloureux*)

Trigeminal neuralgia is characterized by paroxysmal, severe, lancinating, brief (about 30 to 60 seconds), unilateral facial pain in the distribution of one or more branches of the trigeminal nerve (most commonly the second and third divisions). Paroxysms tend to occur in clusters. Trigger points are set off by touching, chewing, talking, or swallowing due to stimulation of the skin, mucosa, or teeth innervated by the ipsilateral trigeminal nerve. Onset is after age 40 in 90% and is more common in women (ratio of 3 to 2). Neurologic exam, including trigeminal sensory and motor exam, is normal. The etiology may be multifactorial and is usually idiopathic but may be due to compression by a redundant artery. Local lesions such as demyelinating lesion (multiple sclerosis), cerebellopontine angle tumors, and schwannomas account for a very small proportion of cases.
Secondary trigeminal neuralgia should be suspected with onset before age 40, with trigeminal sensory or motor abnormalities on exam, or with any other findings referable to the base of the skull or posterior fossa.

Differential diagnosis includes posterior fossa mass lesions such as tumor (meningioma, acoustic neuroma), aneurysm, or arteriovenous malformations (AVM). Trigeminal neuralgia pain may be seen in multiple sclerosis. Trigeminal neuroma and foraminal osteoma are among other causes. Evaluation should include MRI with gadolinium and possibly arteriography.

Treatment of secondary trigeminal neuralgia is aimed at the underlying cause. Idiopathic trigeminal neuralgia is treated medically. Medications that are commonly used are as follows:

1. Carbamazepine is the drug of choice and is effective in 75% to 80%. Start at 50 to 100 mg/day and increase gradually as tolerated to 1 to 1.2 g/day in divided doses. Serum levels of 8 to 12 mg% should be achieved.
2. Imipramine or amitriptyline starting at 25 to 50 mg orally at bedtime and gradually increasing to 150 mg.
3. Phenytoin 300 to 500 mg per day to achieve therapeutic levels.
4. Baclofen starting at 5 mg orally three times a day and increasing gradually to 20 mg orally four times a day.
5. Clonazepam starting at 0.5 mg orally twice a day and increasing to 0.5 to 10 mg/day in two or three divided doses.
6. Other drugs have been used such as divalproex sodium, pimozide, gabapentin, and lamotrigine.
7. Combination approaches have utilized phenytoin with carbamazepine or imipramine. Baclofen has also been used with phenytoin or carbamazepine.

TRIGEMINAL NEURALGIA

8. When pain has been controlled, medications should be tapered periodically because spontaneous remissions can occur.
9. A useful technique in the midst of a severe attack, is the administration of intravenous fosphenytoin at a dose of 250 mg.

Surgical therapy is reserved for intractable pain unresponsive to drug treatment and includes the following:

1. Local neurolysis and nerve block is associated with a risk of painful anesthesia and persistent paresthesias as well as recurrence.
2. Percutaneous radiofrequency thermocoagulation of the trigeminal ganglion can be done under local anesthesia. Painful anesthesia and recurrences are less common.
3. Trigeminal rhizotomy. It is used less often than previously.
4. Microsurgical vascular decompression of the trigeminal root entry zone.
5. Several new procedures have shown promise in patients with refractory cases. These procedures include percutaneous trigeminal nerve compression and stereotactic radiosurgery with the gamma knife.

TRINUCLEOTIDE REPEAT EXPANSION

Triple repeat is a heterogeneous group of neurogenetic disorders. The mechanism of repeat expansion is unknown but may be related to unequal crossing over during meiosis. The size of the repeat expansion can change from parent to offspring, and increases across generation account for the clinical phenomena of anticipation. Several disorders show unstable repeat triplets (Table 69).

TABLE 69
TRINUCLEOTIDE REPEAT DISORDERS

Disorder	Abnormal Protein	Repeat Expansion
1. Fragile X syndrome	FMR1	CGG
2. Spinobulbar muscular dystrophy (Kennedy's syndrome)	Androgen receptor	CAG
3. Myotonic dystrophy	Myotinin kinase	CTG
4. Huntington disease	Huntingtin	CAG
5. SCA 1	Ataxin	CAG
6. SCA 2	Unidentified	CAG
7. SCA 3 (Machado-Joseph Disease)	Unidentified	CAG
8. SCA 6	Unidentified	CAG
9. SCA 7	Unidentified	CAG
10. DRPLA	Unidentified	CAG
11. Friedreich's ataxia	Frataxin	GAA

A = Adenine; C = cytosine; DRPLA = dentatorubral-pallido-luysian atrophy;
G = guanine; SCA = spinocerebellar ataxia; T = thiamine.

TUMORS (see also Paraneoplastic Syndromes, Radiation Injury, Spinal Cord)

The presence of tumor within the nervous system is often suspected by the development of subacute or acute focal symptoms. Some tumors, particularly metastases or carcinomatous meningitis, may result in multifocal signs. The combination of location, patient demographics, and neuro-imaging often suggests the most likely histopathology (see Table 70 and Figure 42).

BRAIN

Although primary brain tumors occur about five times more often in adults than in children, the central nervous system (CNS) is the second most

TABLE 70

HISTOLOGICAL CLASSIFICATION

Neuroepithelial tumors
  Astrocytic tumors:
    Diffuse astrocytoma
    Astrocytoma
    Anaplastic astrocytoma
    Glioblastoma multiforme
    Juvenile pilocytic astrocytoma
    Subependymal giant cell astrocytoma
  Oligodendroglial tumors:
    Oligodendroglioma
    Anaplastic oligodendroglioma
  Ependymal tumors:
    Ependymoma
    Myxopapillary ependymoma
    Anaplastic ependymoma
    Subependymoma
  Choroid plexus tumors:
    Choroid plexus papilloma
    Choroid plexus carcinoma
  Neuronal tumors:
    Ganglioglioma
    Gangliocytoma
  Primitive neuroectodermal tumors:
    Medulloblastoma
    Pineoblastoma
    Neuroblastoma

Meningeal Tumors
  Meningioma
  Papillary meningioma
  Anaplastic meningioma

Nerve sheath tumors:
  Schwannoma (neurilemmoma)
  Neurofibroma
  Neurofibrosarcoma
Tumors of blood vessel origin:
  Hemangioblastoma
  Hemangiopericytoma
Germ cell tumors:
  Germinoma
  Embryonal carcinoma
  Choriocarcinoma
  Teratoma
Malignant lymphomas:
  Hodgkin's disease
  Non-Hodgkin's lymphoma
Malformative tumors:
  Craniopharyngioma
  Epidermoid cyst
  Dermoid cyst
  Neuroepithelial (colloid) cyst
  Lipoma
Regional tumors:
  Chordoma
  Glomus jugulare tumor
  Chondroma
Metastatic tumors:
  Carcinoma
  Sarcoma
  Lymphoma

From Cohen ME: In Bradley WG, Baroff RB, Fenichel GM, Marsden CD, eds: *Neurology in clinical practice*, Boston, Butterworth-Heinemann, 1991.

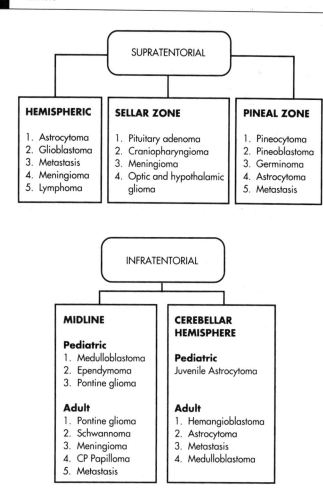

FIGURE 42

Tumors by location.
Illustration continued on opposite page

common site for childhood malignancies. Metastases account for the majority of CNS tumors in adults. Approximately 20% of all patients with systemic cancer have CNS involvement at some time during their illness.

Symptoms and signs of CNS neoplasm may be generalized and non-localizing, usually as a result of diffuse edema, hydrocephalus, or increased intracranial pressure. Headaches are variable and may resemble tension or migraine headaches. Most headaches are ipsilateral to the

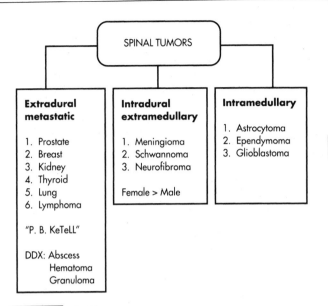

FIGURE 42 —Cont'd
From AAN: Contemporary neuropathology, vol 6, *Basic neurosciences,* AAN Courses 1993; courtesy of JC Goodman.

tumor. With increased intracranial pressure a bifrontal or bioccipital headache is common, regardless of tumor location. Seizures occur more often with slow-growing tumors and with tumors in the frontal and parietal lobes. Vomiting occurs most consistently with posterior fossa masses. Localizing symptoms and signs depend on tumor location. Frontal lobe masses may be silent or, if anterior and midline, may produce changes in personality and memory. Third ventricle and pineal region tumors often produce ventricular and aqueductal obstruction leading to hydrocephalus. Brainstem tumors produce cranial neuropathies, long-tract signs, and hydrocephalus resulting from compression of the aqueduct.

Once suspected, the diagnosis of a brain tumor is usually confirmed by neuroimaging, either CT scan or MRI. Hemorrhage occurs most often with glioblastoma multiforme and metastatic tumors, especially renal cell, melanoma, and choriocarcinoma. Calcification occurs more commonly with oligodendrogliomas and meningiomas. Skull x-rays or CT with bone windows are useful in evaluating bony metastasis; angiography defines vascular anatomy.

Available treatment modalities include debulking surgery, radiation therapy, chemotherapy, and combinations of the three. The late effects of CNS irradiation include radiation necrosis, myelopathy, intellectual deterioration, endocrinopathies, and oncogenesis (see also Chemotherapy, Radiation).

SPINAL CORD

Tumors of the spinal cord and its coverings account for approximately 15% of all CNS tumors. Extradural cord tumors arise from the vertebral bodies and epidural tissues or are metastatic lesions to the epidural space. Intradural tumors are either intramedullary (arising within the substance of the cord) or extramedullary (arising from the leptomeninges or nerve roots). Myelography with CT scanning has been the traditional procedure of choice in the evaluation of spinal cord masses and allows for the simultaneous collection of spinal fluid. Myelography with CT can demonstrate the presence of spinal block, but the upper extent of that may require a second spinal puncture (for example, cervical tap). MRI can differentiate solid from cystic intramedullary tumors and defines whether lesions are intradural or extradural.

Clinical manifestations of spinal masses include local back or radicular pain, myelopathy, sensory complaints, and sphincter dysfunction. On plain radiographic films these masses may produce widening of the interpeduncular distance or of the neural foramina, as well as scalloping of the vertebral bodies. The loss of a pedicle and signs of bone destruction are associated with malignant extradural lesions. Since the majority of spinal tumors are benign and produce symptoms by compression rather than by invasion, surgery is the treatment of choice for most masses.

METASTATIC DISEASE

Metastases to the brain parenchyma are often found at the gray-white matter junction and are typically well demarcated with a zone of surrounding edema. They are usually carcinomas rather than sarcomas or lymphomas. Cancers most commonly associated with metastases vary according to site as follows:

Skull and dura: Breast, prostate, multiple myeloma.
Brain: Lung, breast, colorectal, renal, melanoma.
Leptomeninges: Breast, lung, melanoma, colorectal, lymphoma, leukemia.
Epidural (spinal cord): Lung, breast, prostate, lymphoma, sarcoma, renal.

EPIDURAL SPINAL CORD COMPRESSION

Spinal cord compression represents a neurologic emergency. The diagnosis should be suspected in anyone with a known tumor and back pain who seeks medical attention with segmental or myelopathic signs. Diagnosis can be suspected from the presence of bony destruction if present on plain radiographic films; confirmation can be obtained by MRI, myelography, or occasionally, bone scan. Treatment usually consists of radiotherapy and a regimen of high-dose corticosteroids: load with dexamethasone 100 mg IV, then maintain dexamethasone 24 mg qid (PO or IV) for 3 days; steroids are then tapered over 12 days, decreasing the dose every 2 days (12 mg qid, then 8 mg qid, then 4 mg qid, then 2 mg qid, then 1 mg qid, then 0.5 mg qid). Indications for possible surgery include the following:

1. Occurrence of metastases in a previously irradiated area.
2. Spinal instability.
3. Bony compression of neural structures.
4. Deterioration during radiotherapy, despite administration of high-dose corticosteroids.
5. The need for biopsy when the diagnosis is unclear.

The entire spinal cord should be imaged because 15% to 25% of patients present with two or more lesions.

REFERENCES

Cohen ME: In Bradley WG, Daroff RB, Fenichel GM, Marsden CD, eds: *Neurology in clinical practice,* ed 2, Boston, Butterworth-Heinemann, 2000.
Patchell RA, ed: *Neurol Clin* 9(4); 817–824, 1991.

ULNAR NERVE (see also Peripheral Nerve)

Entrapment at the elbow results from compression of the ulnar nerve as it courses in the elbow joint under the aponeurosis connecting the two heads of the flexor carpi ulnaris. It commonly results from extrinsic compression, from leaning on the elbow (especially in patients with a shallow ulnar groove), or from malpositioning of the arms on operating room tables or the arm rests of wheelchairs. "Tardy ulnar palsy" occurs following an elbow fracture or in association with arthritis, ganglion cysts, lipomas, or neuropathic (Charcot) joints. Symptoms include elbow pain, sensory loss and paresthesias of the fifth and ulnar half of the fourth digits and ulnar aspect of the hand, and wasting of the hypothenar and intrinsic hand muscles. There may be a claw-hand deformity. Marked weakness of the flexor carpi ulnaris suggests that the lesion is above the elbow. There may be tenderness or enlargement of the ulnar nerve (palpable in the epicondylar groove); Tinel's sign may be present at the elbow.

Differential diagnosis includes C8 or T1 radiculopathy, syringomyelia, ALS, lower trunk brachial plexopathy (Pancoast syndrome), and peripheral polyneuropathy. Nerve conduction studies may show conduction block or slowing across the elbow; EMG may show denervation.

Treatment involves removing exacerbating factors by padding the elbow or armchair rests. If this fails, or if motor involvement is found on physical examination or EMG, surgical decompression may be indicated. There is no clear advantage of more complex procedures (such as ulnar nerve transposition) over simple slitting of the aponeurosis of the flexor carpi ulnaris. However, transposition may be indicated in patients with fibrosis from joint disease.

Entrapment at the wrist or hand (Guyon's canal) consist of variable involvement of the deep and superficial branches of the ulnar nerve to the hand, with sparing of the dorsal cutaneus branch that supplies sensation to the dorsal ulnar sensory distribution. The same etiologic factors as for the elbow apply. The EMG and nerve conduction studies should demonstrate involvement of the hand ulnar motor fibers with sparing of sensory function to the dorsal hand.

ULTRASONOGRAPHY

The carotid and vertebral arteries and their branches can be evaluated with ultrasound, that is, sound with frequency higher than 20,000 Hertz. *B-mode* (brightness modulation) is based on the transmission of ultrasound through tissues and reflection from tissue interfaces. This imaging technique produces a real-time two-dimensional picture of examined extracranial vessels in longitudinal or transverse view. It allows measurement of vessel diameter and reveals the presence of stenosis or occlusion. High-resolution scans can also determine plaque morphology, such as ulceration, calcification, or hemorrhage. In *Doppler ultrasonography*, the ultrasound is reflected off moving targets (erythrocytes). Increased blood flow velocity in a narrowed segment of arterial lumen (stenosis) is associated with higher frequency shift, which correlates with flow velocities. The best result in vascular ultrasonography can be obtained by combination of these two techniques, *duplex ultrasonography*. It combines the advantages of B-mode with exact sampling of the site, and systolic, diastolic, and mean velocities are measured in Doppler mode. Carotid duplex ultrasonography has an excellent accuracy for detection of stenotic process compared with angiography. For arteries with more than 50% stenosis, sensitivity is approximately 94% to 100%; for occlusions, sensitivity is 80% to 96% and specificity is 95%. However, these results vary considerably with the experience of the ultrasonographer. Examination of vertebral arteries allow determination of flow direction (for example, subclavian steal syndrome), but morphologic evaluation is not always possible.

Blood flow velocities in the major intracranial arteries can be examined by *transcranial doppler* (TCD). TCD has established value in detection of stenosis >65% in the major basal intracranial arteries, assessing collateral flow, evaluating and monitoring vasospasm after subarachnoid hemorrhage, detecting arteriovascular malformations, and assessing patients with brain death. The accuracy of TCD also depends highly on operator skill and experience. TCD may also be used for intraoperative monitoring during carotid endarterectomy and cardiac surgery and in testing cerebrovascular reactivity and hemodynamic reserve.

REFERENCES

Babikian VL et al: *J Neuroimaging* 10:101–115, 2000.
Beletsky VY, Kelley RE: *J La State Med Soc* 148:467–473, 1996.

UREMIA

Uremia refers to the constellation of signs and symptoms associated with renal failure, regardless of the cause. The presentation varies from patient to patient, depending upon the remaining renal function and the rapidity at which the function is lost. With glomerular filtration rate about 20% to 35% of normal, azotemia occurs. The likely toxins are byproducts of protein and amino acid metabolism such as urea, guidino compounds, aliphatic amines, tyrosine, and phenylalanine.

A. Uremic encephalopathy correlates with *rate of progression of uremia*, as opposed to the absolute blood urea nitrogen and creatinine levels.

Clinical features: Clouding of consciousness may be associated with hallucinations, increased reflexes, and increased tone (may be asymmetric). Asterixis, myoclonus and chorea, stupor, seizures, and coma are signs of terminal uremia.

Evaluation: EEG is characterized by low voltage slowing early; later there may be a generalized paroxysmal slowing. Triphasic waves or epileptiform activity are not uncommon. CSF protein level may be elevated, and aseptic meningitis may occur, accompanied by stiff neck and marked pleocytosis.

Management: Dialysis, supportive care, and antiepileptic drugs.

B. Seizures in renal failure are usually generalized but may be focal. They may occur in the setting of uremic encephalopathy, hypertensive crisis, coexistent electrolyte disturbance, or drug toxicity. Purely uremic seizures often respond to dialysis. When anticonvulsants are required, dosage must be adjusted for glomerular filtration rate. *Diminished renal clearance requires decreased dosages of carbamazepine, phenobarbital, and gabapentin*. Changes in clearance and protein binding lead to decreased total phenytoin levels with an increased unbound fraction. These changes necessitate *free-fraction monitoring for optimal control*. Anticonvulsants with low protein binding affinity are sometimes preferable in patients on hemodialysis.

C. Peripheral neuropathy (distal, symmetric sensorimotor polyneuropathy type) is common in advanced renal failure and can result in flaccid paralysis. It is often painful and may be associated with restless leg syndrome. Abnormal nerve conduction studies may precede clinical symptoms and signs. The neuropathy stabilizes or improves with hemodialysis. The greatest improvement seems to occur with renal transplantation. Tricyclics or anticonvulsants may alleviate pain.

D. Myopathy: Patients with chronic renal failure often have symmetric proximal weakness with atrophy and painful stiffness. Serum creatine kinase (CK) and aldolase levels are usually normal, but EMG shows myopathic changes, sometimes due to secondary hyperparathyroidism. Rarely, ischemic myopathy occurs with elevated levels of serum CK, severe weakness, and gangrenous skin lesions.

E. Tetany that does not respond to calcium may occur.

REFERENCES

Bachman D et al: *Seizure* 5:239–542, 1996.
Burn DJ et al: *J Neurol Neurosurg Psychiatry* 65:810–821, 1998.
Fraser CL, Arieff AL: *Ann Intern Med* 109:143, 1988.
Ruff RL et al: *Neurol Clin* 6:575, 1988.

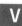

VASCULITIS

Vasculitis refers to a clinicopathologic process characterized by inflammation of the blood vessels. Vasculitides can be primary (idiopathic) or secondary, that is, related to rheumatologic disease, malignancy, drugs, or infections.

PRIMARY VASCULITIDES
Isolated Angiitis of the CNS
The clinical picture of this rare disorder is nonspecific and includes recurrent headaches, encephalopathy, confusion, or focal signs such as hemiparesis or aphasia with subacute to acute onset.

CSF usually shows lymphocytic pleocytosis and elevated protein. In contrast to temporal arteritis, the erythrocyte sedimentation rate (ESR) is usually only mildly elevated. Angiography can show beading of large- and medium-sized vessels. Biopsy of the nondominant temporal lobe including a specimen of leptomeninges is usually recommended before initiation of treatment. Treatment is with high-dose prednisone, usually combined with cyclophosphamide.

Temporal Arteritis (Giant Cell Arteritis)
Temporal arteritis occurs almost exclusively in patients over the age of 55 years and is the most common of the three granulomatous vasculitides, with an estimated incidence of approximately 24 cases per 100,000 people. It mainly affects the extracranial arteries of the head and tends to spare the intracranial vessels. The superficial temporal and the ophthalmic arteries are commonly involved. Physical examination often shows tender, tortuous, thickened, and pulseless temporal arteries. Involvement of the extracranial carotids and vertebrals is also relatively common and can lead to strokes in about 7% of the patients. More proximal vessels, including the aorta and the coronary arteries, can also be affected. The most common

presenting symptoms are headaches and constitutional symptoms. Jaw claudication can be present in as many as 40% of the patients and is secondary to ischemia of the muscles. Amaurosis fugax is less common (10% of patients) but is likely to progress to blindness if left untreated. Polymyalgia rheumatica is seen in more than half of the patients with temporal arteritis. Proximal myalgias and morning stiffness are the hallmark of this condition. ESR is very high in almost all cases. Only 3% of the patients may have a normal ESR. Angiography can demonstrate luminal irregularities and alternating stenosis and dilatation. Histologic confirmation should be obtained, but treatment should be initiated immediately on the basis of the clinical suspicion with high-dose prednisone for 1 month and a subsequent slow taper. The ESR can be used to monitor the disease activity.

Takayasu's Arteritis (TA)

TA most frequently affects young women of Asian and South American descent. It affects the tunica media of large- and medium-sized arteries, primarily the aortic arch and its proximal branches. The carotids are more commonly affected than the vertebral arteries. The intracranial arteries are typically spared. Generalized symptoms (malaise, fever, weight loss, night sweats) may be the initial presenting symptoms. Visual changes are the most common neurologic symptom. Syncope and dizziness are also very common. More than half of the patients may experience focal neurologic deficits such as hemiparesis or aphasia. Seizures can occur and may be associated with the induction of hypoperfusion through postural changes. Physical examination will reveal pulse deficits and multiple vascular bruits in most cases.

Angiography is essential for the diagnosis of TA. Treatment is with high-dose oral steroids. If response to the steroids is poor, then methotrexate or cyclophosphamide can be considered. The ESR is not as reliable a parameter to follow as with temporal arteritis.

The prognosis of the disease is relatively good with an 80% 5-year survival rate. Aggressive surgical and/or angioplastic procedures may improve prognosis significantly in certain cases.

SECONDARY VASCULITIDES
Systemic Lupus Erythematosus (SLE)

Neurologic involvement in SLE is quite common. The reported incidence is in the range of 25% to 75%. The spectrum of neurologic symptoms is very broad and includes headaches, encephalopathy, seizures, myelitis, optic neuritis, cerebral ischemia, cranial and peripheral neuropathies, movement disorders, and seizures. *Seizures are the most common neurologic problem.* The underlying CNS pathology is rarely that of vasculitis. More often, a noninflammatory vasculopathy is observed. Treatment of severe CNS manifestations is with high-dose IV steroids, followed by oral prednisone taper. Cyclophosphamide can be used if steroids fail. Azathioprine can be used as maintenance treatment.

Polyarteritis Nodosa

The disease usually develops in the fifth or sixth decade of life and affects men almost twice as often as women. It is a chronic disease that causes patchy necrosis in the walls of medium- and small-sized arteries. Many of the patients are seropositive for hepatitis B or C. The most frequently affected organs are the kidney, the heart, and the liver. The peripheral nervous system is affected in 50% to 60% of the patients. Painful mononeuritis multiplex is very common, but polyneuropathies, plexo-pathies, and radiculopathies can also occur. CNS involvement typically occurs later with an incidence of <30%. Patients usually present with changes in mental status and seizures. Cerebral ischemia can occur but is uncommon. The diagnosis is based on angiography and/or tissue biopsy. Steroids combined with cyclophosphamide is the treatment of choice.

Wegener's Granulomatosis

This condition involves granulomatous, necrotizing vasculitis of the small arteries and veins, mainly affecting the upper and lower respiratory tract and also associated with glomerulonephritis. Up to 50% of the patients will have skin or eye involvement. Besides the constitutional symptoms, the most common neurologic manifestations are peripheral and cranial neuropathies. Strokes and seizures are less common. The c-ANCA titers are sensitive and specific for active Wegener's. ESR is usually markedly elevated. Diagnosis is based on biopsy of respiratory tract or renal tissues. Treatment is with cyclophosphamide, initially combined with prednisone; azathioprine can be used in those who cannot tolerate cyclophosphamide.

Churg-Strauss Syndrome

This is a granulomatous vasculitis affecting mainly the lung. There is a strong association with severe asthma and peripheral eosinophilia. Mononeuritis multiplex may occur, but it is not common. Treatment is with steroids, if needed combined with cyclophosphamide.

Sjögren's Syndrome

This syndrome is a chronic inflammatory and autoimmune disorder prima-rily affecting lacrimal and salivary glands and causing dry mouth (xerosto-mia) and dry eyes (xerophthalmia). Headaches, aseptic meningitis, myelopathy, mononeuritis multiplex, and focal deficits are among the neurologic complications, but these are altogether uncommon.

Cogan's Disease

This is a rare disease of the young. It presents with interstitial keratitis, vestibular and auditory dysfunction, encephalomyelitis, and polyneuropathy.

Herpes Zoster Ophthalmicus Hemiplegia

This usually presents weeks or months after herpes zoster ophthalmicus. Involvement of the ipsilateral anterior and middle cerebral arteries causes contralateral hemiparesis.

Behçet's Disease

This disease is a rare vasculitic disorder that affects many organs and is characterized by recurrent oral and genital ulcers, uveitis, and nondeforming arthritis. It affects mostly young patients and is more common in eastern Mediterranean countries and in Japan.

Neurologic symptoms occur in approximately 10% of cases and include headache, meningitic syndrome, and a multiple sclerosis-like picture. In cases with uveitis and/or CNS symptoms, high-dose prednisone is used in conjunction with azathioprine or cyclosporine.

REFERENCE

Moore PM: *Curr Rheumatol Rep* 2:376–382, 2000.

VENOUS THROMBOSIS

Cortical vein thrombosis results in headache, seizures, and focal signs. Subarachnoid hemorrhage resulting from rupture of congested veins or extension of hemorrhagic infarction, as well as papilledema, may also occur. Superior sagittal sinus thrombosis is the most common type, and, if the parieto-occipital portion is involved, may produce elevated intracranial pressure, somnolence, and cranial nerve (CN) VI palsy. Contrast-enhanced CT scan shows a "negative delta" sign, which is characterized by opacification of the sinus wall with noninjection of the clot inside the sinus, in about 30% of cases. MRI or magnetic resonance venography may be diagnostic with asymmetry. Venous phase angiography usually shows a filling defect. Other signs of parasagittal stroke or hemorrhage, or both, may be present because of propagation of the thrombus into surrounding cortical veins. Thrombosis may also involve the cavernous sinus (usually as a result of facial or orbital infection; involvement is characterized by facial pain, proptosis, and involvement of CN III, IV, V, and VI) and the superior petrosal (as a result of otitis media; facial pain is prominent), inferior petrosal (Gradenigo's syndrome with retro-orbital pain and CN VI palsy), lateral petrosal (increased intracranial pressure and ear pain), or internal jugular (as a result of catheters or pacemakers, with involvement of CN IX, X and XI). Vein of Galen thrombosis in neonates after trauma or infection may result in extensor posturing, fever, tachycardia, tachypnea, and death. Survivors may develop bilateral choreoathetosis.

Causes of venous thrombosis include the following:

1. Trauma: Injury, neck surgery, indwelling IV lines.
2. Infection: Middle ear, sinuses, meningitis.
3. Endocrine: Pregnancy, contraceptives.
4. Volume depletion: Hyperosmolar coma, inflammatory bowel disease, diarrhea, postpartum, postoperative.
5. Hematologic: Polycythemia vera, disseminated intravascular coagulation, sickle cell disease, cryofibrinogenemia, paroxysmal nocturnal

  hemoglobinuria, thrombocytosis, antithrombin III deficiency, transfusion reaction.
6. Impaired cerebral circulation: Arterial occlusion, congenital heart disease, congestive heart failure, anesthesia in seated position, sagittal sinus webs.
7. Neoplasm: Leukemia, lymphoma, meningeal spread, meningioma.
8. Other: Wegener's granulomatosis, polyarteritis nodosa, Behçet's syndrome, Cogan's syndrome, homocystinuria.

Results of lumbar puncture, if not contraindicated by mass effect, are nonspecific and may reveal increased pressure and increased levels of protein, polymorphonuclear leukocytes (if infection is present), and red blood cells (if hemorrhage has occurred).

  Management includes treatment of the underlying cause and supportive care. Anticoagulation therapy is usually employed if there is no major hemorrhage or bleeding disorder. Intracranial hypertension should be controlled (see also Intracranial Pressure).

REFERENCE

Ameli A, Bazaar MG: *Neurol Clin* 10:87, 1992.

VERTIGO

Vertigo is defined as perception of *movement* of self or surrounding or an unpleasant distortion of *orientation* with respect to gravity. Disorders causing vertigo are formulated in terms of distortion or mismatch of vestibular, visual, and somatosensory inputs. Careful questioning can better delineate the patient's perceptions and help differentiate vertigo from other forms of dizziness that result from disturbances of cardiovascular, visual, or motor function.

  Examination: Blood pressure measurement (lying and standing), hearing screen and otoscopy, general neurologic examination with special attention to past pointing, ophthalmoscopy, ocular motor examination, and characterization of nystagmus; responses to specific maneuvers (if deemed safe), including tragal compression, rapid head turns, valsalva, rotation in chair, hyperventilation, and postural testing. The latter is performed by abruptly moving the patient from a sitting to a lying position, with the head hanging 45 degrees over the end of the examining table and rotated 45 degrees to one side. This is repeated with the head rotated to the opposite side. The development of vertigo and the time of onset, duration, and direction of the fast phase of nystagmus are noted.

CAUSES

l. Physiologic: Resulting from sensory distortion (e.g., change in refraction) or intersensory mismatch (such as motion sickness or height vertigo).

II. Pathologic: Based on localization within vestibular pathways.
   A. Labyrinths: Otitis media, endolymphatic hydrops, otosclerosis, cupulolithiasis, viral infection, perilymph fistula, trauma, drug toxicity (e.g., from antibiotics).
   B. Vestibular nerve and ganglia: Carcinomatous meningitis, herpes zoster.
   C. Cerebellopontine angle: Acoustic neuroma, glomus, or other tumor; demyelination, vascular compression.
   D. Brainstem and cerebellum: Infarct, hemorrhage, tumor, viral infection, migraine, Arnold-Chiari malformation.
   E. Hemispheric connections: Temporal or parietal dysfunction (e.g., seizure).
   F. Systemic and metabolic: Anemia, intoxication (such as ethanol, anticonvulsants, diuretics, and other medications), vasculitis (e.g., Cogan's syndrome of deafness, interstitial keratitis, and systemic vasculitis), metabolic derangement (e.g., thyroid disease).
III. Other causes of vertigo. Psychogenic vertigo has features of rotational or linear movement rather than isolated lightheadedness. It often begins gradually, is associated with anxiety, and terminates abruptly. Forced hyperventilation may provoke vertigo. When a patient complains of severe rotational vertigo without nausea or nystagmus, a psychogenic cause is suggested.

SPECIFIC FORMS

Acute peripheral vestibulopathy (other terms include viral labyrinthitis, vestibular neuronitis, and peripheral vestibulopathy) is associated with spontaneous vertigo, nystagmus (fast phase away from the lesion), and nausea or vomiting, or both, lasting hours to days. The environment seems to move in the direction of the fast phase (away from the lesion). There is a subjective sense of self-motion in the direction of the fast phase. The patient may fall to the side of the lesion during Romberg testing. Past pointing is to the side of the lesion. Symptoms and signs may be brought on by hurried movement ("positioning") but not necessarily by maintaining a particular position ("positional").

Hearing is usually normal. A variable residual deficit of one peripheral vestibular system (labyrinth, nerve, or both) may persist. With a unilateral fixed deficit, central compensatory mechanisms intervene and vertigo and nystagmus decrease and may resolve. Acute peripheral vestibulopathy may recur (see below). Bacterial suppurative ear infection should be excluded.

Perilymph fistula is usually due to spontaneous rupture of the inner ear membranes with resultant vertigo that may be aggravated by changes in position. It is associated with a fluctuating hearing loss. The fistula may occur during strenuous activity or Valsalva maneuver. The patient may hear a "pop" in the ear at the moment of rupture. The attacks are discrete and short-lived. The therapy is bed rest. If this fails, surgery may be required.

V

VERTIGO

Central vestibular vertigo resulting from lesions of the vestibular nuclei or vestibulocerebellar pathways have vertigo and nystagmus, often accompanied by diplopia, dysarthria, weakness, sensory loss, involvement of cranial nerves V and VII, and pathologic reflexes. Acoustic neuromas are usually associated with hearing loss, tinnitus, and occasionally, involvement of other cranial nerves, including VII and V.

Drug-induced vertigo is due to effects on the peripheral end-organ or nerve and may be due to aminoglycosides, furosemide, ethacrynic acid, anticonvulsants (phenytoin, phenobarbital, carbamazepine, and primodone), some antiinflammatory agents, salicylates, and quinine. Drugs may produce only dysequilibrium when the damage is bilateral but can produce vertigo when the damage is asymmetric. Some agents also produce hearing loss.

Meniere's disease that results from endolymph hydrops is characterized by severe episodic vertigo, vomiting, fluctuating or progressive hearing loss, distortions of sound, tinnitus, and pressure or fullness in the ears. Recovery is usually within hours to days. The interval between attacks often ranges from weeks to months. Low-salt diet and diuretics are considered most helpful. Surgical therapy (endolymphatic drainage or vestibular nerve section) may give lasting relief but should be considered only as a last resort. Newer treatments include intratympanic injections of corticosteroids or gentamicin; the latter may be a less invasive alternative to surgery.

Benign paroxysmal positional vertigo is a symptom that usually indicates benign peripheral (end-organ) disease. Vertigo and nystagmus, often with systemic symptoms such as nausea and vomiting, occur when certain positions of the head are assumed, such as lying down on the back or side. Symptoms are usually transient (<60 seconds). Latency is usually several seconds but may be as long as 30 to 45 seconds. Signs and symptoms include fatigue after onset and do not recur until there is a change in position. Nystagmus is most commonly torsional toward (upper pole) the undermost ear during positional testing. With repetitive maneuvers, signs and symptoms lessen (habituate). Therapy consists of repetitive positioning exercises to stimulate central compensation or a liberatory maneuver. Elderly patients compensate more slowly. Vestibular suppressant medications generally do not help in completely alleviating symptoms.

Laboratory studies: Brain imaging (CT, MRI) with attention to posterior fossa and temporal bone; MR angiography with attention to vertebrobasilar circulation; caloric and rotational testing quantify vestibular function. Audiogram and auditory evoked potentials detect associated cochlear or brainstem dysfunction.

Management: Generally, management during acute vertigo includes bed rest, avoiding sudden head movements, clear fluids or light diet if tolerated, and reassurance. Vestibular suppressant medications such as antihistamines and benzodiazepines (see Table 71) and antiemetics may be useful in acute peripheral vestibulopathy, in acute brainstem lesions near

TABLE 71

MEDICATIONS USEFUL IN TREATING SYMPTOMS OF ACUTE VERTIGO

Drug	Dosage	Route
Dimenhydrinate (Dramamine)	50–100 mg q 4–6 hr	PO, IM, IV, PR
Diphenhydramine (Benadryl)	25–50 mg tid to qid	PO, IM, IV
Meclizine (Antivert)	12.5–25 mg bid to qid	PO
Promethazine (Phenergan)	25 mg bid to qid	PO, IM, IV, PR
Hydroxyzine (Atarax, Vistaril)	25–100 mg tid to qid	PO, IM

IM, Intramuscular; IV, intravenous; PO, by mouth; PR, by rectum.

the vestibular nuclei, and for prevention of motion sickness. These agents are of no benefit in chronic vestibulopathies. After the acute phase (approximately 1 to 3 days), a graded program of exercises hastens the adaptive recalibration of the vestibular system to provide better ocular motor and postural control and reduce vertigo.

REFERENCES

Baloh RW: *J Am Geriatr Soc* 40:713–721, 1992.

Brandt T, Steddin S, Daroff RB: *Neurology* 44:796–800, 1994.

Sharpe JA, Barber HO, eds: *The vestibulo-ocular reflex and vertigo,* New York, Raven, 1993.

VESTIBULO-OCULAR REFLEX

The vestibulo-ocular reflex (VOR) generates eye movements that compensate for head movements. Head movements, voluntary or caused by locomotion, are sensed by the semicircular canals and otolith organs (utricle and saccule). Signals from the vestibular end-organs are combined with visual information in brainstem vestibular and ocular motor centers to create the appropriate control signals sent to the extraocular muscles. Adequate vestibular function results in eye rotations nearly equal and opposite to head movements and maintenance of a stable image on the retina, allowing high visual acuity. Overall vestibular function involves cerebral cortical centers and a spinal cord relay and processing of sensory input and motor outflow. Thus, vestibular disorders (peripheral or central) can result in eye movement abnormalities or more subtle disorders of postural control and spatial orientation (see Table 72).

VOR testing: After integrity of the neck is assured, bedside testing of the VOR is best accompanied in the following ways: (1) Rapid, passive head rotations (unpredictable, high-acceleration) are applied while the patient fixes his or her gaze on a stationary target. The examiner watches for a corrective saccadic eye movement which occurs after the head rotation only if the VOR has not adequately maintained gaze. (2) A more continuous high-frequency, low-amplitude head oscillation is applied while the examiner views the optic disc with an ophthalmoscope. If the VOR is intact, the disc image should appear stable to the observer.

V

VESTIBULO-OCULAR REFLEX

TABLE 72
LOCALIZATION OF VESTIBULAR DYSFUNCTION

	Peripheral	Central
History	Sudden onset; episodic; duration several days; intense vertigo; marked exacerbation with head movement; auditory symptoms (often unilateral); neurologic symptoms absent	Insidious onset; continuous; duration up to months; mild dysequilibrium; little or no exacerbation with head movement; no associated auditory symptoms; associated neurologic or vascular symptoms
Examination	Neurologic signs absent; *spontaneous nystagmus:* rotatory component, not vertical; *positional nystagmus:* latency before onset (≤ 45 sec), habituates, conjugate, uniplanar, attenuates with visual fixation	Associated neurologic or vascular signs; *spontaneous nystagmus:* horizontal or vertical, less often rotatory; *positional nystagmus:* immediate onset, no habituation, may change direction with different head positions, no change with visual fixation

Head rotation in comatose patients with a normal VOR results in compensatory controversive eye movements (see Calorics).

Quantitative evaluation of the VOR involves measuring eye movement responses to controlled head perturbations and calculating the VOR *gain*, which is defined as eye velocity divided by head velocity.

REFERENCE

Leigh RJ, Brandt T: *Neurology* 43:1288–1295, 1993.

VISUAL FIELDS

The visual fields can be conceptualized as an "island of vision in the sea of blindness." The peak of the island represents the point of highest acuity, the fovea. The optic disc (blind spot) is a bottomless pit in the midst of the island. Visual field testing is performed with stimuli of various sizes, colors, and intensities. There are various kinds of manual and computerized types of perimetry, but confrontation is the mainstay of clinical testing.

The characteristic features of visual field deficits have high localizing value (see Figure 43).

1. Retinal nerve fiber bundle lesions cause defects originating from the blind spot and respecting the horizontal meridian.
2. Optic disc lesions and retinal vascular occlusions often produce defects that respect the nasal horizontal meridian.

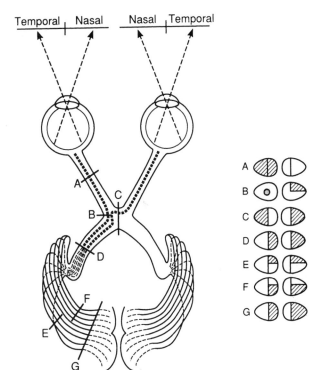

Temporal | Nasal   Nasal | Temporal

FIGURE 43

Diagram showing the effects on the fields of vision produced by lesions at various points along the optic pathway.

3. Optic nerve lesions produce monocular field defects that do not respect the vertical midline. Arcuate defects occur with segmental lesions of the optic nerve.

4. Cecocentral deficits suggest an optic nerve lesion. Junctional scotoma in the contralateral field is confirmatory and is due to von Willebrand loop involvement.

5. Chiasmal lesions produce bitemporal hemianopias.

6. All retrochiasmal lesions cause contralateral homonymous hemianopia or quadrantanopia, which increases in congruence (similarity between the eyes) as the lesions approach the occipital lobe. The visual field defects respect the vertical midline.

7. Visual acuity is not affected by unilateral lesion posterior to the chiasm.

8. Parietal lobe lesions may be associated with smooth pursuit and opto-kinetic nystagmus asymmetry and visual field defects.

9. Occipital lobe hemianopias are associated with macular sparing.
10. Homonymous hemianopsia and alexia without agraphia are caused by dominant occipital lobe lesion extending to the splenium of corpus callosum.

REFERENCES

American Academy of Ophthalmology: *Basic and clinical science course: neuro-ophthalmology*, 1997–1998, 71.
Galetta SL: *Neurosurg Clin N Am* 10:563–577, 1999.

WILSON'S DISEASE

Wilson's disease, also known as hepatolenticular degeneration, is an autosomal recessive disorder of copper metabolism. There is a defect of hepatic copper excretion due to a mutation in the gene on chromosome 13 for a copper-transporting adenosine triphosphatase (ATP7B). Age at onset is usually between 10 and 40 years. It presents with behavioral or personality changes, dysarthria, ataxia, and abnormal movements (chorea, athetosis, tremor, or rigidity). Hepatic dysfunction is identifiable in nearly all patients, and cirrhosis may be apparent early in the course. Other clinical features include hemolytic anemia, joint symptoms, renal stones, cardiomyopathy, pancreatic disease, and hypoparathyroidism. Kayser-Fleischer (KF) rings are present in more than 90% of patients and are virtually pathognomonic. There is brownish discoloration at the corneal limbus, consisting of copper deposits in Descemet's membrane; this may be visible only under slit lamp examination. "Sunflower" cataracts may occur.

The diagnosis is made by observation of the KF rings, low serum level of ceruloplasmin, elevated 24-hour urinary copper excretion, and increased level of copper in liver biopsy specimen. Serum copper measurement is often normal. Although the diagnosis may be relatively easy, Wilson's disease must be suspected in children and younger adults who come to medical attention with unknown hepatic or CNS syndromes.

Treatment consists of chelation with D-penicillamine. Initial dosages are about 0.5 g per day in children and 1 g per day in divided doses for adults. A low-copper diet to minimize acute worsening caused by mobilization of copper store is helpful. Pyridoxine, 25 mg per day, is given to counter the antimetabolite effect of penicillamine. Acute or delayed hypersensitivity reaction to penicillamine develops in up to 20% of patients receiving treatment but may be overcome in some cases with a reduced dose and concomitant administration of corticosteroids. Trientine (a chelator) and zinc salts, which block GI penicillamine, may help. Patients with advanced disease may require liver transplantation. Levodopa may be of some benefit in reversing neurologic symptoms not improved by penicillamine.

REFERENCES

Danks DM: In Scriver CR et al, eds: *The metabolic basis of inherited disease*, ed 6, New York, McGraw-Hill, 1989.

Pfeil SA, Lynn DJ: Wilson's disease: copper unfettered. *J Clin Gastroenterol* 29(1):22–31, 1999.

Z

ZOSTER

Varicella-zoster virus is the infective organism in varicella (chicken pox) and herpes zoster (shingles). Varicella is usually a benign disease of childhood. Rare complications include meningoencephalitis, acute cerebellar ataxia, transverse myelitis, and Reye's syndrome. Although full recovery from the first two is common, rare permanent deficits include paresis, seizures, or cognitive changes.

Herpes zoster (literally; girdle) represents latent virus reactivation. It is most frequent in those with weakened cell-mediated immunity, particularly the elderly and immunocompromised. At particular risk are patients with lymphoma who have had radiation and splenectomy and patients with AIDS (who usually develop disseminated disease). Typically, zoster presents with pain in a single or several adjacent dermatomes; pain may precede the vesicular eruption by up to 3 weeks. Pain is described as sharp, lancinating, and associated with itching, dysesthesia, and allodynia (increased skin sensitivity).

Associated findings include altered sensation in the involved dermatome; fewer then 5% have segmental weakness. The CSF may show an elevated protein and a mild lymphocytic pleocytosis. *Diagnosis* is established by typical rash, Tzanck smear, direct immunofluorescence, viral culture, or comparison of acute and convalescent titers. Demonstration of the presence of varicella-zoster DNA (by polymerase chain reaction [PCR] analysis) and/or of antibodies in CSF to the virus is a strong evidence of the infection in the appropriate clinical setting. Serum antibody analysis is of no value. Histologically, zoster is characterized by lymphocytic inflammation and vasculitis resulting in neuronal loss in ganglia. The process may spread to leptomeninges and adjacent spinal cord.

COMPLICATIONS OF THE PERIPHERAL NERVOUS SYSTEM
Zoster

Varicella-zoster virus may become latent along the entire neuraxis. The most common sites of reactivation are thoracic and trigeminal dermatomes. When zoster affects the cranium (20% of cases), 90% are in the trigeminal distribution and 60% of these will involve the first division—herpes zoster ophthalmicus. Complications include corneal involvement, internal or external ophthalmoplegia, iridocyclitis, and optic neuritis (rare). The prognosis for improvement of ocular motor disturbance is excellent, whereas return of lost vision is minimal. The Ramsay-Hunt syndrome denotes zoster of the geniculate ganglion, presenting with painful vesicles on the tympanic membrane and external auditory canal, a peripheral CN VII palsy, and variable CN VIII dysfunction. Thoracic zoster may occasionally produce arm weakness (zoster paresis), whereas lumbar reactivation may be associated with leg weakness and bowel/bladder dysfunction.

Rarely the pain occurs in the absence of any rash (zoster sine herpete), leading to considerations of carcinomatous, lymphomatous or diabetic radiculopathies. Analysis of PCR of varicella DNA in CSF and blood mononuclear cells, and antibody titer in CSF are usually diagnostic. Treatment for varicella-zoster infection consists of acyclovir (800 mg five times a day), famciclovir (500 mg tid), or valacyclovir; pain management is essential but frequently difficult due to residual pain despite multiple medications.

Postherpetic Neuralgia

Postherpetic Neuralgia is persistent dysesthesias and hyperpathia persisting beyond healing of the zoster vesicles (usually beyond 2 months). The pain has three components: (1) A constant, deep burning pain; (2) paroxysms of shooting pain; (3) sharp pains after light stimulation (allodynia). Pathologically, it is associated with a localized small- and large-fiber sensory neuropathy and may result from reorganization of inputs to the second order neurons. Postherpetic neuralgia is rare in patients under 50, but occurs in up to 50% of patients over 60 and in 75% of those over 70. It resolves within 1 month in 90% of patients and in half of the remainder by 2 months, but may last up to 1 year. Only about 2% of patients have persistent pain, which may last for months or years. Antiviral treatments tend to reduce incidence of the postherpetic neuralgia. Tricyclic antidepressants (amitriptyline/nortriptyline 25 to 75 mg PO qd) and anticonvulsants, such as carbamazepine (400 to 1200 mg PO qd), phenytoin (300 to 400 mg PO qd), Gabapentin, prednisone (40 to 60 mg qd 3 to 5 days), topical aspirin in chloroform, and capsaicin 0.75% ointment 5 times per day for at least 4 weeks may be used. Topical lidocaine (ointment or skin patch) may also help.

COMPLICATIONS OF THE CENTRAL NERVOUS SYSTEM

Occasionally, after reactivation of varicella-zoster virus in either an immunocompetent or immunocompromised patient, the virus spreads into the spinal cord and brain. CNS complications of zoster include myelitis, encephalitis, large-vessel granulomatous arteritis, small-vessel encephalitis, meningitis, and ventriculitis. Myelitis usually occurs 1 to 2 weeks after rash development and may be confirmed by CSF PCR of varicella DNA; the illness is mostly severe in immunocompromised patients. Varicella-zoster can cause encephalitis as a result of large- or small-vessel vasculopathy. Large-vessel (granulomatous) arteritis occurs predominantly in immunocompetent patients and presents with focal deficits (stroke; ischemic or hemorrhagic). Small-vessel encephalitis is the most common complication of CNS varicella-zoster and is seen in immunocompromised patients. Deep-seated ischemic or demyelinating lesions may manifest as headache, fever, vomiting, mental status changes, seizures, and focal deficits. A few cases of ventriculitis and meningitis have occurred in immunocompromised patients. The treatment for CNS complications is with IV acyclovir; steroids are used for antiinflammatory effects.

Acute zoster is treated symptomatically in the normal host. Oral acyclovir accelerates cutaneous healing but has no affect on acute neuritis or postherpetic neuralgia. In the immunocompromised, parenteral acyclovir is more effective than vidarabine in preventing dissemination and accelerating cutaneous healing. Corticosteroids may reduce acute pain and the risk of postherpetic neuralgia, but evidence of effectiveness is inconclusive.

Z

ZOSTER

REFERENCES

Gilden DH et al: *N Engl J Med* 342(9):635–645, 2000.

Terrence CF, Fromm GH: In Olesen J, Tfelt-Hansen P, Welch KMA, eds: *The headaches*, chapter 114, New York, Raven Press, 1993.

INDEX

Note: Page numbers followed by f refer to figures; page numbers followed by t refer to tables.

A

Abducens nerve (VI) palsy, 278–279
Abetalipoproteinemia, 220
Abscess
 brain, 1–2, 7
 epidural, 3
Absence status epilepticus, 132, 132t
Acalculia, 3
Acid maltase deficiency, 246f, 247
Acidosis
 metabolic, 116
 respiratory, 115–116
Aciduria, organic, 218, 219t
Acquired immunodeficiency syndrome (AIDS), 5–8
 CSF in, 63t
 early, 5–6
 encephalitis in, 124
 late, 6–8
 midstage, 6
Acromegaly, myopathy in, 245
Action tremor, 365–366
Acute disseminated encephalomyelitis, CSF in, 62t
Acyl coenzyme A dehydrogenase deficiency, myopathy in, 246f, 248
Addison's disease, myopathy in, 245
Adenoma, pituitary, 307–308
Adenylate deaminase deficiency, 249
Adrenal insufficiency, myopathy in, 245

Adrenoleukodystrophy, 89
Agnosia, 4
Agraphia, 4–5
Akathisia, neuroleptic-induced, 259
Akinetic mutism, 79
Alcohol use, 8–10
 myopathy with, 250
 withdrawal from, 9
Alexander disease, 89
Alexia, 3, 10–11
Alkalosis
 metabolic, 116
 respiratory, 115
Alper's disease, 91
Alprazolam, 23t
Alzheimer's disease, 93–96
 diagnosis of, 94, 95t–96t
 genetic factors in, 94t
 treatment of, 94, 96
Amantadine, in Parkinson's disease, 293
Amaurosis fugax, 11–12, 11t
Amblyopia, nutritional, 10
Aminoacidurias, 92
Amitriptyline, 23t
Amnesia, 362
Amyotrophic lateral sclerosis, 18t, 19, 221–222
Anarithmetria, 3
Aneurysm, 12–13, 13f
Angiitis, 376
Angiography, 14–17, 15f, 16f
Angioid streaks, 334
Angioma, 17
Anisocoria, 321, 323t, 324
Anosodiaphoria, 4

Anosognosia, 4
Anterior cord syndrome, 346, 348
Anterior inferior cerebellar artery, 53
Antibiotics
  in brain abscess, 2
  in meningitis, 213t
Antibodies, 18–22, 18t, 20t
  anti-glycoprotein, 18t, 20
  anti-glycosphingolipid, 18t
  anti-Hu, 20–21, 20t, 289t
  antineuronal, 289t
  anti–RNA-binding protein, 18t
  anti-sulfatide, 22
Anticholinesterase agents, in myasthenia gravis, 236–237
Anticoagulation, in stroke, 189–190
Antidepressants, 22–24, 23t
Antidiuretic hormone, inappropriate secretion of, 355–356
Antiepileptic drugs, 134t–136t, 136t, 139t–141t, 142t, 143
Anti-ganglioside antibodies, 18–19, 18t
Anti-Hu antibody, 20–21, 20t, 289t
Antiplatelet agents, in stroke, 190–191
Antipsychotics, 258–260
Anti-sulfatide antibodies, 22
Aphasia, 24–26, 25t, 26t
Aphemia, 26t
Apneustic breathing, 76
Apoplexy, pituitary, 309
Apraxia, 26–27
Argyll Robertson pupil, 323t, 325
Arithmetic skills, impairment of, 3
Arnold–Chiari malformation, 85
Arrhythmias, 109
Arteriovenous malformation, 17
Arteritis, 376–377
Arthritis, rheumatoid, 335–336
Aseptic meningitis
  CSF in, 62t
  with chemotherapy, 64

Aspirin, in stroke, 190–191
Astereognosis, 4
Asterixis, 27
Ataxia, 28–29, 52, 351–353
  with chemotherapy, 64
Ataxia-telangiectasia, 257
Ataxic breathing, 76
Athetosis, 29
Atrial fibrillation, 109
Attention deficit–hyperactivity disorder, 29–31
Audiologic testing, 165–166
Auditory agnosia, 4
Autism, 31
Autoantibodies, 18–22, 18t, 20t, 289t. *See also* Antibodies.
Autonomic dysfunction, 31–34
  classification of, 32t
  diagnosis of, 33–34
Autonomic dysreflexia, 37–38
Avellis' syndrome, 183t

B

Babinski–Nageotte syndrome, 183t
Babinski's sign, 331–332
  in infant, 70t
Baclofen, in spasticity, 345
Balint's syndrome, 27
Bassen–Kornzweig disease, 220
Becker muscular dystrophy, 230
Becker's disease, 253t, 254
Behçet's disease, 379
Bell's palsy, 152
  during pregnancy, 313
Benedikt's syndrome, 182t
Benign childhood epilepsy with centrotemporal spikes, 129
Benign paroxysmal positional vertigo, 382
Benzodiazepines, 34–35
Benztropine, in Parkinson's disease, 293
Bethanechol, in bladder dysfunction, 37t
Binswanger's disease, 96

Bladder
  dysfunction of, 35–38, 36t, 37t
  neuroanatomy of, 35, 35f
Bleeding. *See also* Hemorrhage.
  after lumbar puncture, 63
Blepharospasm, 153
Blood pressure, in autonomic
  dysfunction, 33, 34
Botulinum toxin, in spasticity,
  346
Bourneville's disease, 256
Bovine spongiform
  encephalopathy, 99
Brachial plexus, lesions of, 38–39,
  38f, 314
Brain
  abscess of, 1–2, 7
  congenital malformation of,
  83–85
  herniation of, 166–169, 167t,
  168t
    after lumbar puncture, 63
  tumors of, 368–372, 368t,
  369f–270f
Brain death, 39–40
  electroencephalography in,
  111–112
Brainstem auditory-evoked
  potentials, 145–146
Brancher enzyme deficiency, 248
Breathing, in coma, 75–76
Broca's aphasia, 25t
Brown–Sequard syndrome, 348
Brown–Vialetto–van Laere
  syndrome, 41
Bulbar palsy, 40–41
Bupropion, 23t
Bypass surgery, 192

C
Calcification, cerebral, 41–42
Calcium, 112t, 114
California encephalitis, 123
Callosal apraxia, 27
Caloric testing, 42–43
Canavan disease, 89

Cancer, 368–373, 368t
  brain, 368–372, 368t,
  369f–270f
  chemotherapy-related neurologic
  complications in, 64–65,
  65t
  during pregnancy, 316
  metastatic, 372
  radiation-induced, 328
  sensory neuronopathy with,
  20–21, 20t
  spinal cord, 372
Carbamazepine
  in epilepsy, 135t, 137t, 139t
  in spasticity, 346
Carbidopa, in Parkinson's disease,
  293
Cardiac syncope, 354
Cardiopulmonary arrest, 43
Carnitine deficiency, myopathy in,
  246f, 248
Carnitine palmityltransferase
  deficiency, myopathy in, 246f,
  248
Carotid endarterectomy, 192
Carpal tunnel syndrome, 43–44
  during pregnancy, 313
Cauda equina, 44–45, 45t
Caudal vermis syndrome, 53
Cavernous angioma, 17
Central core disease, 250
Central (transtentorial) herniation,
  166, 167t, 168t
Central neurogenic
  hyperventilation, 75–76
Central pontine myelinolysis, 10
Central vestibular vertigo, 382
Cerebellar arteries, 52–53
Cerebellar ataxia, 352, 353
Cerebellar hemorrhage, 56
Cerebellar tonsillar herniation,
  167, 167t
Cerebellar tremor, 366
Cerebellum, 45–54, 46f
  blood supply of, 52–53
  cellular organization of, 47

Cerebellum (*Continued*)
  cortical input of, 47–49, 48t
  disorders of, 51–52, 53–54
  infarction of, 54
  interneurons of, 49
  neocerebellum of, 48t, 51
  spinocerebellum of, 48t, 50–51
  vestibulocerebellum of, 48t, 50
Cerebral angiography, 14–17, 15f, 16f
Cerebral calcification, 41–42
Cerebral cortex, 55, 55f
Cerebral hemorrhage, 54–58, 55f–56f
Cerebral necrosis, radiation therapy–induced, 326
Cerebral palsy, 58–59
Cerebral salt wasting syndrome, 309–310
Cerebrospinal fluid (CSF), 59–64. *See also* Lumbar puncture.
  appearance of, 59–60
  cytology of, 60–61, 60t
  disease-specific profiles of, 62t–63t
  formation of, 59
  glucose in, 60t, 61
  in syphilis, 357, 358
  protein in, 60t, 61
Cerebrum, radiation therapy-induced injury to, 326–327
Cervical radiculopathy, 329
Cestan–Chenais syndrome, 183t
Charcot–Marie–Tooth disease, 263–264
  during pregnancy, 314
Chediak–Higashi syndrome, 90, 257
Chemotherapy, neurologic complications of, 64–65, 65t
Cherry red spot, 334
Cheyne–Stokes respiration, 75
Chiari–Frommel syndrome, 308
Child neurology, 65–70. *See also* Infant.
  Denver Development Screening Test in, 66f

Child neurology (*Continued*)
  developmental milestone evaluation in, 70t
  general examination in, 65–66, 66f–69f, 69t–70t
  head circumference evaluation in, 67f–69f
  neurologic examination in, 66–68
  patient history in, 65
  reflex evaluation in, 69t–70t
Childhood, degenerative diseases of, 89–92
Childhood absence epilepsy, 129–130
Chlorpromazine, in spasticity, 346
Chorea, 71–73
Chorea gravidarum, 314–315
Chromosomal disorders, 73–74
Chronic daily headache, 165
Chronic inflammatory demyelinating polyradiculoneuropathy, 267–268
  during pregnancy, 314
Chronic paroxysmal hemicrania, 161
Chronic progressive external ophthalmoplegia, 280
Churg–Strauss syndrome, 378
Cingulate (subfalcine) herniation, 167, 167t
Circular nystagmus, 274
Citalopram, 23t
Claude's syndrome, 182t
Clonazepam, in epilepsy, 136t, 137t, 140t
Cluster headache, 161
  treatment of, 164–165
Cockayne's syndrome, 90
Cogan's disease, 378
Cogwheel rigidity, 337
Coma, 74–80
  brainstem function in, 74–75
  breathing patterns in, 75–76
  causes of, 76–80
  clinical course of, 78

Coma (*Continued*)
electroencephalography in, 111
emergency management of, 75t
Glasgow coma scale in, 76, 77t
prognosis for, 79–80
sensorimotor evaluation in, 76, 77t
vs. akinetic mutism, 79
vs. locked-in syndrome, 79
vs. vegetative state, 78–79
Complex partial status epilepticus, 132t, 142
Complex regional pain syndrome, 80–81
Complex repetitive discharges, on EMG, 119–120
Compound motor action potential (M wave), 117–118
Computed tomography (CT), 81–83, 82t
in brain abscess, 2
in cerebral hemorrhage, 56
in hemorrhage, 82t, 83
in stroke, 82t, 187
Conduction aphasia, 25t
Confusional state, 83
Conjugate eye deviations, 155
Constructional apraxia, 27
Conus medullaris, 44–45, 45t
Convergence-retraction nystagmus, 274
Cortical atrophy, in alcoholism, 10
Corticobasal ganglionic degeneration, 291
Corticosteroids, in myasthenia gravis, 237
Cramp, 85–87
Cramp potential, on EMG, 120
Cranial nerve(s), 87t–88t
II, 281–283
III, 279–280, 323t
in stroke, 182t–184t
IV, 279
VI, 278–279
VII, 87t, 150–153, 151f
VIII, 166

Craniocervical junction, dysfunction of, 88
Craniopharyngioma, vs. pituitary adenoma, 308–309
Craniosynostosis, 88–89
Creutzfeldt–Jakob disease, 98–99
Crossed adductor reflex, in infant, 70t
Cryptococcal meningitis, in AIDS, 7, 63t
CSF. See Cerebrospinal fluid (CSF).
CT. See Computed tomography (CT).
Cushing's syndrome, 308
Cyanocobalamin deficiency, 269

D
Dantrolene sodium, in spasticity, 345–346
Davidoff–Dyke–Masson syndrome, 59
Debranching enzyme deficiency, 246f, 247–248
Decerebrate posturing, 337
Decorticate posturing, 337
Dejerine–Klumpke palsy, 39
Dejerine–Sottas disease, 264
Delirium tremens, 9
Dementia, 92–99, 94t, 95t–96t. See also Alzheimer's disease.
dialysis, 103
diffuse Lewy body, 97
frontotemporal, 97–98
in AIDS, 7–8
vascular, 96–97, 97t
Demyelinating disease, 99–100
Denny–Brown, hereditary sensory neuropathy of, 264
Denver Development Screening Test, 66f
Dermatomes, 101f, 102f
Desipramine, 23t
Detrusor areflexia, 37
Detrusor hyperreflexia, 36
Diabetic ketoacidosis, 156
Diabetic neuropathy, 265–266

Diagonal nystagmus, 274
Dialysis, 103
Diazepam, in spasticity, 345
Diffuse Lewy body dementia, 97
Diphtheria toxoid vaccine, 176
Diplopia
    after lumbar puncture, 64
    testing for, 148–150
Disequilibrium, 104
    dialysis, 103
Disseminated intravascular
        coagulation, 103–104
Dissociated nystagmus, 272–273
Distal myopathy, 233, 234t
Distal sensory polyneuropathy,
        265–266
    in AIDS, 8
Divalproex sodium, in epilepsy, 135t
Dizziness, 104–105
L-Dopa, in Parkinson's disease, 293
Dopaminergic agents, in
        Parkinson's disease, 292–293
Doppler ultrasonography, 374
Down's syndrome (trisomy 21), 73
Doxepin, 23t
Drugs. See also specific drugs.
    chemotherapeutic, neurologic
        complications of, 64–65,
        65t
    headache with, 161–162
    porphyria with, 312t
Duchenne muscular dystrophy,
        229–230
Duchenne–Erb palsy, 38–39
Dysarthria, 52, 105
Dysautonomia, familial, 265
Dyskinesia, 105
Dysmetria, saccadic, 275
Dysphagia, 106
Dystonia, 106–108
    neuroleptic-induced, 259
Dystonia-plus syndrome, 107

E

Eastern equine encephalitis, 123
Eclampsia, 318

Edward's syndrome (trisomy 18),
        73
EEG. See Electroencephalography
        (EEG).
Ekbom syndrome, 332
Elbow, ulnar nerve entrapment at,
        373–374
Electrocardiography (ECG),
        108–109
Electroencephalography (EEG),
        109–112
    in brain abscess, 2
    in brain death, 111–112
    in coma, 111
    in diffuse encephalopathy, 111
    in epilepsy, 110–111
    in focal brain lesions, 111
    normal, 109–110
    sleep, 110
Electrolytes, 112–116, 112t
Electromyography (EMG),
        118–121
    in myasthenia gravis, 236
    insertional activity on, 119
    motor unit action potential on,
        120–121
    spontaneous activity on,
        119–121
Electroretinography, 144
Elliptic nystagmus, 274
Emery–Dreifuss muscular
        dystrophy, 231–232
EMG. See Electromyography
        (EMG).
Empty sella syndrome, 309
Encephalitis, 122–125
    AIDS, 124
    nonviral, 124–125
    viral, 122–124
Encephalomyelitis
    disseminated, acute, 62t
    postinfectious, 125
Encephalopathy, 125–126
    asterixis in, 27
    dialysis, 103
    electroencephalography in, 111

Encephalopathy (Continued)
  hypoxic-ischemic, 125–126
  in AIDS, 7–8, 63t
  in infancy, 218–220, 219t
  radiation therapy–induced, 326
  uremic, 375
  with chemotherapy, 64
Endocrine myopathy, 245–246
Endovascular therapy, 192
Entacapone, in Parkinson's
    disease, 293
Epidemic encephalitis, 123–124
Epidural abscess, 3
Epidural hemorrhage, 58, 350
Epilepsy, 127–143
  classification of, 127–129
  cryptogenic, 130
  differential diagnosis of, 129
  drugs for, 134t–136t, 137t,
      138t–141t, 142t, 143
  during pregnancy, 317
  electroencephalography in,
      110–111
  idiopathic, 129–130
  symptomatic, 130–131
Erectile dysfunction, 177–178
Ergotamine, in headache,
    162–164, 163t
Essential tremor, 366
Ethosuximide, in epilepsy, 135t,
    137t, 139t
Eulenberg's disease, 254
Evoked potentials, 144–148, 145f
Extraocular muscles, 148–150,
    149f, 149t, 150f
  disorders of, 277–281
Eye(s)
  gaze palsy of, 155
  in coma, 75
  in Graves' disease, 158–159
  nystagmic movements of, 273t,
      275–276
  oscillary movements of,
      275–276
Eye muscles. See Extraocular
    muscles.

F
F wave, 117–118, 117t
Fabry's disease, 258
Facial myokymia, 153
Facial nerve (VII), 87t, 150–153,
    151f
Facioscapulohumeral muscular
    dystrophy, 230–231
Fahr disease, 91
Familial dysautonomia, 265
Fasciculation potentials, 120
Fatal familial insomnia, 99
Fatty acid oxidation disorder, 219t
Febrile seizures, 131–132
Felbamate, in epilepsy, 136t,
    137t, 140t
Fibrillation potentials, 119
Finger agnosia, 155–156
Fishman's formula, 61
Fistula, perilymph, 381
Flu vaccine, 175
Fluoxetine, 23t
Foix–Chavany–Marie syndrome,
    318–319
Folate deficiency, 269–270
Fontanel, 153
Forbes–Cori disease, 246f,
    247–248
Foster Kennedy syndrome, 282
Foville's syndrome, 182t
Fragile X syndrome, 73, 368,
    368t
Friedreich's ataxia, 352–353
Froin's syndrome, 60
Frontal lobe, 154
Frontotemporal dementia, 97–98
Fungal meningitis, CSF in, 62t

G
Gabapentin, in epilepsy, 136t,
    137t, 141t
Gag reflex, in infant, 69t
Gait
  ataxic, 28–29, 52, 64, 351–353
  disorders of, 154
Galactosemia, 220

Gangliosides, antibodies against, 18–19, 18t
Gaucher's disease, 90
Gaze palsy, 155
Gaze-evoked nystagmus, 272
Gegenhalten, 337
Generalized convulsive status epilepticus, 132t, 142
Generalized tonic-clonic status epilepticus, 132, 132t, 133t
Gerstmann's syndrome, 155–156
Gerstmann–Straussler–Scheinker disease, 99
Gestational distal polyneuropathy, 314
Giant cell arteritis, 376–377
Gilles de la Tourette's syndrome, 361–362
Glasgow coma scale, 76, 77t
Global aphasia, 25t
Glossopharyngeal neuralgia, 156
Glucose, 156–157
   in CSF, 60t, 61
Glutaric aciduria, 92
Glycogen, metabolism of, 247f
Glycogenoses, 246–248, 246f, 247f
Glycolysis, 247f
Glycoprotein, antibodies against, 18t, 20
Glycoprotein degradation disorder, 219t
Glycosphingolipids, antibodies against, 18t
Granulomatosis, Wegener's, 378
Graves' ophthalmopathy, 158–159
Guillain-Barré syndrome, 266–267
   autoantibodies in, 18t, 19
   CSF in, 62t
   during pregnancy, 314

H

H wave, 117t, 118
Hachinski scale, 96, 97t
Hallervorden–Spatz disease, 91

Hallucinations, 159–160
   olfactory, 276–277
Head circumference
   evaluation of, 67f–69f
   in children, 68f, 69f
   in infant, 67f
   small, 220–221
Headache, 160–165
   after lumbar puncture, 61, 63
   during pregnancy, 316–317
   treatment of, 162–165, 163t
Hearing, 165–166
Heart disease, in stroke, 187–188
Heart rate, in autonomic dysfunction, 33
Hematoma, MRI in, 209t
Hematomyelia, 351
Heme, synthesis of, 310f
Hemicraniectomy, 192
Hemifacial spasm, 153
Hemispheric syndrome, 53
Hemodialysis, 103
Hemorrhage
   cerebral, 56–58, 55f
   computed tomography in, 82t, 83
   epidural, 58, 350
   subarachnoid, 12–13, 57, 350–351
      CSF in, 62t
      during pregnancy, 315–316
      syncope with, 354–355
   subdural, 57–58, 350
Hepatolenticular degeneration, 386
Hereditary motor and sensory neuropathy, 263–264
Hereditary sensory and autonomic neuropathy, 264–265
Herniation syndromes, 166–169, 167t, 168t
Herpes simplex encephalitis, 122–123
   CSF in, 62t
Herpes zoster ophthalmicus hemiplegia, 378

Hiccups, 169
Hoffmann sign, 332
Hoffman's syndrome, 361
Holmes–Adie syndrome, 323t, 325
Homocystinuria, 220
Horizontal gaze palsy, 155
Horner's syndrome, 169–171, 170f, 323t
Hunter syndrome, 90
Hunt–Hess scale, in aneurysm, 12–13
Huntington disease, 91, 171, 368, 368t
Hurler syndrome, 90
Hydrocephalus, 172–173, 173f
Hydrocephalus ex vacuo, 172
Hypercalcemia, 112t, 114
Hyperglycemia, 156–157
  nonketotic, 218, 219t
Hyperkalemia, 112t, 113
  periodic paralysis with, 253t, 295–296, 295t
Hypermagnesemia, 112t, 114–115
Hypernatremia, 112t, 113
Hyperosmia, 276
Hyperparathyroidism, myopathy in, 245
Hyperreflexia, 331
Hypertension
  during pregnancy, 318
  intracranial, 178–179
Hyperthyroidism, 359–360
  myopathy in, 245
Hyperventilation, 173–174
Hyperventilation syndrome, 105
Hypocalcemia, 112t, 114
Hypoglycemia, 156
Hypoglycorrhachia, 157
Hypokalemia, 112t, 113
  periodic paralysis with, 295–296, 295t
Hypomagnesemia, 112t, 114
Hyponatremia, 112–113, 112t
Hypoparathyroidism, myopathy in, 245
Hypophosphatemia, 112t, 115

Hypopituitarism, myopathy in, 245
Hyporeflexia, 330–331
Hypotension
  intracranial, 179
  orthostatic, 33, 34
Hypothyroidism, 220, 360–361
  myopathy in, 245
Hypotonia, 51–52
  in infancy, 174–175, 174t
Hypovolemia, 354
Hypoxic-ischemic encephalopathy, 125–126
Hysterical tremor, 366

I
Ideational apraxia, 27
Ideomotor apraxia, 26–27
IgM monoclonal gammopathy, 18t, 20
Imipramine, 23t
  in bladder dysfunction, 37t
Immune deficiency. See also Acquired immunodeficiency syndrome (AIDS).
  encephalitis in, 124
Immunization, 175–176
Immunoglobulin, intravenous, in myasthenia gravis, 237
Impotence, 177–178
Inclusion body myositis, 244
Incontinentia pigmenti, 257
Infant. See also Child neurology.
  birth injury in, 314
  hypotonic, 174–175, 174t
  lactic acidosis in, 218, 219t
  length of, 67f
  neurometabolic diseases in, 218–220, 219t
  reflexes in, 69t–70t
  urea cycle disorder in, 218, 219t
  weight of, 67f
Infarction, cerebellar, 54
Infection. See also Abscess and specific infections.
  in sickle cell disease, 342
  in transplant patient, 362–364

Inflammatory demyelinating polyneuropathy, 266–268
Inflammatory myopathy, 243–245, 244t
Influenza vaccine, 175
Insomnia, 343–344
Intention tremor, 366
Interneurons, 49
Internuclear ophthalmoplegia, 280–281
Intra-arterial thrombolysis, in stroke, 191–192
Intracranial pressure
  decrease in, 179
  increase in, 178–179
Ischemia, 180–200. See also Stroke.
  optic nerve, 282

J

Jackson's syndrome, 184t
Juvenile myoclonic epilepsy of Janz, 130

K

Kearns–Sayre syndrome, 249, 249t
Kennedy's syndrome, 368, 368t
Klinefelter's syndrome (XXY), 73
Klippel–Trenaunay–Weber syndrome, 257
Klüver–Bucy syndrome, 359
Knapsack paralysis, 38–39
Kocher–Debre–Semelaigne syndrome, 361
Krabbe's disease, 89
Kuru, 99

L

La Crosse virus encephalitis, 123
Labor. See also Pregnancy.
  neonatal palsy with, 314
Lactate dehydrogenase deficiency, 246f, 247
Lactic acidosis, in infant, 218, 219t
Lacunar syndromes, 194–195, 195t

Lambert–Eaton myasthenic syndrome, 200–202
Lamotrigine, in epilepsy, 136t, 137t, 140t
Landau reflex, 70t
Landouzy–Dejerine dystrophy, 230–231
Latent nystagmus, 271
Lead-pipe rigidity, 337
Learning disabilities, 202
Leigh's disease, 91
Length, of infant, 67f
Lennox Gastaut syndrome, 130
Leukodystrophy, metachromatic, 89
Leukoencephalopathy, radiation therapy–induced, 327
Levetiracetam, in epilepsy, 137t, 141t
Levodopa, in Parkinson's disease, 293
Lid nystagmus, 274
Limb-girdle muscular dystrophy, 232–233
Limbic system, 203
Limb-kinetic apraxia, 27
Lipidoses, 90, 246f, 248
Lipofuscinosis, neuronal, 90, 219t
Locked-in syndrome, 79
Lumbar puncture, 59–64, 60t. See also Cerebrospinal fluid (CSF).
  complications of, 61, 63–64
  contraindications to, 64
Lumbar radiculopathy, 329–330
Lumbosacral plexus, 203, 204f
Lung cancer, sensory neuronopathy with, 20–21, 20t
Lyme disease, 205–206
  CSF in, 63t
Lymphoma, in AIDS, 6

M

M wave (compound motor action potential), 117–118
Machiafava–Bignami syndrome, 10

Macrocephaly, 206–207
Macula, cherry red spot of, 334
Mad cow disease, 99
Magnesium, 112t, 114–115
Magnetic resonance imaging
    (MRI), 207–212
    advantages of, 211
    clinical uses of, 210–211
    disadvantages of, 211–212
    in brain abscess, 2
    in hematoma, 209t
    in stroke, 187
    intraoperative, 212
    technical parameters in,
        207–210, 208t, 209t
Malformation
    of brain, 83–85
    of spine, 83–85
Maple syrup urine disease, 219t,
    220
Marcus–Gunn pupil, 324–325,
    324f
McArdle's disease, 246, 246f
Measles vaccine, 176
Median nerve, compression of,
    43–44
Meige's syndrome, 107
Melanosis, neurocutaneous, 257
MELAS (mitochondrial
    encephalomyopathy with
    lactic acidosis and strokelike
    episodes), 91, 249, 249t
Melkersson–Rosenthal syndrome,
    152
Melkersson's syndrome, 152
Memory, 212–213
Meniere's disease, 382
Meningitis, 213–216, 213t, 214t,
    215t
    CSF in, 62t
    in AIDS, 7
    syphilitic, 7, 356
    with chemotherapy, 64
Menkes' disease, 91
Mental status testing, 216–218,
    217f

Meralgia paresthetica, during
    pregnancy, 313–314
MERRF (myoclonic epilepsy with
    ragged red fibers), 249, 249t
Metabolic acidosis, 116
Metabolic alkalosis, 116
Metabolic diseases, of childhood,
    218–220, 219t
Metabolic myopathy, 246–248,
    246f, 247f
Metachromatic leukodystrophy, 89
Methotrexate, neurologic
    complications of, 65t
Methylmalonic acidemia, 92
Microcephaly, 220–221
Midbrain pupil, 323t, 325
Migraine headache, 160–161
    CSF in, 62t
    treatment of, 162–165, 163t
Millard–Gubler syndrome, 183t
Miller–Fisher syndrome,
    autoantibodies in, 18t,
    19–20
Mitochondrial disorders, myopathy
    in, 249, 249t
Mitochondrial encephalopathy with
    lactic acidosis and strokelike
    episodes (MELAS), 91, 249,
    249t
Möbius' syndrome, 152
Mollaret's meningitis, 216
Monoamine oxidase inhibitors, 23t
Monoclonal gammopathy, 18t, 20
Mononeuritis multiplex, in AIDS, 8
Mononeuropathy, 261
Moro reflex, 69t
Morphine, 286–287, 286f, 287f
Morvan's disease, 264–265
Motor neuron disorders, 221–224,
    222t
    atypical, 223–224, 223t
    autoantibodies in, 18t, 19
    radiation therapy–induced,
        327–328
Motor unit action potential,
    118–121, 120–121

Motor-evoked potentials, 144
Moyamoya disease, 196–197
MRI. See Magnetic resonance imaging (MRI).
Mucopolysaccharidoses, 90–91
  encephalopathy in, 219t
Multifocal motor neuropathy, 18–19, 18t
Multiple sclerosis, 224–226
  CSF in, 62t
  during pregnancy, 315
  evoked potentials in, 147–148
Multiple system atrophy, 291
Multisystem triglyceride storage disorder, myopathy in, 248
Muscle(s)
  athetosis of, 29
  cramps of, 85–87
  diseases of, 227t–228t. See also specific diseases.
  dystonia of, 106–108
  fiber types of, 227t
  strength of, 226t
Muscular dystrophy, 229–235
  Becker, 230
  congenital, 233, 235
  Duchenne, 229–230
  Emery–Dreifuss, 231–232
  facioscapulohumeral, 230–231
  limb-girdle, 232–233
  oculopharyngeal, 233
  scapuloperoneal, 231
Mutism, akinetic, 79
Myasthenia gravis, 235–238
  diagnosis of, 236
  during pregnancy, 315
  nystagmus in, 274
  ocular, 237–238
  treatment of, 236–238
Myelin-associated glycoprotein, antibody against, 18t, 20
Myelography, 238
Myelopathy, 348–349
  in rheumatoid arthritis, 336
  in sickle cell disease, 342
  radiation therapy–induced, 327

Myelopathy (Continued)
  vacuolar, 8
  with chemotherapy, 65
Myoclonic epilepsy with ragged red fibers (MERRF), 91, 249, 249t
Myoclonus, 239–241
  ocular, 275
  treatment of, 241
Myoedema, 361
Myoglobinuria, 242–243
Myokymia
  facial, 153
  oblique, superior, 275
Myokymic discharges, on EMG, 120
Myopathy, 243–254
  alcoholic, 10
  congenital, 250–251
  distal, 233, 234t
  endocrine, 245–246
  hypothyroid, 361
  in renal failure, 375–376
  inflammatory, 243–245, 244t
  metabolic, 246–248, 246f, 247f
  mitochondrial, 249, 249t
  nemaline, 250–251
  thyrotoxic, 360
  toxic, 250, 250t
  with chemotherapy, 65
Myophosphorylase deficiency, 246, 246f
Myotomes, 251t–252t
Myotonia, 252–254, 253t
Myotonia congenita, 253t, 254
Myotonic discharges, on EMG, 120
Myotonic dystrophy, 252–254, 253t, 368, 368t
  during pregnancy, 314

N
Narcolepsy, 344
Narcotic analgesia, 286–287, 286f, 287f

Necrosis, cerebral, radiation therapy-induced, 326
Neglect, 254–255
Nemaline myopathy, 250–251
Neonatal seizures, 131–132
Neonatal status epilepticus, 143
Neoplastic meningitis, CSF in, 62t
Nerve conduction study, 117–121, 117t
Neuralgia
  glossopharyngeal, 157–158
  postherpetic, 388
  trigeminal, 367–368
Neuralgic amyotrophy, 39
Neuroaxonal dystrophy, 90
Neurocutaneous melanosis, 257
Neurocutaneous syndromes, 255–258
Neurofibromatosis
  type 1, 255
  type 2, 255–256
Neuroleptic malignant syndrome, 260
Neuroleptics, 258–260
  extrapyramidal side effects of, 259–260
Neurometabolic diseases, of childhood, 218–220, 219t
Neuromyotonia, 86
  on EMG, 120
Neuronal lipofuscinosis, 90, 219t
Neuronal tissue transplantation, 192–193
Neuropathy, 260–268
  diabetic, 265–266
  hereditary, 263–265
  in hypothyroidism, 361
  in renal failure, 375
  lumbosacral plexus, 203
  of lower extremity, 298, 303f–306f
  of upper extremity, 296–298, 299f–302f
  treatment of, 268
  with chemotherapy, 65
Neurosarcoidosis, 338–339

Neurosyphilis, 356–358
Niacin deficiency, 270
Nicotinic acid deficiency, 270
Niemann–Pick's disease, 90
Nociception, 284–287
Nonketotic hyperglycemia, 218, 219t
Normal pressure hydrocephalus, 172
Nortriptyline, 23t
Nothnagel's syndrome, 182t
Noxious stimuli, response to, in coma, 76
Nutritional amblyopia, 10
Nutritional deficiency syndrome, 269–270
Nystagmus, 52, 270–274, 273t
  acquired, 271
  congenital, 271
  downbeat, 272, 273t
  optokinetic, 283–284
  treatment of, 274
  upbeat, 272, 273t

O
Oblique myokymia, superior, 275
Occipital lobe, 274–275
Ocular bobbing, 275
Ocular dipping, 275
Ocular flutter, 275
Ocular myoclonus, 275
Oculomotor apraxia, 27
Oculomotor nerve (III) palsy, 279–280, 323t
Oculopharyngeal dystrophy, 233
Oculosympathetic paresis, 169–171, 170f
Olfaction, 276–277
Olivopontocerebellar atrophy, 353
One-and-a-half syndrome, 182t, 281
Opalski's syndrome, 277
Ophthalmoplegia, 277–281
Optic disc, swelling of, 281–282
Optic nerve (II), 281–283

Optic neuritis, 282
    CSF in, 62t
    visual evoked potentials in, 148
Optic neuropathy, 282
Optokinetic nystagmus, 283–284
Orthostatic hypotension
    in autonomic dysfunction, 33,
        34
    treatment of, 34
Orthostatic tremor, 366
Osler–Weber–Rendu syndrome,
    257
Osteomalacia, myopathy in, 246
Oxcarbazine, in epilepsy, 137t,
    141t
Oxybutynin, in bladder
    dysfunction, 37t

P
Paget's disease, 284
Pain, 284–287
    in sickle cell disease, 342
    treatment of, 285–287, 286f,
        287f
Palatal myoclonus, 239
Pallidotomy, in Parkinson's disease,
    294
Palmar grasp reflex, in infants, 69t
Pancerebellar syndrome, 53–54
Pancoast's syndrome, 39
Papilledema, 281–282
Parachute response, in infant, 70t
Paramyotonia congenita, 253t,
    254
Paraneoplastic sensory
    neuronopathy, 20–21, 20t
Paraneoplastic syndromes, 20–21,
    20t, 288–290, 289t
Paratonia, 337
Parietal lobe syndromes, 290
Parinaud dorsal midbrain
    syndrome, 182t, 323t, 325
Parkinsonian tremor, 366
Parkinsonism, 290–291
    neuroleptic-induced, 259
    secondary, 291

Parkinson's disease, 292–294
Paroxetine, 23t
Parsonage–Turner syndrome, 39
Pavor nocturnus, 345
Pelizaeus–Merzbacher disease, 89
Penicillamine, in Wilson's disease,
    386
Penicillin, in syphilis, 357
Perilymph fistula, 381
Periodic alternating nystagmus,
    272
Periodic paralysis, 295–296, 295t
    hyperkalemic, 253t, 295–296,
        295t
    hypokalemic, 295–296, 295t
    normokalemic, 296
Peripheral neuropathy. See
        Neuropathy.
Peroxisomal disorder, 219t
Pertussis vaccine, 176
Phakomatoses, 255–258, 334
Phantom limb pain, 285
Phenobarbital, in epilepsy, 134t,
    137t, 138t
Phenylketonuria, 90, 220
Phenytoin
    in epilepsy, 134t, 137t, 138t
    in spasticity, 346
Phosphate, 112t, 115
Phosphoglycerate kinase
    deficiency, 246, 246f
Phosphoglycerate mutase
    deficiency, 246f, 247
Physiologic nystagmus, 272
Physiologic tremor, 365–366
Pineal tumor, pupil in, 325
Ping-pong gaze, 275
Pituitary apoplexy, 309
Pituitary gland, 307–310
    tumors of, 307–309
Placing reflex, in infant, 70t
Plantar grasp reflex, in infant, 70t
Plasmapheresis, in myasthenia
        gravis, 237
Poliomyelitis vaccine, 176
Polyarteritis nodosa, 378

Polymyalgia rheumatica, 244–245
Polymyositis, 243–244, 244t
Polyneuropathy, 260–261
    diabetic, 265–266
Pompe's disease, 246f, 247
Pontine hemorrhage, 56
Porphyria, 310–313, 310f, 311t
    drug-induced, 312t
    during pregnancy, 314
    treatment of, 313
Positron emission tomography
    (PET), 306–307
Posterior inferior cerebellar artery,
    52–53
Potassium, 112t, 113
Pregnancy, 313–318
    autoimmune disorders in, 315
    cerebrovascular disease in,
        315–316
    eclampsia in, 318
    epilepsy in, 317
    mononeuropathy in, 313–314
    movement disorders in,
        314–315
    neoplasms in, 316–317
    obstetrical palsy in, 314
    plexopathy in, 314
    polyneuropathy in, 314
Preolivary syndrome, 184t
Presyncope, 104
Pretectal afferent pupillary defect,
    325
Primidone, in epilepsy, 134t,
    137t, 139t
Prion diseases, 98–99, 124–125
Progressive multifocal
    leukoencephalopathy, 6–7
Progressive supranuclear palsy,
    290–291
Prolactinoma, 308
Protein, in CSF, 60t, 61
Protriptyline, 23t
Pseudobulbar palsy, 318–319
Pseudotumor cerebri, 319
Psychogenic dizziness, 105
Psychosis, treatment of, 258–260

Ptosis, 320–321
Pupils
    drug effects on, 322t
    examination of, 321–325, 323t
        in autonomic dysfunction, 33
        in coma, 74
    light reflex pathway of, 324f
Pure-tone threshold testing, 165
Purkinje cells, 47, 49
Putamenal hemorrhage, 54
Pyknolepsy, 129–130
Pyridostigmine, in myasthenia
    gravis, 236–237
Pyridoxine deficiency, 220, 269R

R
Rabies, 123
Rabies vaccine, 176
Radiation injury, 326–328
    cerebral, 326–327
    peripheral, 328
    spinal, 327–328
Radiculopathy, 328–330
    cervical, 329
    diagnosis of, 329
    lumbar, 329–330
Ramsay–Hunt syndrome, 152
Raymond–Cestan syndrome, 182t
Raymond's syndrome, 183t
Reading inability, 10–11
Rebound nystagmus, 273
Red blood cells, in CSF, 60–61,
    60t
Reflex sympathetic dystrophy,
    80–81, 285
Reflex syncope, 354
Reflexes, 330–332, 330t, 331t
    in infants, 69t–70t
Relative afferent pupillary defect,
    324–325, 324f
Renal failure, 375–376
Repetitive stimulation study, 118
Respiratory acidosis, 115–116
Respiratory alkalosis, 115
Respiratory heart rate variation, in
    autonomic dysfunction, 33

Restless legs syndrome, 332
Retina, 333–335, 335t
   in sickle cell disease, 342
Retinitis pigmentosa, 333
Retinovitreal syndromes, 334
Rhabdomyolysis, myoglobinuria in, 242–243
Rheumatoid arthritis, 335–336
Rigidity, 337
Riley–Day syndrome, 265
Rinne's test, 165
RNA-binding proteins, antibodies against, 18t
Romberg sign, 337
Rostral vermis syndrome, 53
Rotary nystagmus, 272
Rubella vaccine, 176
Rubral tremor, 366

S
Saccades, 275
St. Louis encephalitis, 123
Salt wasting syndrome, cerebral, 309–310
Sanfilippo syndrome, 91
Sarcoidosis, 338–339
   CSF in, 62t
   myopathy in, 244
Scapuloperoneal dystrophy, 231
See-saw nystagmus, 272
Seizures, 127–143. See also Epilepsy.
   CSF in, 63t
   in renal failure, 375
   in sickle cell disease, 342
   with chemotherapy, 64
Selective serotonin reuptake inhibitors, 23t
Selegiline, in Parkinson's disease, 292–293
Sepsis, 339
Sertraline, 23t
Sheehan's syndrome, 316
Shunt, 339–341, 340f
Sickle cell disease, 197–198, 341–342

Sildenafil, 177
Simple partial status epilepticus, 132t, 142
Simultanagnosia, 4
Single photon emission computed tomography (SPECT), 306–307
Singultus, 169
Sjögren's syndrome, 378
Sleep disorders, 343–345
Sleep electroencephalography, 110
Sleep terrors, 345
Sodium, 112–113, 112t
Somatosensory-evoked potentials, 146–147
Spasm, hemifacial, 153
Spasmodic torticollis, 107
Spasmus nutans, 275–276
Spasticity, 345–346
Sphingolipidosis, 219t
Spinal artery, disorders of, 350–351
Spinal block, CSF in, 63t
Spinal cord, 346–351, 347f
   compression of, 372–373
   cross section of, 348f
   hemorrhage in, 350–351
   radiation therapy–induced injury to, 327–328
   syringomyelia of, 349–350
   trauma to, 350
   tumors of, 372
   vascular syndromes of, 350–351
Spinal shock, 346
Spine
   congenital malformation of, 83–85
   degenerative disease of, 349–350
Spinobulbar muscular dystrophy, 368, 368t
Spinocerebellar ataxia, 368, 368t
Spinocerebellar degeneration, 351–353

Spondylosis, 349
Square-wave jerks, 275
Status epilepticus, 132, 132t, 133t, 142–143
Stepping reflex, in infant, 70t
Stiff-person syndrome, 86
Stroke, 180–200
    after radiation therapy, 328
    anatomy of, 180, 181f, 185f
    anticoagulation in, 189–190
    antiplatelet agents in, 190–191
    classification of, 180
    clinical evaluation of, 187–188
    computed tomography in, 82t
    cranial nerve effects in, 182t–184t
    differential diagnosis of, 186, 193–194
    during pregnancy, 316
    in AIDS, 7
    in moyamoya disease, 196–197
    in sickle cell disease, 197–198, 342
    in young patient, 188
    laboratory evaluation of, 187–188
    lacunar, 194–195, 195t
    mechanism of, 186
    natural history of, 186–187
    prognosis for, 193
    recovery from, 193
    rehabilitation after, 193
    risk factors for, 186–187
    surgical treatment of, 192–193
    syndromes with, 182t–184t
    thalamic, 195–196
    thrombolytic therapy in, 191–192
    treatment of, 188–189
    vascular anatomy of, 180, 181t
    venous thrombosis in, 198–199
    with chemotherapy, 64
Sturge–Weber syndrome, 257
Subacute sclerosing panencephalitis, 124
    CSF in, 62t
Subarachnoid hemorrhage, 12–13, 57, 350–351
    CSF in, 62t
    during pregnancy, 315–316
    syncope with, 354–355
Subdural hemorrhage, 57–58, 350
Subthalamic nucleus stimulation, in Parkinson's disease, 294
Suck reflex, in infant, 69t
Sulfatide, antibody to, 22
Sulfite oxidase deficiency, 218, 219t
Superior cerebellar artery, 53
Superior oblique myokymia, 275
Surgery, in Parkinson's disease, 293–294
Swallowing, dysfunction of, 106
Syncope, 104, 353–355
Syndrome of inappropriate antidiuretic hormone secretion, 355–356
Syphilis, 356–358
    meningeal, 7, 356
Syringomyelia, 349–350
Systemic lupus erythematosus, 377

T
Tabes dorsalis, 357
Tactile agnosia, 4
Takayasu's arteritis, 377
Tapia's syndrome, 184t
Tardive dyskinesia, neuroleptic-induced, 259
Taste, 358–359
Tay–Sachs disease, 90
Telangiectasias, 17
Temporal arteritis, 376–377
Temporal lobe, 359
Temporal lobe epilepsy, 130–131
Tensilon test, 236
Tension-type headache, 161
Tetanus, 86–87
Tetanus toxoid vaccine, 176
Tetany, 86

Thalamic hemorrhage, 54, 56
Thalamic syndromes, 195–196
Thiamine deficiency, 269
Thomsen's disease, 253t, 254
Thrombolytic therapy, in stroke, 191–192
Thymectomy, in myasthenia gravis, 237
Thyroid gland, 359–361
Thyrotoxic crisis, 359
Thyrotoxic myopathy, 245
Tiagabine, in epilepsy, 140t
Tic douloureux, 367–368
Ticlopidine, in stroke, 191
Tics, 361–362
Tigabine, in epilepsy, 137t
Tissue plasminogen activator, in stroke, 191–192
Tolcapone, in Parkinson's disease, 293
Tolosa–Hunt syndrome, 280
Tolterodine, 36–37
Tonic neck reflex, in infant, 69t
Tonic pupil syndrome, 323t
Topiramate, in epilepsy, 137t, 140t
Torticollis, spasmodic, 107
Tourette's syndrome, 361–362
Toxic myopathy, 250, 250t
Toxoplasmosis, in AIDS, 6, 63t
Transient global amnesia, 362
Transient ischemic attack, 180, 186. See also Stroke.
    treatment of, 189
Transplantation, 362–365
Trazodone, 23t
Tremor, 52, 365–366
    thyrotoxic, 360
Tricyclic antidepressants, 23t
Trigeminal neuralgia, 367–368
Trihexyphenidyl, in Parkinson's disease, 293
Trinucleotide repeat expansion, 368, 368t
Trisomy 13, 73
Trisomy 18, 73

Trisomy 21, 73
Trochlear nerve (IV) palsy, 279
Tromner sign, 332
Tuberculosis, in AIDS, 7
Tuberculous meningitis, CSF in, 62t
Tuberous sclerosis, 256
Tumors, 368–373, 368t
    brain, 368–372, 368t, 369f–270f
    during pregnancy, 316
    metastatic, 372
    radiation-induced, 328
    sensory neuronopathy with, 20–21, 20t
    spinal cord, 372
Tuning fork tests, 165
Turner's syndrome (XO syndrome), 74

U
Ulnar nerve, 373–374
Ultrasonography, 374
    in stroke, 187
Uncal (lateral) herniation, 166, 167t, 168t
Uncinate fits, 277
Urea cycle disorder, in infant, 218, 219t
Uremia, 375–376
Urine, myoglobin in, 242–243241
Uvea, 334, 335t

V
Vaccines, 175–176
Vacuolar myelopathy, in AIDS, 8
Valproate, in epilepsy, 137t
Valproic acid, in epilepsy, 135t, 139t
Varicella-zoster virus infection, 387–389
    in AIDS, 8
Varices, 17
Vascular dementia, 96–97, 97t
Vasculitis, 376–379
    secondary, 377–379

Vasovagal syncope, 354, 355
Vegetative state, 78–79
Venezuelan equine encephalitis, 123
Venous angioma, 17
Venous thrombosis, 379–380
  cerebral, 198–199. See also Stroke.
Ventriculoperitoneal shunt, 339–341, 340f
Vernet's syndrome, 183t
Vertical gaze palsy, 155
Vertigo, 380–383, 383t
Vestibular nystagmus, 271
Vestibulocochlear nerve (VIII), 166
Vestibulo-ocular reflex, 383–384, 384t
Vestibulopathy, peripheral, acute, 381
Viral encephalitis, 122–124
Vision loss, with chemotherapy, 64
Visual agnosia, 4
Visual fields, 384–386, 385f
Visual-evoked potentials, 144–145
Vitamin A deficiency, 269
Vitamin B$_1$ deficiency, 269
Vitamin B$_6$ deficiency, 269
Vitamin B$_{12}$ deficiency, 269
Vitamin D deficiency, 270
Vitamin E deficiency, 270
Voluntary nystagmus, 274
Von Hippel–Landau disease, 256

W

Wallenberg's syndrome, 183t
Weber's syndrome, 182t
Weber's test, 165

Wegener's granulomatosis, 378
Weight, of infant, 67f
Wernicke–Korsakoff syndrome, 98, 269
Wernicke's aphasia, 25t
West Nile virus encephalitis, 123–124
West's syndrome, 130
White blood cells, in CSF, 60–61, 60t
Wilson's disease, 91–92, 386
  during pregnancy, 315
Withdrawal syndrome, with neuroleptic discontinuation, 259–260
Worster–Drought syndrome, 319
Wrist, ulnar nerve entrapment at, 374
Writer's cramp, 107
Writing inability, 4–5
Writing tremor, 366
Wyburn–Mason syndrome, 257

X

Xanthochromia, 60
Xeroderma pigmentosa, 256
XO syndrome, 74
XXX syndrome, 73
XXY syndrome, 73
XYY syndrome, 73

Y

Yohimbine, 178

Z

Zellweger syndrome, 91
Zonisamide, in epilepsy, 137t, 140t

NIH STROKE SCALE

A. ITEM	B. Score (circle one)	C. ITEM	D. Score (circle one)
1.a. Level of consciousness: — Alert — Drowsy — Stuporous — Coma	0 1 2 3	**5b. Left arm:** — Normal (extends arms 90 degrees for 10 seconds without drift) — Drift — Some effort against gravity — No effort against gravity — No movement	9 untestable 0 1 2 3 4
1.b. Ask patient the month and their age: — Answers both correctly — Answers one correctly — Both incorrect	 0 1 2	**6. Motor: 6a. Right leg:** — Normal (leg 30 degrees for 5 seconds) — Drift — Some effort against gravity — No effort against gravity — No movement	9 untestable 0 1 2 3 4
1.c. Ask patient to open and close eyes and squeeze and let go: — Obeys both correctly — Obeys one correctly — Both incorrect	 0 1 2	**6a. Left leg:** — Normal (leg 30 degrees for 5 seconds) — Drift — Some effort against gravity — No effort against gravity — No movement	9 untestable 0 1 2 3 4
2. Best gaze (only horizontal eye movement): — Normal — Partial gaze palsy — Forced deviation	 0 1 2	**7. Limb Ataxia:** — No ataxia — Present in one limb — Present in two limbs	 0 1 2
3. Visual Field testing: — Normal — Partial hemianopia — Complete hemianopia — Bilateral hemianopia (blind)	 0 1 2 3	**8. Sensory (Use pinprick to test arms, legs, trunk and face — compare side to side:** — Normal — Mild to moderate decrease — Severe to total	 0 1 2
4. Facial Paresis (Ask patient to show teeth, raise eyebrows and squeeze eyes shut: — Normal symmetrical — Flat nasolabial fold — Partial paralysis — Complete paralysis	 0 1 2 3	**9. Best Language (describe picture, name items, read sentences):** — Normal aphasia — Mild to moderate — Severe aphasia	 0 1 2
5. Motor: 5a. Right arm: — Normal (extends arms 90 degrees for 10 seconds without drift) — Drift — Some effort against gravity — No effort against gravity — No movement	9 untestable 0 1 2 3 4	**10. Dysarthria:** — Normal articulation — Mild to moderate slurring — Near complete — Intubated	 0 1 2 9 untestable
		11. Inattention or extinction: — Normal — Extinction to one sensory modality — Severe hemineglect	 0 1 2

TOTAL (B+D) =